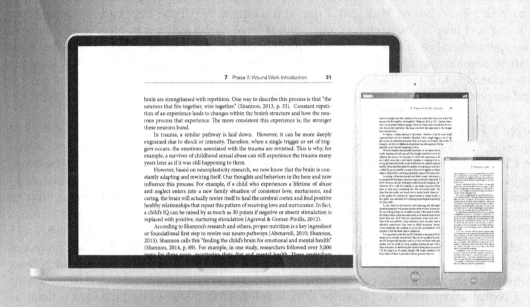
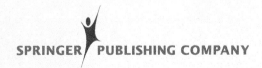

Karen Bauce, DNP, MPA, RN, NEA-BC, is associate dean for Graduate Online Programs and assistant clinical professor in the MSN Online Program at Sacred Heart University in Fairfield, Connecticut, where she teaches a variety of courses, including research. She received her BSN from the University of Connecticut, MPA from New York University, and DNP from Oakland University in Rochester, Michigan. Prior to teaching at SHU, she held various senior-level nursing and hospital management positions at large health systems in New York City, and also spent several years as a collaborative practice consultant working with hospitals and their staff to develop and implement models of shared decision making. Dr. Bauce has traveled internationally to learn about nursing practice in other countries and has published on culture and empowerment. She is a frequent contributor to Dr. Joyce J. Fitzpatrick's publications.

Joyce J. Fitzpatrick, PhD, MBA, RN, FAAN, FNAP, is Elizabeth Brooks Ford Professor of Nursing, Frances Payne Bolton School of Nursing, Case Western Reserve University (CWRU) in Cleveland, Ohio, where she was dean from 1982 to 1997. She is also adjunct professor, Department of Geriatrics, Icahn School of Medicine, Mount Sinai Hospital, New York, New York. She earned a BSN (Georgetown University), an MS in psychiatric–mental health nursing (The Ohio State University), a PhD in nursing (New York University), and an MBA (CWRU). She was elected a fellow in the American Academy of Nursing (AAN; 1981) and a fellow in the National Academies of Practice (1996). She received the *American Journal of Nursing* Book of the Year Award 20 times. Dr. Fitzpatrick received the American Nurses Foundation Distinguished Contribution to Nursing Science Award for sustained commitment and contributions to development of the discipline (2002). She was a Fulbright Scholar at University College Cork, Cork, Ireland (2007–2008) and was inducted into the Sigma Theta Tau International Research Hall of Fame (2014). In 2016, she was named a Living Legend of the AAN. Dr. Fitzpatrick's work is widely published in nursing and health care literature with more than 300 publications, including more than 80 authored/edited books. She served as a coeditor of the *Annual Review of Nursing Research* series, volumes 1 to 26, and she currently edits the journals *Applied Nursing Research, Archives of Psychiatric Nursing,* and *Nursing Education Perspectives,* the official journal of the National League for Nursing.

NURSING RESEARCH CRITIQUE

A Model For Excellence

KAREN BAUCE, DNP, MPA, RN, NEA-BC

JOYCE J. FITZPATRICK,
PHD, MBA, RN, FAAN, FANP

Editors

SPRINGER PUBLISHING COMPANY

Springer Publishing Company, LLC
11 West 42nd Street
New York, NY 10036
www.springerpub.com

Acquisitions Editor: Joseph Morita
Compositor: diacriTech, Chennai

ISBN: 978-0-8261-7509-0
ebook ISBN: 978-0-8261-7541-0

18 19 20 21 22 / 5 4 3 2 1

The author and the publisher of this Work have made every effort to use sources believed to be reliable to provide information that is accurate and compatible with the standards generally accepted at the time of publication. Because medical science is continually advancing, our knowledge base continues to expand. Therefore, as new information becomes available, changes in procedures become necessary. We recommend that the reader always consult current research and specific institutional policies before performing any clinical procedure. The author and publisher shall not be liable for any special, consequential, or exemplary damages resulting, in whole or in part, from the readers' use of, or reliance on, the information contained in this book. The publisher has no responsibility for the persistence or accuracy of URLs for external or third-party Internet websites referred to in this publication and does not guarantee that any content on such websites is, or will remain, accurate or appropriate.

Library of Congress Cataloging-in-Publication Data
Names: Bauce, Karen, editor. | Fitzpatrick, Joyce J., 1944- editor.
Title: Nursing research critique : a model for excellence / Karen Bauce,
  Joyce J. Fitzpatrick, editors.
Description: New York, NY : Springer, [2018] | Includes index.
Identifiers: LCCN 2017052257| ISBN 9780826175090 | ISBN 9780826175410 (ebook)
Subjects: | MESH: Nursing Research | Evaluation Studies as Topic | Models, Nursing
Classification: LCC RT81.5 | NLM WY 20.5 | DDC 610.73072—dc23
LC record available at https://lccn.loc.gov/2017052257

Contact us to receive discount rates on bulk purchases.
We can also customize our books to meet your needs.
For more information please contact: sales@springerpub.com

Printed in the United States of America.

CONTENTS

CONTRIBUTORS

Karen Bauce, DNP, MPA, RN, NEA-BC, Associate Dean, Online Nursing Programs, Sacred Heart University College of Nursing, Fairfield, Connecticut

Linda Cook, DNP, MPH, APRN, NNP-BC, CNL, Program Director, MSN Clinical Nurse Leader Track, Clinical Assistant Professor of Nursing, Sacred Heart University College of Nursing, Fairfield, Connecticut

Mary A. Dolansky, PhD, RN, FAAN, Associate Professor, Director of the QSEN Institute, Frances Payne Bolton School of Nursing, Case Western Reserve University, Cleveland, Ohio

Emerson E. Ea, DNP, PhD, APRN, CNE, Clinical Associate Professor, Director, Undergraduate Program, New York University Rory Meyers College of Nursing, New York, New York

Deborah B. Fahs, DNP, FNP B-C, Assistant Professor, Yale University School of Nursing, New Haven, Connecticut

Anne Folte Fish, PhD, RN, FAHA, Associate Professor of Nursing, University of Missouri–St. Louis, St. Louis, Missouri

Joyce J. Fitzpatrick, PhD, MBA, RN, FAAN, Elizabeth Brooks Ford Professor of Nursing, Frances Payne Bolton School of Nursing, Case Western Reserve University, Cleveland, Ohio

Selena A. Gilles, DNP, ANP-BC, CCRN, Clinical Assistant Professor, New York University Rory Meyers School of Nursing, New York, New York

Rebecca Witten Grizzle, PhD, RN, NP-C, Clinical Assistant Professor, Sacred Heart University College of Nursing, Fairfield, Connecticut

Margaret A. Harris, PhD, RN, Associate Professor, Oakland University School of Nursing, Rochester, Michigan

Patricia Keresztes, PhD, RN, CCRN, Associate Professor of Nursing, Saint Mary's College, Notre Dame, Indiana

Elizabeth A. Madigan, PhD, RN, FAAN, Chief Executive Officer, Sigma Theta Tau International, Indianapolis, Indiana

Nadine M. Marchi, DNP, RN, CNE, CRRN, McGregor Fellow and Instructor, Frances Payne Bolton School of Nursing, Case Western Reserve University, Cleveland, Ohio

Margaret McCarthy, PhD, RN, FNP-BC, Assistant Professor, New York University Rory Meyers College of Nursing, New York, New York

Annette Peacock-Johnson, DNP, RN, Associate Professor of Nursing, Saint Mary's College, Notre Dame, Indiana

Joseph D. Perazzo, PhD, RN, Assistant Professor, College of Nursing, University of Cincinnati, Cincinnati, Ohio

Andrew P. Reimer, PhD, RN, CFRN, Assistant Professor, Frances Payne Bolton School of Nursing, Case Western Reserve University, Cleveland, Ohio

Jacqueline Rhoads, PhD, ACNP-BC, ANP-BC, FAANP, Professor Distance Learning Programs, CAEPH Instructional Training Center for Applied Environmental Public Health, Tulane University, New Orleans, Louisiana

Julie Schexnayder, DNP, CRNP, PhD Student, Frances Payne Bolton School of Nursing, Case Western Reserve University, Cleveland, Ohio

Anita Ayrandjian Volpe, DNP, APRN, Director, Surgical Outcomes, Research, and Education, Department of Surgery, New York–Presbyterian/Queens, New York, New York

FOREWORD

I graduated from an RN–BSN program prior to the incorporation of evidence-based practice (EBP) content in nursing curricula. As students, we practiced nursing as our expert faculty had taught us. I graduated with a baccalaureate degree with limited research knowledge and skills and felt like an imposter when I critiqued research conducted by doctorally prepared nurses. As a lifelong learner who is curious about all of the possibilities of being a nurse, I pursued graduate nursing degrees, which empowered me to be one of the nurses who was appraising, generating, translating, and implementing evidence for nursing practice and education.

I believe that the start of all scholarship and research begins with a spirit of inquiry. It is this spirit that lays the foundation for questioning how we practice, spawns creative ideas, examines interventions critically, and seeks new solutions as to how we practice. We are challenged to step outside of our comfort zones, to embrace and engage in scholarship. As professionals, all nurses are ethically mandated and have an obligation and duty to question authority, access knowledge, and apply evidence to practice to provide the best care for our patients.

EBP is not an option for professional nursing practice. Nurses practice from a base of evidence. Engaging in scholarly inquiry—whether it is searching the literature, critiquing the evidence, or generating the research—is imperative to how we practice as professionals. There will be challenges of integrating evidence-based changes into patient care, but there will be triumphs as well. Nurses have a wealth of practice experience to support our clinical decision making and these decisions must be informed by evidence. Although the research literature abounds with obstacles to engaging in scholarly inquiry, it is our responsibility to seek the "best" available evidence to promote quality and safety to achieve optimal patient outcomes.

As nursing students transition into professional practice, they have to be able to navigate, adapt, and change practice in partnership with other health care professionals. To be a knowledgeable consumer of research who functions in a partnership role, the baccalaureate graduate needs to be able to critically appraise research evidence. The ability to identify and judge the strengths and weaknesses of a research study and establish the soundness of the evidence are critical first steps in determining whether the findings are ready for practice implementation. Professional accountability is promoted through research.

Both nationally and globally, nurses are in a unique position to transform nursing practice as part of the interprofessional health care team and as leaders in an ever-changing complex health care environment. EBP is the norm for health care providers in the planning and implementation of patient care. Assuming a lead role in EBP requires that nurses enhance their abilities and competence through critical thinking, logical reasoning, decision making, independent judgment, and effective communication. Nurses can bring to this research dialogue clinically relevant questions and insights into patient care problems; the impetus for direct change is most often initiated by those at the patient's bedside.

Nurses are no longer bystanders in the scholarship of research. There is a growing body of evidence supporting how nurses practice; however, without critical evaluation and translation into practice, the science of nursing will not grow and be recognized by other disciplines, health care providers, or the public. The ability to critique research well is a skill that needs to be honed and practiced. Like any technical skill, this cognitive skill requires repetition and reinforcement to gain the necessary confidence and competence to challenge research findings, ask the next question, or translate and implement evidence in practice. It is not enough to simply know the language of the research process. Being a professional means asking the difficult questions, challenging the ideas others take for granted, and suggesting new ideas based on sound evidence.

Transitioning to a leadership role in EBP means acquiring the necessary research appraisal knowledge and skills. A strength of this text is that it includes a broad range of research examples from both qualitative and quantitative paradigms in different practice settings to allow students to gain that appraisal expertise. Practice evidence needs to be evaluated and critiqued to make the evidence actionable. This much-needed text provides exemplar critiques that are accessible to those students and nurses who are enhancing their research skill set, engaging in scholarly inquiry, and developing as professionals and leaders in health care reform.

Barbara Patterson, PhD, RN, ANEF
Professor, Widener University
Chester, Pennsylvania
Distinguished Scholar, National League for Nursing/Chamberlain Center for the
Advancement of the Science of Nursing Education
Washington, DC

PREFACE

The ability to evaluate and critically analyze research literature is essential for members of a practice profession guided by evidence. Determining any research study's usefulness and application to nursing practice results from a systematic appraisal of methodological rigor, which leads to an overall assessment of strengths and limitations. Although all research studies have limitations, nurses must be able to place them in an appropriate context so that potentially valuable implications for practice are not overlooked.

The impetus for this book was the result of our collective years of experience teaching an introductory research course to BSN and MSN students. Students struggle with understanding the fundamental differences between quantitative and qualitative research methodology and their underlying paradigms, as well as the actual critique process. Even when provided with a template that identifies specific components of a research study to address, students remain challenged. Furthermore, current nursing texts describe the elements of critique, but none *demonstrate* the process as applied by experienced nursing faculty and researchers to a wide variety of research studies.

After reviewing existing guides and consulting with our colleague Dr. Rebecca Witten Grizzle, from Sacred Heart University, Fairfield, Connecticut, we developed a new framework to assist students in the critique process. Dr. Witten Grizzle's years of teaching research to BSN and MSN students have given her unique insight into their learning needs and we are grateful for her contributions to our critique template.

This book is organized into two parts: the first provides critiques of 11 quantitative research studies utilizing various methodologies, such as a randomized controlled trial and correlational and cross-sectional descriptive studies; the second part includes three qualitative studies. We included far more quantitative research because it seems to be especially challenging for students to critique, while at the same time it is easier to understand its implications for practice. The research problems and phenomena of interest addressed in the studies reflect concerns of nurses in contemporary practice, such as compassion fatigue, use of opioids for pain management, and geriatric falls in nursing homes. In addition, two of the studies address global health issues—childhood immunization in the Philippines and betel nut chewing among Palauans.

We believe that nursing students as well as their faculty will find this book a useful adjunct to course content. Students are provided with 14 exemplars of critical analysis of research literature, reinforcing critique as an essential skill for acquiring knowledge for evidence-based practice. We are thankful to all of the chapter authors for their contributions as well as to the lead authors of the original research studies, who recognized the importance of this book and appreciated being part of the process.

Karen Bauce
Joyce J. Fitzpatrick

INTRODUCTION

Karen Bauce and Joyce J. Fitzpatrick

Nursing students, including both undergraduate and beginning graduate students, and experienced practitioners are often intimidated at the prospect of critiquing a research study, particularly one that includes any form of statistical analysis. As professionals who use current evidence for best practice, nurses must be able to thoughtfully and critically evaluate research findings. Only then can a determination be made as to what might contribute to best practice in any particular nursing specialty.

We developed our critique template as a way to evaluate quantitative and qualitative research that is understandable for students and nurses who are not experienced in the research process. The specific questions included in the template address the major components of a research study. Overall, the completed critique helps the student and nurse arrive at a conclusion about the relative strengths and limitations of the study being evaluated. In addition, after following this process, the student can decide the overall merits of the study, including whether the study was warranted and adds to the scientific knowledge base of the discipline.

The template that we developed is included in Table I.1. First, the student will find a brief overall summary of the critique of the article. This summary includes the key highlights of the extensive critique that follows. It serves to orient the student to the strengths of the research. Next, the title of the study is critiqued. Most journals require titles that are 10 to 12 words, succinct and yet descriptive enough to identify the main focus of the study, for example, the population that was of interest and the intervention if one has been used in the research. At times, the title also includes the nature of the study, for example, pilot or exploratory study, quantitative or qualitative research, or mixed methods. Author credentials are evaluated, including whether they have expertise in research methodology and/or the clinical area of study. Many research reports now include multiple authors and thus the collective expertise of the authors should be considered. At times, there are clinicians and researchers who work together in launching research. Most published studies include a brief biographical statement about the authors, including most often their place of employment. The author credentials often are judged based on the degrees listed and employment status. If further evaluation is desired, the student can pursue the authors' other publications, either through the university home page, which often lists curriculum vitae and publications, or through an Internet search of the authors' other publications. Author credentials also can be assessed by reviewing the cited publications in the article to determine whether the authors have published other papers on the topic.

The abstract is an important component of any research report. Very often, only the abstract is available on Internet searches; thus, the abstract should be sufficiently inclusive of the key study components so that the reviewer can quickly determine whether the study is of interest or relevant. There are varying journal requirements for abstracts, with some journals specifying the exact structure of the abstract when reporting a research study and other journals specifying only the maximum word count; they expect the researcher to know what components of the research report need to be included. The abstract should never include references and should be concise (fewer than 200 words). It should entice the reader to read the full report and to evaluate the overall relevance of the research reported.

The study introduction is the next component evaluated. The introduction should be clear in its description of the phenomena or problem of interest in the research. Most important, the introduction section of a research report should answer the "so what" question. In other words, what difference will this study make to the existing knowledge and why is this study important? The study significance will also be addressed later in the research report, but certainly the introduction should give the reader and evaluator a sense of the importance of the study.

The study objective and research aims are the next component to be evaluated. Often this component is stated as the study purpose. The research aims and objectives must be clear and concise and follow logically from the research problem identified in the introduction; they should be explicitly stated. The study purpose is followed by the significance section. The researcher is expected to clearly indicate the significance of the study to nursing and health care, and it should be clear how the significance flows from the study purpose. Often, due to the journal's page constraints, there is not a specific section of the article that is labeled "significance," but the reviewer should be able to discern the implied significance. For example, it should be clear that there is a compelling care for the need to address a specific gap in knowledge about a nursing/health care phenomenon of interest, and whether the study will contribute to new knowledge development.

The background of the study often includes the conceptual and/or theoretical framework that guided the study. If it is not explicitly included, the reviewer should evaluate the implied conceptual and/or theoretical framework. Often, due to page limitations in research and/or clinical journals, this section of the research is not included. If it is included, there should be clear theoretical/conceptual definitions of the concepts. The background section is often combined with the literature review section in a research report. The literature review should include only primary sources and should be as current as possible. Some journals specify that only literature within the past 5 years should be cited unless using classical sources or sources necessary to understand the study measures. The search strategy often is included and should be evaluated to determine whether it also is relevant to the study variables. The literature review should be structured so as to be logically presented, leading up to the most recent research. The reviewer should evaluate the relevance of the literature reviewed to the research aims and the comprehensiveness of the literature review. The summary of the literature review should include a rationale for the study. The researcher should explicitly state how the present study will extend prior knowledge and fill a gap in the literature. If this is a follow-up or replication study, this should be stated. The rationale should lead directly to the research questions and/or hypotheses. These should include the variables of interest in the study, be explicit and clearly stated, and be logically related to the study purpose of research aim/ objective.

A major component of any research report is the methods section. The research design, for example, qualitative or quantitative, or mixed methods, should be clearly stated. Further, more detail regarding the specifics of the design should be given; for example, if it is a qualitative study design, and the author should note the particular qualitative methodology used (descriptive, phenomenology, etc.). If the design is quantitative, the researcher should describe the method in detail, for example, cross-sectional descriptive, quasi-experimental, experimental, and so on. The evaluator should know whether there is consistency between the design chosen and the paradigm that guides the study, whether this is the best choice of design to address the research problem, and whether there is rigor in the design.

Each research report includes some description of the setting in which the study took place or the setting in which the data were collected. The reviewer would evaluate whether the setting was clearly described and whether biases were introduced as a result of a particular setting. For example, if the setting was only an academic medical center, then the report might have a bias in the responses of nurses to a particular issue unless the research problem of interest is specific regarding nurses employed in academic medical centers.

Using the standard structure of research reporting, following the description of the setting, the researcher describes both the sampling plan and the sample. The sampling plan should be clearly specified and should represent the population of interest and be consistent with the research aims. Further, the evaluator should assess the sufficiency of the sample size to adequately address the research questions and/or hypotheses. In quantitative research, the explication of the sample sufficiency most often is in the form of a power analysis. In qualitative research, the research argues for data saturation in justifying the sample size.

Next, the researcher should specify the variables of interest in the study. These variables should be clearly presented with operational definitions if quantitative measures are used. The variables should be consistent with the theoretical concepts of the study. And if the design includes independent and dependent variables, these points should be noted in the report.

The methods of data collection of any research report would be expected to include specific details that would make the research replicable. The measurements and instruments used in quantitative studies should be described and the psychometrics (validity and reliability) of instruments should be addressed, both in the literature and explicitly related to the current study. The variables measure is expected to address the underlying theoretical concepts or phenomena of interest. In addition, in this section of the research report, ethical issues, including the institutional review board (IRB) approval for protection of human rights, should be included. The reviewer is expected to evaluate the appropriateness of the data-collection methods for the research design and indicate the presence of bias as noted. If there is an intervention, the fidelity of the intervention is addressed in the critique.

Evaluation of the data-analysis section of a research report with a quantitative design often presents challenges for the novice reviewer of research, particularly if he or she does not have knowledge of statistics. The statistical tests that have been used should be evaluated for their appropriateness and for the detail in which they are presented. The analysis should be comprehensive and should be chosen to answer the research questions and/or test the hypotheses. In a qualitative study, the methodology for analysis also should be clearly and explicitly described, including how themes were identified and whether the analysis is trustworthy and credible.

Following the description of the data analysis, the researcher presents the study results. First, the sample size and the sample characteristics are presented, with the characteristics most often presented in table format. The findings should be clearly presented in relation to each research question/hypothesis with all outcome variables addressed. The tables are presented to add information to the text and provide a snapshot of the key study results. They should not duplicate what is presented in the text. Statistical significance of the study findings is noted in the results section of the report. It is important that this section include the reporting of results without interpretation of the findings as the interpretation is included in the discussion section.

The discussion section should be comprehensive and include attention to all of the study findings, linking these findings to previous research in the area. The discussion of the results, however, must not go beyond the specific study reported, but rather include interpretation of its own results for this one study as related to the literature. This section of the report also includes information about the generalizability/transferability of study findings.

All research studies have limitations, sometimes based on aspects inherent in the methodology and at times due to constraints of time and resources available. The researcher is expected to identify the specific limitations of his or her study, and the evaluator assesses the accuracy and inclusiveness of the limitations identified.

In research journals, there may not be a section of the report dedicated to the implications of the study findings for research; this component is often overlooked. Clinical or education journals often report the implications for clinical practice or education without paying attention to the implications for research. Recommendations for future research are often identified in research reports. If the article is published in a clinical or education journal, there may be recommendations for how the research can be applied. The last section of a research report is the conclusion. This is where the researcher is expected to tie everything together succinctly and summarize the importance of the study.

TABLE I.1. Template for Research Study Critique

Overall Summary
Title
Does the title include the key concepts/variables/phenomenon of interest?
Is it concise (12 words or less) and professionally stated?
Researcher(s) Credibility
Educational credentials?
Prior methodological research experience of the authors (i.e., methodological expertise)?
Subject matter content experience (prior research on the subject matter)?

(continued)

TABLE I.1. Template for Research Study Critique (*continued*)

Abstract
Does it include the key components (objective/aim, background/rationale, methods, results, and conclusion)? Does or does not include references? Is it concise (150–250 words or less)? Does it entice you to read the rest of the article (interesting)?
Introduction/Problem
Is the research problem or phenomenon of interest clearly stated? Is it succinct? Does it answer the "so what" question?
Research Aims/Objectives
Is the research aim/objective clearly stated? Is it concisely written? Does it follow logically from the research problem/phenomenon of interest?
Significance
Is the significance to nursing and health care clearly written? Does the significance follow from the research aim/objective?
Background
Is there a theoretical perspective? Is there an explicit description of a theoretical perspective or conceptual framework? If not, is it implied? Are there clear theoretical/conceptual definitions of the concepts?
Literature Review
Primary sources only? Current (within the past how many years)? Is the search strategy included? Is literature relevant to the research aims/objectives? Is it chronologically presented (old to current)? Is it comprehensive? If not, is sufficient background literature provided?
Rationale for the Study
Is there a gap in the literature that this study will fill (will it extend prior knowledge)? Is the rationale clearly stated? Is this a follow-up or replication study?
Research Question(s) and/or Hypotheses
Are these explicitly and clearly stated? Do they include the variables/phenomenon of interest? Do they follow from the research aim/objective?
Methods
Research Design/Paradigm
Is the research design clearly stated? Is there consistency between the research design and paradigm? Is this the best choice of design to address the research problem/phenomenon of interest? Is there rigor in the design?

(*continued*)

TABLE I.1. Template for Research Study Critique (*continued*)

Setting
Is the setting clearly described?
What biases are introduced as a result of selecting this particular setting?
Sampling Plan and Sample
Is the sampling plan clearly identified?
Does it represent the population of interest?
Is the sampling plan consistent with the research aim/objective?
Is the sample size sufficient (e.g., power analysis or data saturation)?
Variables
Are variables clearly identified?
Are variables operationally defined and consistent with theoretical concepts?
Are independent and dependent variables identified, if applicable?
Method of Data Collection
What are the methods of data collection?
Are validity and reliability clearly addressed for prior research and current study, if applicable?
Do the measures/instruments address the underlying theoretical concepts or phenomenon of interest?
Were human rights protected?
Are other ethical issues identified?
Is the data-collection method appropriate for the research design?
Is there bias in the data collection?
What is the fidelity of intervention addressed, if applicable?
Data Analysis
Are data analysis techniques described (e.g., statistical tests, methodology for qualitative analysis)?
Does the analysis answer the research question?
Is it appropriate?
Is the analysis comprehensive? Are themes identified?
Is there bias in the analysis (trustworthiness? credibility?)?
Results
Are sample characteristics described and fully reported?
Are findings presented related to the research aim/objective?
Are all outcome variables addressed, if applicable?
Are results clearly presented in text and/or tables/figures?
Is significance of results reported, if applicable?
Discussion of Results
Do the authors link the findings to previous research studies?
Are the conclusions comprehensive, yet within the data?
Do the authors interpret the results in the discussion?
Are the findings generalizable or transferable?
Limitations
Identified?
Accurate?
Inclusive?

(continued)

TABLE I.1. Template for Research Study Critique (*continued*)

Implications
Are there implications for practice, education, research?
Are there implications for clinical significance?
Recommendations
Recommendations for future study/study replication?
Conclusion
Is it succinct and does it tie everything together?

Each chapter includes a research study, published in a nursing or health care journal, and a research critique conducted by an experienced nurse researcher. We received permission to reprint the published studies as required. The format is to present the study and the critique side by side so that the inexperienced reviewer (most often students in their first research class) can follow logically and quickly ascertain the dimension of each critique that the experienced researcher evaluated. We expect that this research template, used alongside the accompanying studies and contributors' critiques, will assist students and nurses to develop beginning proficiency in this essential skill, which is at the core of evidence-based practice.

QUANTITATIVE STUDIES

MATERNAL AND PATERNAL KNOWLEDGE AND PERCEPTIONS REGARDING INFANT PAIN IN THE NICU

1

Victoria Vazquez, RN, MS, is a student at the University of Connecticut School of Nursing.

Xiaomei Cong, PhD, RN, is an associate professor in the University of Connecticut School of Nursing and also serves as a participating faculty in the University of Connecticut Institute for Systems Genomics. Dr. Cong is a clinical researcher, educator, and neonatal nurse. Her longstanding interest is in the mechanisms of stressful and painful early life experiences associated with health outcomes in vulnerable high-risk preterm infants. Dr. Cong has more than 10 years of clinical research experience.

Angela DeJong, BSN, RN, is a student at the University of Connecticut School of Nursing.

ABSTRACT

Purpose: To investigate parents' knowledge, self-efficacy, and satisfaction about infant pain in the neonatal intensive care unit (NICU).

Design and sample: A survey was conducted, and 80 parents (57 mothers and 23 fathers) participated in the study.

Main outcome variable: A researcher-developed questionnaire composed of three dimensions: parents' knowledge about infant pain, perception of self-efficacy regarding infant pain, and satisfaction with infant pain management.

Results: Most parents had adequate knowledge and moderate to high self-efficacy and were satisfied with infant pain management in the NICU. Mothers and fathers responded differently regarding self-efficacy and satisfaction, and parents' perceptions were correlated with infants' correct age and parents' own age. Most important, most parents wanted to be present and to be given the opportunity to comfort their infant during and after a painful procedure. Parents also preferred to receive formal/written information on infant pain.

KEY WORDS: infant pain; parental attitudes; NICU; education

Infants and their parents are highly impacted by their experiences in the neonatal intensive care unit (NICU). Infants in NICUs may experience 10 to 20 painful procedures per day including heelsticks, peripherally and centrally inserted

Vazquez, V., Cong, X., & DeJong, A. (2015). Maternal and paternal knowledge and perceptions regarding infant pain in the NICU. *Neonatal Network, 34*(6), 337–344. doi:10.1891/0730-0832.34.6.337. Republished with permission of Springer Publishing Company.

intravenous catheters, arterial punctures, lumbar punctures, chest tube insertions, continuous positive airway pressure, and other stressful events,[1-4] all of which are managed with varying degrees of analgesia dependent on institutional protocols and guidelines and health providers' preference; parents of these infants suffer from the NICU experience as well, with a significant portion experiencing and suffering from both acute stress disorders and posttraumatic stress disorders.[5] Parents report that the sources for their elevated stress, anxiety, and depression include unfamiliarity with the NICU environment, lack of awareness of resources, lack of access to their infant, and concern for the discomfort or pain their infant may be experiencing in the NICU.[6-8] However, there has not been much research investigating what parents know about infant pain, what their self-efficacy is regarding infant pain management, and what their level of satisfaction is with the medical teams and bedside nurses' assessment and management of their infant's pain.[9]

Parents need information regarding infant pain, such as complications from infant pain and infant pain relieving practices. However, many parents are not receiving this information.[9] Studies showed that almost a third of parents did not know if their infants had received pain medication and that most parents worried about immediate and future medical complications of their infant being in pain.[9,10] Parents not only want information on how to relieve their infant's pain, but, more importantly, they also need hands-on opportunities to master methods to comfort their infant. In a Franck and colleagues' study,[11] only 18% of parents reported being educated on the signs of infant pain, and 55% were shown methods to comfort their infant; however, parents' stress and anxiety were not alleviated by this type of education. In contrast, in an ethnographic study,[12] as parents had more opportunities to comfort their infant, they gained more confidence and subsequently took more responsibility and initiative in the care of their infant. This active parental behavior and involvement is what decreased parental anxiety. Even though parents desire more opportunities to be involved in infant pain management and research reveals greater parental involvement decreasing parental anxiety, parents report barriers in the NICU, including restrictive visiting hours and even nursing staff who prevent them from engaging in caretaking activities with their infant.[9]

Parental self-efficacy in infant pain assessment and management has been rarely reported. Self-efficacy refers to the personal convictions that people have regarding their ability to successfully execute particular behaviors to produce certain outcomes, and, particularly, self-efficacy can predict and explain individual health behaviors.[13] Parental self-efficacy refers to parents' perception and confidence in their abilities to successfully perform a particular parenting behavior.[14] Lack of parental self-efficacy, that is, an inability to alleviate his or her infant's pain during painful procedures, may hinder the parent from performing nurturing behaviors and increase levels of emotional arousal and anxiety.[14] More research is needed to explore this feature of parental self-efficacy during the early stage of parenting.

One significant aspect that increased parents' satisfaction with the management of their infant's pain was the ability and opportunity to be present during a painful procedure or at least to be present soon afterward to comfort their infant.[11,15,16] Studies found that, although many parents reported they would like to be at the bedside during potentially painful procedures, <25% of parents reported ever being asked if they would like to be present during painful procedures. Parents who were with their infants during painful procedures reported significantly less stress and anxiety than the parents who were not.[11,16]

As parents become more involved in the care of their infant, they may experience less stress and anxiety, become more skilled in the management of their infant's comfort, and have a greater satisfaction regarding their NICU experience. The importance of evaluating parental attitudes regarding infant pain is to promote parental awareness and involvement in the management of their infant's pain. Therefore, this study had two specific aims. The first aim was to describe NICU parents' general knowledge about infant pain, parents' self-efficacy regarding infant pain, and their satisfaction with the assessment and management of their infant's pain. The second aim was to explore the correlations between the survey items and the parental and infant demographic characteristics.

METHODS
Design and Setting

A descriptive survey design was used for this study. The multicenter study was conducted in two level IV NICUs in the northeast United States, with one of the NICUs consisting of two campus sites. One NICU is 56 beds, and the other is a combined 72 beds between the two campuses.

Participants

The target population was mothers and fathers of newborn infants admitted in the NICU. Inclusion criteria were parents >18 years of age, English speaking, having infants in the NICU more than 14 days, and being able to read survey instructions and answer the survey questions.

Instruments

A researcher-designed 24-item survey and the demographic sheet were used for this study. The content of the survey was determined through a literature review pertaining to parental attitudes and feelings related to infant pain in the NICU. The search engines used were PubMed and Cumulative Index to Nursing and Allied Health Literature (CINAHL) using key terms: *mother, father, parents, infant, discomfort, pain, NICU, analgesia,* and *pain management.* A panel of neonatal intensive care experts consisting of one doctor of philosophy (PhD) neonatal nurse researcher, ten NICU bedside registered nurses, three nurse practitioners, and three neonatologists examined the survey for content validity. The 24-item survey consisted of three categories: (a) parents' general knowledge about infant pain, (b) parents' sense of self-efficacy concerning their infant's pain, and (c) parents' satisfaction regarding the assessment and management of their infant's pain. Each survey item was scaled from 1 (*strongly disagree*) to 5 (*strongly agree*). In addition to parents' and infants' demographic information, parents were asked whether they knew their infant had undergone painful procedures during their NICU stay, such as heelsticks, continuous positive airway pressure, intubations, lumbar punctures, and peripheral intravenous line placements.

Data Collection Procedure

The institutional review boards from both study hospitals and the university approved the study. Researchers approached eligible parents and asked if they would like to participate in this anonymous survey study. Once the parents agreed to participate, they received an information sheet, the survey, and the demographic sheet. The researchers were available to answer parents' questions regarding any of the earlier mentioned information. When the parents completed the survey in the NICU, they put the survey in an envelope provided by the researcher. The researchers then collected the envelope and assigned each survey a study ID number, and mother–father dyads were also coded.

Data Analysis

SPSS Version 20 was used to analyze the data. Descriptive analysis methods were conducted to analyze survey data and demographic characteristics. Chi-square analyses were also run to compare responses to survey questions between mothers and fathers. Pearson's correlations were conducted to analyze the association of survey items with demographic information.

RESULTS
Participant Characteristics

There were 80 parents who participated in this study with 57 mothers and 23 fathers (Table 1), and this resulted in 20- or 21-paired responses from mother and father depending on the question. Mothers were 30.6 ± 7.2 years of age, and most were non-Hispanic Caucasian (66.7%), married (52.6%), college educated (82.5%), and full-time employed (61.4%). Fathers were 31.3 ± 8.5 years of age, and most were non-Hispanic Caucasian (56.5%), married (60.9%), college educated (60.9%), and full-time employed (73.9%). The mean gestational age of infants was 29.8 ± 4.2 weeks, and mean postnatal age was 37.4 ± 27.4 days. Most parents (86.4%) had not had an infant previously in the NICU.

Parents' General Knowledge About Infant Pain

Most mothers and fathers agreed that older newborn infants who are full term or have been in the NICU for a longer period of time as well as young infants who are premature and newly admitted to the NICU can feel pain and can express their pain (Table 2). They believed that parents' soft voice is comforting to a baby. Regarding breastfeeding's analgesic capabilities, most mothers (59.6%) and fathers (73.9%) responded "disagree" or undecided. Regarding knowing which procedures are painful for their infant, 59.6% of mothers and 47.8% of fathers stated they agreed that they knew which procedures were potentially painful for their infant.

Parents' Perceived Self-Efficacy at Managing Infant Pain

Most mothers and fathers felt that they could tell when their infant was in pain, but only 61.4% of mothers and 30.4% of fathers believed that they were able to lessen their infant's pain (Table 3). Most mothers and fathers felt confident doing kangaroo care and believed holding their infant was effective in reducing their infant's crying (89.5% of mothers and 72.7% of fathers), but less felt that they could get their infant into a quiet sleep if in pain (52.7% of mothers and 22.7% of fathers). Parents overwhelmingly wanted to be present during a painful procedure (75.9% of mothers and 81.8% of fathers) and to hold their infant as soon as possible after a painful procedure (92.6% of mothers and 77.3% of fathers).

Parents' Satisfaction With Management of Infant Pain

Overall, most mothers and fathers were satisfied with the pain treatment provided by the medical team (88.7% of mothers and 77.3% of fathers), but less felt that the

TABLE 1. Participant Demographic Characteristics

	Mothers (*N* = 57) *n* (%)	Fathers (*N* = 23) *n* (%)
Marital Status		
Single	16 (28.1)	4 (17.4)
Married	30 (52.6)	30 (52.6)
Divorced	1 (1.8)	0 (0.0)
Living together	10 (17.5)	5 (21.7)
Ethnicity		
Caucasian (non-Hispanic)	38 (66.7)	13 (56.5)
African American	6 (10.5)	5 (21.7)
Hispanic	11 (19.3)	4 (17.4)
Mixed/other	1 (1.8)	0 (0.0)
Education		
Some high school	3 (5.3)	2 (8.7)
High school graduate	7 (12.3)	7 (30.4)
Some college	16 (28.1)	4 (17.4)
College graduate	24 (42.1)	8 (34.8)
Graduate school	7 (12.3)	2 (8.7)
Employment		
Full time	35 (61.4)	17 (73.9)
Part time	5 (8.8)	0 (0.0)
Student	1 (1.8)	0 (0.0)
Not working outside of home	16 (28.1)	6 (26.1)
Infant	*M* (SD)	
Gestational age at birth (wk)	29.8 (4.2)	
Postnatal age (d)	37.4 (27.4)	
Corrected age (wk)	35.2 (4.1)	

medication decreased infant pain (75.5% of mothers and 52.2% of fathers; Table 4). Parents felt that the medical team explains well how they manage and treat infant pain, but fewer parents felt that the bedside nurses explain well how they measure (61.4% of mothers and 56.5% of fathers) and manage infant pain (77.2% of mothers and 73.9% of fathers). Most of the parents felt that they could ask the bedside nurses and medical team about their infant's pain. Most mothers and fathers felt written information on infant pain would be helpful.

Chi-square analyses showed that fathers' responses especially disagreed with mothers on the following items: "I am able to lessen my baby's pain," "If my baby seems in pain, I can get him/her into a quiet sleep," "I want to hold my baby as soon as possible after a painful procedure," and "the medication decreases(ed) my baby's pain" ($p < .05$; see Tables 3 and 4).

Significant positive correlations were found between parents' responses and their infants' corrected age on the following items: "a parent's soft voice is comforting to a baby"; "I am able to lessen my baby's pain"; "My baby stops crying when

TABLE 2. Parents' General Knowledge Regarding Infant Pain (Mother $N = 57$, Father $N = 23$)

Questions		Strongly Disagree/ Disagree n (%)	Undecided n (%)	Strongly Agree/ Agree n (%)	x^2 p
1. Older newborn babies feel pain.	Mother	4 (7.2)	3 (5.4)	49 (87.5)	>.05
	Father	1 (4.3)	3 (13.0)	19 (82.6)	
2. Premature babies feel pain.	Mother	5 (8.8)	1 (1.8)	51 (89.5)	>.05
	Father	1 (4.3)	1 (4.3)	21 (91.3)	
3. Babies of any age can show us they are in pain.	Mother	3 (5.3)	5 (8.8)	49 (86.0)	>.05
	Father	0 (0.0)	2 (8.7)	21 (91.3)	
4. A parent's soft voice is comforting to a baby.[a]	Mother	0 (0.0)	2 (3.5)	55 (96.5)	>.05
	Father	0 (0.0)	0 (0.0)	23 (100.0)	
5. Breastfeeding reduces a baby's pain.	Mother	10 (17.5)	24 (42.1)	23 (40.3)	>.05
	Father	7 (30.4)	10 (43.5)	23 (40.3)	
6. I know which procedures are painful for my baby.	Mother	17 (29.8)	6 (10.5)	34 (59.6)	>.05
	Father	10 (43.5)	2 (8.7)	11 (47.8)	

[a]Parents' responses were positively correlated with infants' corrected age, $p < .05$.

I give him or her the pacifier"; "I want to hold my baby as soon as possible after a painful procedure"; "the medical team explains what they are doing to lessen my baby's pain"; "the bedside nurses explain what they do to lessen my baby's pain" ($r = 0.26–0.40$, $p < .05$; see Tables 1–3). In addition, mothers and fathers' responses on several items were negatively correlated with their own age in that older parents felt less satisfaction with pain treatment and communication with the medical team and nurses in the NICU ($r = –0.27 \sim –0.47$, $p < .05$; see Table 4).

DISCUSSION

Although several studies have been conducted regarding parents' perceptions about infant pain, this study is unique in that it compared maternal and paternal responses in knowledge, self-efficacy, and satisfaction regarding infant pain management in the NICU. Most parents were found to have adequate knowledge and moderate to high self-efficacy and to be satisfied with infant pain management. Mothers and fathers responded differently on several items regarding self-efficacy and satisfaction, and parents' perceptions were also correlated with infants' correct age and parents' age. Interestingly and importantly, the vast majority of parents wanted to be present and be given the opportunity to comfort their infant during and after a painful procedure as well as to be given formal/written information on infant pain.

Parental Knowledge of Infant Pain

Parents in this study generally knew that infants can feel pain at all ages but may be not sure as to which procedures are painful and what pain intervention they can provide for alleviating infant pain. For instance, only less than half of the mothers and less than one-third of fathers agreed that breastfeeding can reduce infant pain,

TABLE 3. Parents' Perception of Self-Efficacy Regarding Infant Pain Management (Mother $N = 57$, Father $N = 23$)

Questions		Strongly Disagree/ Disagree n (%)	Undecided n (%)	Strongly Agree/Agree n (%)	$x^2 p$
7. I can tell when my baby is in pain.	Mother	5 (8.8)	10 (17.5)	42 (73.7)	>.05
	Father	1 (4.3)	6 (26.1)	42 (73.7)	
8. I am able to lessen my baby's pain.[a,b]	Mother	7 (12.3)	15 (26.3)	5 (61.4)	6.55 < .05
	Father	4 (17.3)	11 (52.2)	7 (30.4)	
9. I feel confident doing kangaroo/skin-to-skin care.	Mother	2 (3.5)	1 (1.8)	54 (94.7)	>.05
	Father	1 (4.5)	2 (9.1)	19 (86.3)	
10. My baby stops crying when I hold him/her.	Mother	0 (0.0	6 (10.5)	51 (89.5)	>.05
	Father	1 (4.5)	5 (22.7)	16 (72.7)	
11. My baby stops crying when I give him/her the pacifier.[b]	Mother	2 (3.5)	12 (21.1)	43 (75.5)	>.05
	Father	2 (9.0)	7 (31.8)	8 (59.1)	
12. If my baby seems in pain, I can get him/her into a quiet sleep.[a]	Mother	7 (12.3)	20 (35.1)	30 (52.7)	6.11 < .05
	Father	5 (22.7)	12 (54.5)	5 (22.7)	
13. I want to be present during a painful procedure to comfort my baby.	Mother (n = 54)	5 (9.3)	8 (14.8)	41 (75.9)	>.05
	Father (n = 22)	1 (4.5)	3 (13.6)	8 (81.8)	
14. I want to hold my baby as soon as possible after a painful procedure.[a,b]	Mother[c] (n = 54)	3 (5.6)	1 (1.9)	50 (92.6)	6.78 < .05
	Father (n = 22)	1 (4.5)	4 (18.2)	50 (92.6)	

Note: Only 54 mothers and 22 fathers answered Questions 13 and 14 because these items were not included in the survey in one NICU.

[a]The responses between mothers and fathers are significantly different, $p < .05$.

[b]Parents' responses were positively correlated with infants' corrected age, $p < .05$

[c]Mothers' responses were negatively correlated with mothers' age, $p < .05$.

even though existing research has shown that it does.[17,18] With a high percentage of uncertainty with parental responses pertaining to knowledge especially on pain assessment and interventions, it is clear that an educational intervention on infant pain management can be helpful for the parents.

Parents' Perception of Self-Efficacy in Pain Management

Most mothers and fathers felt confident about using comforting techniques, such as kangaroo care, holding, and pacifier, whereas fathers reported having less confidence than mothers in reducing their infant's pain and getting infants into a quiet sleep during a pain situation. No studies have reported different perceptions of self-efficacy among mothers and fathers, although this study revealed the support and education needs of fathers in the NICU. Consistent with other studies, both mothers and fathers expressed a strong desire to be present during and after painful procedures to comfort

TABLE 4. Parents' Satisfaction Regarding Infant Pain Management (Mother $N = 57$, Father $N = 23$)

Questions		Strongly Disagree/ Disagree n (%)	Undecided n (%)	Strongly Agree/Agree n (%)	x^2 p
15. The medical team (MD/NP/PA) treats my baby's pain well.	Mother[c]	0 (0.0)	6 (10.7)	50 (89.2)	>.05
	Father[d]	0 (0.0)	1 (4.3)	22 (95.7)	
16. The medication decreases(ed) my baby's pain.[a]	Mother[c]	1 (1.8)	13 (22.8)	43 (75.5)	6.11 < .05
	Father	0 (0.0)	11 (47.8)	12 (52.2)	
17. The medical team (MD/NP/PA) explains what they are doing to lessen my baby's pain.	Mother[c]	4 (7.0)	6 (10.5)	47 (82.5)	>.05
	Father	1 (4.3)	1 (4.3)	21 (91.3)	
18. The bedside nurses explain how they measure my baby's pain.	Mother[c]	12 (21.1)	10 (17.5)	35 (61.4)	>.05
	Father	6 (26.1)	4 (17.4)	13 (56.5)	
19. The bedside nurses explain what they do to lessen my baby's pain.[b]	Mother[c]	6 (10.5)	13 (22.8)	38 (66.7)	>.05
	Father	3 (13.0)	3 (13.0)	17 (73.9)	
20. I am included in decisions about treating my baby's pain.	Mother	10 (17.5)	4 (7.0)	43 (75.5)	>.05
	Father	4 (17.4)	3 (13.0)	16 (69.6)	
21. I can ask the bedside nurses about my baby's pain.	Mother	0 (0.0)	0 (0.0)	57 (100.0)	>.05
	Father	0 (0.0)	1 (4.3)	22 (95.6)	
22. I can ask the medical team (MD/NP/PA) about my baby's pain.	Mother	1 (1.8)	0 (0.0)	56 (98.3)	>.05
	Father	0 (0.0)	1 (4.3)	22 (95.6)	
23. I am satisfied with the treatment of my baby's pain.	Mother	0 (0.0)	7 (12.3)	50 (87.7)	>.05
	Father	0 (0.0)	5 (21.7)	18 (77.3)	
24. It would be helpful to receive written information on infant pain.	Mother[c]	4 (7.0)	5 (8.8)	48 (84.3)	>.05
	Father	2 (9.1)	1 (4.3)	20 (91.0)	

MD, medical doctor; NP, nurse practitioner; PA, physician assistant.

[a]The responses between mothers and fathers are significantly different, $p < .05$.

[b]Parents' responses were positively correlated with infants' corrected age, $p < .05$.

[c]Mothers' responses were negatively correlated with mothers' age, $p < .05$.

[d]Fathers' responses were negatively correlated with fathers' age, $p < .05$.

their infants; however, significantly less fathers felt confidence in being able to lessen their infant's pain. In a randomized clinical trial, parents from both intervention and control groups wanted to be involved in a painful procedure with their infants.[16] Parents have seen their involvement in infant pain care as a vital role, and they want full involvement as much as possible.[9,16] Similarly, in another study, parents felt that at least one parent needed to remain with their infant during a painful procedure to support and provide comfort.[6] What was not assessed in this study but can be valuable to include in future studies is how many of those parents who voiced a desire to be present during a painful procedure were actually given the opportunity to do so. Franck and colleagues' study reported that only <25% of these parents were actually given the chance to be present during a painful procedure.[16] Parents who are not given the opportunity to comfort their infant when they feel their infant is in pain can experience increased stress from a loss of their parental role and a loss in their ability to protect their infant.[6]

Although it is understood that various procedures that occur in the NICU may need to be done rapidly or as emergently as possible for the safety and welfare of the infant, there are also many procedures that can be delayed for a brief period to allow time for parents to be notified and asked if they would like to be present. Sometimes, parental presence might not be appropriate due to safety concerns. At times, there are emergencies in the NICU that call for rapid intervention. In other situations, procedures need to be sterile or done in the operating room; however, there are many procedures such as heel sticks, suctioning, and nasogastric tube insertions that can be delayed for a short time to allow the parents to be notified and asked if they want to be present. Having more parental presence during procedures may take a shift in unit philosophy, staff habits, and comfort levels, but the changes may be well worth potentially increased staff–parent education, parent satisfaction, and parent–infant bonding, and further studies are needed to examine these potential benefits. The more this is encouraged, the less parents will experience stress and anxiety, and the greater the parents' satisfaction and parent–infant bonding.[12,19] When comparing nurses' and parents' perspectives, it has been found that both nurses and parents in the NICU agree that infants are capable of experiencing pain; however, many neonatal nurses do not agree that parents should be involved with the care and comfort of infants during painful procedures.[20,21] This may be because most nurses feel that parents are emotionally affected by the pain that their infant may be experiencing. Effective communication between the neonatal nurses and NICU parents is needed to address the different perceptions; this communication issue may be solved by providing NICU staff education and training.[21]

Parental Satisfaction With Infant Pain Management

Most parents felt satisfied with pain treatment provided by the medical team and agreed that the team, including nurses, explained what they do to lessen infant pain. The results are congruent with Franck and colleagues' results that a high level of satisfaction was perceived by parents with their infant's pain care.[11] Franck and colleagues also reported that many parents did not know if their infants had received analgesics or sedatives for pain management,[11] so a paradox might exist with high parent satisfaction in the case of potentially inadequate pain management. In this study, even though parents reported a high level of satisfaction, only about half of them felt that the medication decreased their infant's pain. Parents agreed that bedside nurses explain how they measure their infant's pain.

The survey showed that more than 80% to 90% of mothers and fathers were willing to receive written information on infant pain, which is consistent with a previous study saying parents desire more information.[9,16] Parents who have received the written information on infant pain, which taught them about infant pain cues and comforting techniques, felt high satisfaction with the information, were more prepared to take an active role in infant pain care, and were more positive about their role after discharge.[16,22] When giving information to parents regarding pain management, it is important to gauge their readiness for this knowledge. Parents are under a lot of stress in the NICU and often want to know as much as they can about their baby's care. It is important to not overwhelm the parents when offering this information. When distributing our survey, we made sure that parents shared a desire to discuss pain management. We debriefed them after giving the survey to see if parents felt the survey was overwhelming with how much it mentioned infant pain. The parents did not express feelings of being overwhelmed but did express a strong desire to want more information. Parents voiced that they did not always feel included in decisions about the treatment of their baby's pain. These results indicate that there are a sizable number of parents who felt an inability to recognize the signs and symptoms of their infant's pain and how to use skills to decrease their infant's pain. Parents report that, early in their NICU stay, they feel incompetent in terms of many of their parenting tasks and with the parenting role in general, but, as they are able to take on the parenting tasks, they more quickly begin to gain a secure sense of their own abilities to care for their infants.[6,23-25]

In addition, this study revealed that parents' perceptions were correlated with infants' corrected age and with parents' own age, which have not been investigated in previous studies. Parents of infants with older corrected age were more confident about managing their infant's pain and more satisfied with the communication about pain treatment between the parent and the medical team and nurses. Many young premature babies may have a weak cry or less behavioral responses to pain as well as to pain relief interventions because of their prematurity and/or medical condition, such as with intubation. The older the baby is, the more apparent are their pain cues, and parents often find it easier to assess and manage pain in infants with greater gestational and postnatal age. It has been found that the lower the gestational age of the infant at birth, the more negative parental perceptions and experiences were in the area of relationship with the infant.[26] Medical teams and nurses may also be more comfortable in treating neonatal pain in older infants because they are perceived as less vulnerable to the adverse effects of medications.[21] Regarding infant pain management, older mothers and fathers felt less satisfaction with pain treatment and communication with the medical team and nurses in the NICU. This negative correlation may show that older parents are more critical and might seek more explanation from the bedside nurses regarding their baby's care. Interestingly, the correlation showed that younger mothers were more willing to be present during painful procedures and receive written information on infant pain. No other studies have previously shown that parent age may affect their perceptions of infant pain management. Clinicians as well as researchers need to consider the effect of infants' and parents' age on the outcomes when they provide pain treatment and education and conduct research in the NICU.

Infant pain is inevitable in the NICU, but health care providers can include parents in the assessment and management of their infant's pain. Parents have consistently stated through studies that they want more information and to be included more in the care of their infant and, in this case, the management of their infant's pain. Perhaps one area nurses can focus on to encourage parents in the care of their infant is in the use of effective nonpharmacologic pain-relieving strategies, such as breastfeeding and kangaroo care. Because most parents were unclear as to the potential of breastfeeding to reduce infant pain yet felt confident doing kangaroo care, it could be beneficial to educate parents on the connection found between breastfeeding, kangaroo care, and infant analgesia.[2,18,27,28] Clinicians need to be reminded to be sensitive when educating parents on infant pain, gauging the parents' readiness and receptivity. Some parents want to know all there is to know about the NICU, but others might benefit more from small and selective bits of NICU information.[6,9]

CONCLUSION

The findings from this study are in line with the results of previous research, which highlighted that, during the NICU stay, parents encounter difficulties in managing infant pain and want more information and to be involved as much as possible in the care and management of their infant's pain. The more opportunities we afford parents for education and hands-on care pertaining to recognizing signs of infant pain and effective ways to minimize their infant's pain, the more we encourage and facilitate parental competencies, thus encouraging, promoting, and building a vital aspect of their parental role. Limitations of this study were the small sample size of fathers and that the survey mostly included well-educated and English-speaking parents and was conducted in the NICUs at large, urban hospitals. Therefore, representative bias may exist, and further studies are warranted.

DISCLOSURE

The authors have no relevant financial interest or affiliations with any commercial interests related to the subjects discussed within this article. No commercial support or sponsorship was provided for this educational activity.

REFERENCES

1. Anand KJ; and International evidence-Based group for neonatal pain. Consensus statement for the prevention and management of pain in the newborn. *Arch Pediatr Adolesc Med.* 2001;155(2):173–180.
2. Carbajal R, Rousset A, Danan C, et al. Epidemiology and treatment of painful procedures in neonates in intensive care units. *JAMA.* 2008;300(1):60–70.
3. Lago P, Garetti E, Merazzi D, et al.; and Pain Study Group of the Italian Society of Neonatology. Guidelines for procedural pain in the newborn. *Acta Paediatr.* 2009;98(6):932–939.
4. Simons Sh, van Dijk M, Anand KS, Roofthooft D, Van Lingen RA, Tibboel D. Do we still hurt newborn babies? A prospective study of procedural pain and analgesia in neonates. *Arch Pediatr Adolesc Med.* 2003;157(11):1058–1064.
5. Holditch-Davis D, Bartlett TR, Blickman AL, Miles MS. Posttraumatic stress symptoms in mothers of premature infants. *J Obstet Gynecol Neonatal Nurs.* 2003;32(2):161–171.
6. Gale G, Franck LS, Kools S, Lynch M. Parents' Perceptions of their infant's pain experience in the NICU. *Int J Nurs Stud.* 2004;41(1):51–58.
7. Holditch-Davis D, Miles MS. Parenting the Prematurely born child. *Annu Rev Nurs Res.* 1997;15:3–34.
8. Miles MS, Holditch-Davis D, Schwartz TA, Scher M. Depressive symptoms in mothers of prematurely born infants. *J Dev Behav Pediatr.* 2007;28(1):36–44.
9. Franck LS, Oulton K, Bruce E. Parental involvement in neonatal pain management: an empirical and conceptual update. *J Nurs Scholarsh.* 2012;44(1):45–54.
10. Franck LS, Allen A, Cox S, Winter I. Parents' views about infant pain in neonatal intensive care. *Clin J Pain.* 2005;21(2):133–139.
11. Franck LS, Cox S, Allen A, Winter I. Parental concern and distress about infant pain. *Arch Dis Child Fetal Neonatal Ed.* 2004;89(1):f71–f75.
12. Skene C, Franck L, Curtis P, Gerrish K. Parental involvement in neonatal comfort care. *J Obstet Gynecol Neonatal Nurs.* 2012;41(6):786–797.
13. Bandura A. Self-efficacy: toward a unifying theory of behavioral change. *Psychol Rev.* 1977;84(2):191–215.
14. Patrick S, Garcia J, Griffin L. The role of family therapy in mediating adverse effects of excessive and inconsolable neonatal crying on the family system. *Fam Syst Health.* 2010;28(1):19–29.
15. Franck LS, Cox S, Allen A, Winter I. Measuring neonatal intensive care unit-related parental stress. *J Adv Nurs.* 2005;49(6):608–615.
16. Franck LS, Oulton K, Nderitu S, Lim M, Fang S, Kaiser A. Parent involvement in pain management for NICU infants: a randomized controlled trial. *Pediatrics.* 2011;128(3):510–518.
17. Holsti L, Oberlander TF, Brant R. Does breastfeeding reduce acute procedural pain in preterm infants in the neonatal intensive care unit? A randomized clinical trial. *Pain.* 2011;152(11):2575–2581.

18. Shah PS, Herbozo C, Aliwalas LL, Shah VS. Breastfeeding or breast milk for procedural pain in neonates. *Cochrane Database Syst Rev.* 2012;(12):Cd004950.

19. Axelin A, Lehtonen L, Pelander T, Salanterä S. Mothers' different styles of involvement in preterm infant pain care. *J Obstet Gynecol Neonatal Nurs.* 2010;39(4):415–424.

20. Cong X, Delaney C, Vazquez V. Neonatal nurses' perceptions of pain assessment and management in NICUs: a national survey. *Adv Neonatal Care.* 2013;13(5):353–360.

21. Cong X, Mcgrath JM, Delaney C, et al. Neonatal nurses' perceptions of pain management: survey of the United States and China. *Pain Manag Nurs.* 2014;15(4):834–844.

22. Spence K, Henderson-Smart D. Closing the evidence-practice gap for newborn pain using clinical networks. *J Paediatr Child Health.* 2011;47(3):92–98.

23. Fegran L, Fagermoen MS, Helseth S. Development of parent-nurse relationships in neonatal intensive care units—from closeness to detachment. *J Adv Nurs.* 2008;64:363–371.

24. Fegran L, Helseth S, Fagermoen MS. A comparison of mothers' and fathers' experiences of the attachment process in a neonatal intensive care unit. *J Clin Nurs.* 2008;17(6):810–816.

25. Fenwick J, Barclay L, Schmied V. Craving closeness: a grounded theory analysis of women's experiences of mothering in the special Care nursery. *Women Birth.* 2008;21(2):71–85.

26. Tooten A, Hoffenkamp HN, Hall RA, Braeken J, Vingerhoets AJ, van Bakel HJ. Parental perceptions and experiences after childbirth: a comparison between mothers and fathers of term and preterm infants. *Birth.* 2013;40(3):164–171.

27. Cong X, Cusson RM, Walsh S, Hussain N, Ludington-Hoe SM, Zhang D. Effects of skin-to-skin contact on autonomic pain responses in preterm infants. *J Pain.* 2012;13(7):636–645.

28. Yilmaz F, Arikan D. The effects of various interventions to newborns on pain and duration of crying. *J Clin Nurs.* 2011;20(7–8):1008–1017.

MATERNAL AND PATERNAL KNOWLEDGE AND PERCEPTIONS REGARDING INFANT PAIN IN THE NICU

Critique by *Linda Cook, Anita Ayrandjian Volpe, and Karen Bauce*

OVERALL SUMMARY

The paucity of research addressing parental knowledge about infant pain makes this study particularly relevant to nurses assisting parents to become more involved in the care of their infant in the neonatal intensive care unit (NICU). The authors developed their own research instrument to survey mothers and fathers about their general knowledge of infant pain, self-efficacy at managing their infant's pain, and their overall satisfaction with management of infant pain in the NICU. Study findings, which are clearly presented through the use of tables and discussion, have significance for nurses desiring to encourage and facilitate parental involvement and competencies in nonpharmacologic pain-relieving strategies.

TITLE

Does the title include the key concepts/variables/phenomenon of interest?

The title peaks interest and clearly states the experience that was studied, parental knowledge and perception of neonatal pain in the NICU, as well as the subjects under study, mothers and fathers of infants.

Is it concise (12 words or less) and professionally stated?

The authors may consider shortening the title to *Parental Knowledge and Perceptions Regarding Infant Pain in the NICU.*

RESEARCHER(S) CREDIBILITY

Educational credentials?

The first and third authors are MS- and BSN-prepared nurses who were students at a reputable state university at the time the study was published. The second author is PhD prepared as well as a neonatal nurse.

Prior methodological research experience of the authors (i.e., methodological expertise)?

As noted in the reference list, the second author has previous research experience with descriptive survey design to investigate neonatal nurses' perceptions regarding pain assessment and management.

Subject matter content experience (prior research on the subject matter)?

The second author's prior research experience on pain in preterm infants and NICU nurses' practice related to pain management and assessment provide credibility for this study. It would be helpful to know the clinical expertise of the nondoctorally prepared authors in order to establish research credibility/subject content expertise.

ABSTRACT

Does it include the key components (objective/aim, background/rationale, methods, results, and conclusion)?

The abstract distinctly states the purpose of the study, design and sample, outcome and results.

Does or does not include references?

The abstract appropriately does not include references.

Is it concise (150–250 words or less)?

The abstract is succinct containing a total of 138 words, which is less than the 150- to 250-word requirement of an abstract. Keywords are included.

Does it entice you to read the rest of the article (interesting)?

The abstract is thought provoking, provides a clear overview of the study, and would appeal to the professional subscriber of this journal, *Neonatal Network*.

INTRODUCTION/PROBLEM

Is the research problem or phenomenon of interest clearly stated?

The research problem is clearly stated in the introduction. Parents need information related to their infant's pain but are not receiving the information from providers. Parents also want hands-on opportunities to learn comfort measures. We really do not appreciate what parents know about infant pain or their self-efficacy in pain assessment and management because there is insufficient research on the topic. The research problem is significant to neonatal nursing because family-centered care is an important part of the care of the infant in the NICU and parents need to be able to feel they can comfort their infant.

Is it succinct?

The research problem is succinctly stated.

Does it answer the "so what" question?

The research problem speaks to the need for further understanding of parental knowledge, self-efficacy, and satisfaction about NICU pain management so that parents can become more involved and skilled in their infant's pain management, experience less stress, and have a more positive NICU experience.

RESEARCH AIMS/OBJECTIVES

Is the research aim/objective clearly stated?

The study contains two clearly stated research aims in the last paragraph of the Introduction section: assessment of parental knowledge regarding infant pain, parental self-efficacy regarding infant pain, and parental satisfaction regarding the assessment and management of infant pain, as well as exploration of the correlations between 24 survey items and parental and infant demographic characteristics.

Is it concisely written?

The aims are concisely written.

Does it follow logically from the research problem/phenomenon of interest?

> The research aims follow logically from the problem of lack of understanding of parental knowledge and perceptions of infant pain in the NICU.

SIGNIFICANCE

Is the significance to nursing and health care clearly written?

> The significance to nursing is not explicitly stated but can be inferred in the beginning presentation of the background literature. The authors describe the importance of evaluating parental attitudes regarding infant pain in light of research indicating that active involvement in their infant's care and pain management leads to a variety of positive outcomes. The authors also state that nurses should educate parents on nonpharmacologic methods of pain relief, including breastfeeding and kangaroo care.

Does the significance follow from the research aim/objective?

> The significance to nursing and health care follows from the two previously identified research aims.

BACKGROUND

Is there an explicit description of a theoretical perspective or conceptual framework? If not, is it implied?

> There is no theoretical framework identified. There is no stated nursing framework and none is implied.

Are there clear theoretical/conceptual definitions of the concepts?

> The concepts of self-efficacy and parental self-efficacy are clearly defined in the third paragraph of the introduction.

LITERATURE REVIEW

Primary sources only?

> Only primary sources were used.

Current (within the past how many years)?

> The literature review in the introduction presents a discussion of parents' perceptions of their infant's pain and desire to have knowledge on how to comfort their infant during painful procedures. It also touched on parental attitudes regarding infant pain and satisfaction with the medical management of their infant's pain. Of the 28 resources cited, only 13 were published within 5 years of the research study publication date. Two studies from 1997 were included in the review but there was no mention that either one was a seminal study and thus merited inclusion. The authors should make a point of noting the paucity of current literature in the area of parental knowledge and attitudes regarding infant pain.

Is the search strategy included?

> The search strategy or databases used were not identified. The only discussion of a search strategy is related to a literature review that informed the development of the 24-item survey instrument used to measure parental knowledge, self-efficacy, and satisfaction.

Is literature relevant to the research aims/objectives?

> The literature review was relevant to the research aims/objectives.

Is it chronologically presented (old to current)?

> The literature was not presented chronologically yet provides a logical progression of what is known about parental knowledge and attitudes regarding infant pain.

Is it comprehensive? If not, is sufficient background literature provided?

> The literature review was sufficiently comprehensive and permits the reader to grasp what is known and unknown in this area.

RATIONALE FOR THE STUDY

Is there a gap in the literature that this study will fill (will it extend prior knowledge)? Is the rationale clearly stated?

> The gap in the literature can be inferred from the authors' discussion of the limited research done on the topic of parental knowledge and perception of their infant's pain in the NICU. This study could add to that limited knowledge.

Is this a follow-up or replication study?

> This is not a follow-up or replication study.

RESEARCH QUESTION(S) AND/OR HYPOTHESES

Are these explicitly and clearly stated?

> There are no explicit research questions, rather two broad research aims that are clearly stated in the last paragraph of the Introduction section.

Do they include the variables/phenomenon of interest?

> It can be inferred from the research aims that parental general knowledge about infant pain, parental perceived self-efficacy at managing infant pain, and parental satisfaction with management of infant pain are the outcome variables of interest.

Do they follow from the research aim/objective?

> The outcome variables of interest flow logically from the research problem and research aims.

METHODS

Research Design/Paradigm

Is the research design clearly stated?

> A descriptive survey design was used for this study and is clearly stated in the Methods section.

Is there consistency between the research design and paradigm?

The descriptive design of this quantitative study is focused on obtaining information related to parental knowledge and perceptions regarding infant pain from a survey instrument, which is consistent with the positivist approach to understanding phenomena of interest.

Is this the best choice of design to address the research problem/phenomenon of interest?

Given the limited research on parental knowledge and perceptions of infant pain in the NICU, a descriptive design is appropriate as its intent is to further understanding of the phenomenon of interest.

Is there rigor in the design?

There is rigor to the design because it is an appropriate choice, based on the current level of knowledge of the phenomenon of interest.

SETTING

Is the setting clearly described?

The setting is clearly described as two Level IV NICUs in the northeastern United States, one with dual sites. One NICU contains 56 beds, and the other has a combined 72 beds between both campuses.

What biases are introduced as a result of selecting this particular setting?

Limiting the setting to two Level IV urban NICUs in one geographical part of the country introduces bias that prevents the ability to generalize study findings to other NICUs in other locations.

SAMPLING PLAN AND SAMPLE

Is the sampling plan clearly identified?

Although not explicitly identified, the sampling plan appears to be a nonrandom convenience sample consisting of mothers and fathers of newborn infants admitted into the NICUs in the study settings. Inclusion criteria were specified but there is limited information on how participants were originally screened other than the researchers stating that eligible parents were approached for participation.

Does it represent the population of interest?

The sample represents the population of interest, mothers and fathers of newborn infants admitted to the NICU.

Is the sampling plan consistent with the research aim/objective?

The sampling plan is consistent with the two research aims related to understanding parental knowledge and perception of infant pain.

Is the sample size sufficient (e.g., power analysis or data saturation)?

There was no power analysis presented so the reader was unable to determine whether the sample size of 80 parents was sufficient to detect statistically significant differences in correlations between maternal and paternal responses to the survey questions and parental and infant demographic characteristics.

VARIABLES
Are variables clearly identified?
The three outcome variables of interest are clearly identified in the first research aim.

Are variables operationally defined and consistent with theoretical concepts?
Parental self-efficacy is defined theoretically and it is inferred that it is operationally defined as the score on the self-efficacy category in the researcher-developed survey instrument. Although the authors state that each survey item was scaled from 1 (strongly disagree) to 5 (strongly agree), the reader has to assume that higher scores in this category indicate a higher degree of parental self-efficacy. Similarly, it is also inferred that parental knowledge and satisfaction are operationally defined as the scores on the respective survey categories and higher scores indicate a higher degree of knowledge and satisfaction. It would be helpful if the authors provided definitional terms for infant pain and pain management and clarified what is meant by infants' corrected age. The authors do not describe the process for determining the survey's content validity, other than to state it was evaluated by a panel of neonatal intensive care experts, and there is no indication that the survey questions were tested prior to use in this study.

Are independent and dependent variables identified, if applicable?
The three dependent outcome variables of interest are identified in the first research aim.

METHOD OF DATA COLLECTION
What are the methods of data collection?
There is minimal information about data collection other than a reference to the authors collecting surveys completed by parents in the NICU and placed in envelopes provided by the researchers. The time frame for collecting data is unknown as is the response rate, that is, number of surveys returned versus distributed.

Are validity and reliability clearly addressed for prior research and current study, if applicable?
Validity and reliability of the researcher-designed 24-item survey instrument used to measure parental knowledge, self-efficacy, and satisfaction are not addressed other than the authors stating that content validity was assessed by a panel of neonatal intensive care experts. This makes it difficult for the reader to determine whether the survey is an appropriate measure of the outcomes of interest.

Do the measures/instruments address the underlying theoretical concepts or phenomenon of interest?
In the absence of information about the validity and reliability of the researcher-designed instrument, it cannot be determined whether the concepts of self-efficacy, parental knowledge, and parental satisfaction are actually being measured.

Were human rights protected?
The institutional review boards from the university and both study hospitals approved the study.

Are other ethical issues identified?
The authors do not describe where parents completed the demographic sheet and questionnaire, which may introduce concerns about privacy, and do not indicate whether they contained any personal identifying information.

Is the data-collection method appropriate for the research design?

The use of a survey for data collection is appropriate for descriptive quantitative research.

Is there bias in data collection?

Utilizing a research-developed survey without addressing its validity and reliability introduces bias in the data collection.

DATA ANALYSIS

Are data analysis tecniques described (e.g., statistical tests, methodology for qualitative analysis)?

Data analysis is clearly described and utilized appropriate statistical test measurements. Tables display participant demographic characteristics and parental responses to survey questions and are self-explanatory.

Does the analysis answer the research question?

The data analysis does address the research aims, providing information on parental perceptions of infant pain and differences between maternal and paternal responses.

Is it appropriate?

The analysis was appropriate for this descriptive study.

Is the analysis comprehensive? Are themes identified?

The analysis was comprehensive and discussed in detail all outcome variables, themes, and differences between maternal and paternal responses.

Is there bias in the analysis (trustworthiness? credibility?)?

One source of possible bias in the analysis is related to the lack of information on the validity and reliability of the researcher-developed survey used to collect data on maternal and paternal attitudes and feelings about infant pain. Without this information, it is difficult to know whether and how well the survey measures the outcome variables of interest.

RESULTS

Are sample characteristics described and fully reported?

Sample characteristics are appropriately described and displayed in Table 1.

Are findings presented related to the research aim/objective?

Findings are presented in detail in relation to the two research aims.

Are all outcome variables addressed if applicable?

The authors address parental knowledge about and self-efficacy of infant pain, as well as satisfaction with management of their infant's pain in the NICU.

Are results clearly presented in text and/or tables/figures?

All four tables clearly present study findings.

Is significance of results reported, if applicable?

> Significant results are reported in the discussion of results and noted in Tables 2 to 4. It would be helpful, particularly for the novice reader of research studies, if the authors referred to statistically significant differences rather than areas of especial disagreement between maternal and paternal responses on survey items. In addition, explaining the meaning of a significant positive or negative correlation between parental responses and demographic characteristics would further enhance understanding of the results.

DISCUSSION OF RESULTS

Do the authors link the findings to previous research studies?

> There is appropriate linkage to the findings from previous research studies throughout the Discussion section with the authors emphasizing that the current study is unique in its differentiation between maternal and paternal responses.

Are the conclusions comprehensive, yet within the data?

> The discussion is comprehensive and does not extend beyond what is supported by the data.

Do the authors interpret the results in the discussion?

> The authors interpret the results in the Discussion section, acknowledging the inevitability of infant pain in the NICU as well as parental desire to be involved in comfort measures.

Are the findings generalizable or transferable?

> The generalizability/transferability of the findings is limited as the participant population was a convenience sample of English-speaking individuals with a high level of education, the sample size of fathers was small, and the study was conducted in two Level IV urban NICUs in one geographical part of the country. The authors address bias from the small sample size of fathers in the Conclusion section.

LIMITATIONS

Identified? Accurate? Inclusive?

> The authors describe a few generic study limitations while omitting others, such as the absence of power analysis and reliability and validity testing of the researcher-developed survey instrument.

IMPLICATIONS

Are there implications practice, education, research?
Are there implications for clinical significance?

> There is no defined section for implications, which are briefly discussed within the last paragraph of the discussion and in the conclusion. The authors identify an opportunity for nurses to facilitate and increase parental involvement in the assessment and management of their infant's pain in the NICU through education and hands-on care. The authors also refer to a need for further studies without providing additional detail.

RECOMMENDATIONS

Recommendations for future study/study replication?

The authors recommend further studies without providing any detail as to how they would be designed to improve on the current study.

CONCLUSION

Is it succinct and does it tie everything together?

The conclusion is quite brief but reminds the reader of parental difficulties in managing infant pain and their desire for greater education and hands-on care.

CULTURAL COMPETENCE AND PSYCHOLOGICAL EMPOWERMENT AMONG ACUTE CARE NURSES

2

Karen Bauce, DNP, RN, NEA-BC,
is an adjunct professor at Sacred Heart University, School of Nursing.
Previously she was a health care consultant at Bridgeport Hospital,
Bridgeport, Connecticut, where she designed and implemented the
structures and processes for collaborative professional practice.

Suha Al-Oballi Kridli, PhD, RN,
is an associate professor at Oakland University, School of Nursing. She received her Bachelor degree
from the University of Jordan and her Master and Doctoral degrees from the University of Missouri-
Columbia. Her research interest is in the areas of health beliefs and practices of Middle Eastern
population and childhood obesity.

Joyce J. Fitzpatrick, PhD, RN, FAAN,
is an Elizabeth Brooks Ford professor of nursing at the Frances Payne Bolton School of Nursing, Case
Western Reserve University in Cleveland, Ohio.

ABSTRACT

Increased cultural diversity of patients requires that nurses manage differences
in health beliefs, practices, and expectations. It has been suggested that cultural
competence is fundamentally nursing competence because it reflects the nurse's
ability to provide individualized patient care regardless of the patient's social
or cultural background. Psychological empowerment has been identified as an
important contributor to professional nursing practice and may influence the
provision of culturally competent care. The purpose of this study was to describe
the relationship between cultural competence and psychological empowerment
among acute care nurses in one urban hospital in southern Connecticut. Schim and
colleagues' Cultural Competence Model was used as the theoretical framework.

KEY WORDS: cultural competence, cross-cultural nursing, psychological
empowerment, empowerment, nurses

Nurses care for culturally diverse patients. Current challenges in care are related to
lack of awareness or knowledge of cultural differences, communication difficulties
due to language differences, ethnocentrism and prejudice in caregivers, and lack

Bauce, K., Kridli, S. A., & Fitzpatrick, J. J. (2014). Cultural competence and psychological empowerment
among acute care nurses. *Online Journal of Cultural Competence in Nursing and Healthcare, 4*(2), 27–38.
doi:10.9730/ojccnh.org/v4n2a3. Reprinted with permission.

of organizational support to meet the needs of diverse patients (Taylor & Alfred, 2010). The U.S. Census Bureau (2010) projects continued significant increases in racial and ethnic diversity over the next four decades, therefore the provision of culturally congruent care has become a priority (Taylor & Alfred, 2010). Because nurses provide most of the direct health care services in an organization, they are expected to be knowledgeable about the diverse health beliefs and practices of their patients in an effort to plan and implement culturally appropriate interventions.

Empowerment is often discussed in the literature in the context of factors that influence the nurse's ability to make autonomous decisions based on professional judgment and expertise (Laschinger & Wong, 1999). A common theme found in several definitions of empowerment is that individuals require power in order to do their work in a meaningful way (Laschinger, Gilbert, Smith, & Leslie, 2010). It is assumed that empowered nurses will provide better care, resulting in better patient outcomes (Laschinger et al., 2010). Psychological empowerment, as conceptualized by Spreitzer (1995), reflects an individual's intrinsic task motivation to positively influence his job and workplace. There is empirical support for psychological empowerment as an essential component of positive patient outcomes (Laschinger, Finegan, Shamian, & Wilk 2004; Purdy, Laschinger, Finegan, Kerr, & Olivera, 2010).

A literature review resulted in no published studies regarding the effect of psychological empowerment on cultural competence or cultural competence on psychological empowerment. The purpose of this study, therefore, was to describe the relationship between cultural competence and perceptions of psychological empowerment among acute care nurses.

THEORETICAL FRAMEWORK

The theoretical rationale for this study is based on the Cultural Competence Model, developed by Schim and Miller (1999) and subsequently revised (Schim, Doorenbos, Benkert, & Miller, 2007), using the analogy of a three-dimensional (3-D) jigsaw puzzle (Figure 1) to represent the four pieces of provider level competence. The four constructs include (a) cultural diversity, which varies in quantity and quality across place and time and includes not only differences in race and ethnicity but also differences in language, religion, gender, sexual orientation, and socioeconomic class; (b) cultural awareness, which includes knowledge and recognition of the various factors that contribute to differences in and between groups; (c) cultural sensitivity, or attitudes (CAS) about oneself and willingness to become more culturally knowledgeable and skillful; and (d) cultural competence behaviors (CCBs), which involves a set of behaviors demonstrated in response to cultural diversity, awareness, and sensitivity (Schim et al., 2007).

Schim and colleagues (2007) theorize that all four constructs are required, but are not individually sufficient to achieve culturally competent care. In addition, the development of cultural competence is an ongoing process that is informed by each cross-cultural encounter. The goal is not complete mastery of cultural competence, but rather matching provider competencies to meet the needs of specific populations and individuals who are the recipients of care (Schim et al., 2007).

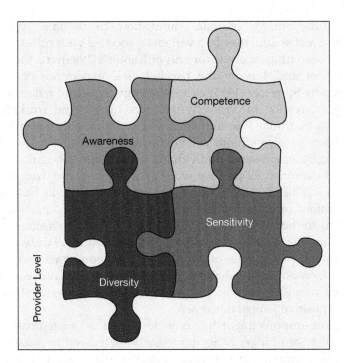

FIGURE 1. Provider level of three-dimensional cultural competence puzzle model. Adapted from Schim et al. (2007, p. 105). Reprinted with permission.

LITERATURE REVIEW

Research regarding variables associated with cultural competence has demonstrated a positive correlation between level of educational attainment and cultural competence, and prior training and cultural competence (Schim, Doorenbos, & Borse, 2005; Schim, Doorenbos, & Borse, 2006). Nurses who have obtained a BSN or higher academic degrees are more likely to score higher on measures of cultural awareness and sensitivity (Schim et al., 2006). Greater experience with culturally diverse patient populations has not been linked with cultural competence among nurses (Schim et al., 2005), which may indicate that clinical encounters alone are insufficient to minimize cultural dissonance.

Taylor and Alfred's (2010) study of nurses' perceptions of organizational supports needed for culturally competent care identified several challenges, including language barriers, lack of knowledge of cultural differences, minimal training programs, and the absence of explicit organizational expectations. Nurses' communication difficulties and insufficient knowledge of cultural differences created misunderstandings with patients and their families that made care more challenging. However, the authors concluded that even with the availability of adequate interpreter services and educational programs, nurses may not incorporate training into patient care in the absence of explicit organizational expectations for cultural competence, accountability, and support for behavioral change.

Although several researchers (Salman et al., 2007; Schim et al., 2005; Taylor & Alfred, 2010) suggest that training and education may enhance cultural competence, there is little empirical research that demonstrates the effectiveness of such training in improving clinical outcomes or identifies the requirements for sustainability.

Furthermore, the nurse's personal motivation to become culturally aware, knowledgeable, and skillful may be a variable associated with cultural competence.

Empirical research has focused primarily on Kanter's (1999) structural determinants of empowerment and less on the psychological experience of empowerment, conceptualized by Spreitzer (1995) as a set of cognitions that reflect an individual's intrinsic task motivation to positively influence his job and workplace. Spreitzer (1995) theorizes that unless an individual is psychologically receptive, social, and structural empowering conditions will not be fully realized.

Psychologically empowered individuals report high job satisfaction and less job strain, and demonstrate positive work performance (Spreitzer, 1995). Faulkner and Laschinger (2008) found psychological empowerment to be associated with nurses' perceptions of respect, and Laschinger et al. (2004) reported psychological empowerment to be a significant predictor of job satisfaction, productivity, effectiveness, and decreased intent to leave the organization. Purdy et al. (2010) also found that nurses' perceptions of psychological empowerment were significantly associated with empowered behaviors, job satisfaction, and nurse-assessed quality of care, which provides support for psychological empowerment as an essential component of positive patient outcomes.

Psychological empowerment has been identified as a predictor of innovative behavior (Knol & van Linge, 2009; Spreitzer, 1995), as well as a mediator between structural empowerment and innovative behavior (Knol & van Linge, 2009). Knol and van Linge (2009) suggest that psychologically empowered nurses believe they are autonomous and have an impact on their immediate work environment, and as a result may be more likely to be creative and engage in innovative behaviors. They further suggest that psychological empowerment may be important for stimulating and managing organizational change.

Leggat, Bartram, Casimir, and Stanton's (2010) research indicated that psychological empowerment mediated the relationship between high-performance work systems and nurses' perceptions of the quality of patient care. The mediating effect of psychological empowerment on other outcome variables important for nursing practice (e.g., burnout and organizational commitment) has been previously reported (Hochwalder, 2007; Avolio, Zhu, Koh, & Bhatia, 2004).

In summary, cultural competence of nurses is influenced by level of educational attainment and cultural diversity training, as well as explicit organizational expectations for cultural competence. In addition, psychological empowerment enhances nurses' work effectiveness and job satisfaction, which lead to positive patient outcomes.

RESEARCH METHODS
Design

A quantitative descriptive correlational design was used to examine the relationship between cultural competence and perceptions of psychological empowerment among acute care registered nurses. The setting for the study was a 425-bed licensed acute care urban hospital in southern Connecticut. Data were collected over an 8-week period.

Sample

A nonprobability convenience sampling strategy was used to obtain participants for this study. The accessible population ($n = 593$) consisted of acute care nurses working at the study facility. Inclusion criteria for the sample consisted of nurses working a minimum of 24 hours weekly and willingness to participate in the study.

Sample size was determined from power analysis, using a power level of 0.80. A small effect size of 0.20 to 0.30 (Burns & Grove, 2009) was assumed because this study represented a new area of research. With an alpha level of significance = 0.05, a minimum of 83 nurse participants were needed to detect statistically significant differences.

Following institutional review board approval from the study facility and the Human Rights Review Committee at Oakland University in Rochester, Michigan, survey questionnaires were given to nurse managers, who informed nurses where the questionnaires were located on their units. Completed and returned questionnaires indicated nurses' consent to participate in the study. The researcher collected completed questionnaires on a weekly basis over an 8-week period. A final sample of 120 nurses was obtained, indicating a 20% response rate.

Instruments

Cultural competence was measured using the Cultural Competence Assessment (CCA) Questionnaire, a 26-item instrument designed to measure cultural diversity experience, awareness and sensitivity, and competence behaviors. The CCA can be applied to a wide range of health care disciplines, cultural groups, and education levels (Schim, Doorenboos, Miller, & Benkert, 2003). Cultural diversity experience is measured by respondents' answer to a single question asking about specific racial or ethnic groups encountered in the workplace in the past 12 months. The item score is a count of the number of groups checked, with higher numbers indicating a greater diversity experience. The CCA has two subscales: the first subscale includes cultural awareness (knowledge) and CAS, and is measured with a 7-point Likert-scale with responses ranging from "strongly agree (7) to strongly disagree (1)." A "no opinion" response option is included but not scored. The second subscale for CCB is also measured with a 7-point Likert-like response set, with categories ranging from "always (7) to never (1)." A "not sure" response option is included but not scored. The items in each subscale are summed, with higher scores indicating higher levels of knowledge, more positive attitudes, and greater self-reported frequency of competence behaviors. In this study, the CAS and CCB subscale scores were added as an indicator of total cultural competence (S. M. Schim, personal communication, December 11, 2011). Demographic items on the CCA include questions about age, prior cultural diversity training, self-identified race or ethnicity, and level of education. The researcher added three additional demographic questions pertaining to gender, number of hours worked per week, and number of years worked in the nursing field.

The Cronbach alpha coefficient for the total CCA has been reported in previous studies at over 0.80 (Schim et al., 2006). In a study among acute care nurses, Cronbach alpha for the CCA was 0.89; 0.76 for the CAS subscale; and 0.93 for the CCB subscale (Schim et al., 2005). Content and face validity of the CCA were initially established by a panel of expert reviewers and also supported in contrasted group validity tests (Schim et al., 2003). An examination of concurrent validity between Campinha-Bacote's (1999) Inventory for Assessing the Process of Cultural Competence Among Healthcare Professionals (IAPCC) and the CCA revealed that scores from the CCA moderately correlated ($r = 0.66$) with those from the IAPCC (Schim et al., 2003).

Psychological empowerment was measured using the Psychological Empowerment Questionnaire (PEQ) (Spreitzer, 1995), a 12-item instrument that uses a 7-point Likert scale to measure the four subconstructs (meaning, competence, self-determination, impact) of psychological empowerment in the workplace. There are three items per dimension, and responses range from "very strongly agree (7) to very strongly disagree (1)." Items from each of the four subscales are added to measure total empowerment, with higher scores indicating higher degrees of psychological empowerment. Each subscale total is divided by three to indicate the average score of that subscale.

Cronbach alpha coefficients for the PEQ have ranged from 0.85 to 0.93 for the four subscales, and 0.85 for the total score (DeCicco, Laschinger, & Kerr, 2006). Faulkner and Laschinger (2008) reported Cronbach alphas ranging from 0.86 to 0.91 for the four subscales, and 0.89 for the total scale. Second-order confirmatory factor analysis to assess convergent and discriminant validity of the four subconstructs of psychological empowerment has indicated that each of the four dimensions represent different aspects of empowerment and contribute to the overall construct (Spreitzer, 1995). Spreitzer (1995) has reported that validity estimates for the dimensions are typically around 0.80 across a wide range of work environments, employees, and cultures.

DATA ANALYSIS

Data analysis was completed using the Statistical Program for Social Sciences software (Version 19.0). An apriori alpha level of significance was set at 0.05. Surveys with more than 10% missing data ($n = 9$) were excluded from analysis. The final sample size ($n = 120$) was sufficiently powered to detect a small effect ($r = .25$). Descriptive statistics were computed to characterize the study sample. A Pearson's product-moment correlation coefficient was calculated to determine statistical significance between cultural competence and perception of psychological empowerment. Cronbach alpha reliability coefficients were computed for the major study variables.

RESEARCH RESULTS

Demographic characteristics of the nurses in the study sample are described in Table 1. A majority of the participants were female (92.6%) with a mean age of 45.4 (SD 12.19). Most of the nurses were White (81.8%), but the sample also included Black/African American, Hispanic/Latino, and Asian. Mean years working as an RN was 17.01 (SD 13.40), and mean number of hours worked per week was 35.6 (SD 5.8). Sixty percent held a bachelor's or graduate level degree, and 91% had participated in cultural diversity training.

Descriptive statistics and Cronbach alpha reliability analyses related to the CCA and PEQ are presented in Table 2. Cronbach alpha for the total CCA in this study, as measured by the combined CCA and CCB subscales was 0.86, and the total PEQ alpha was 0.84. All of the subscale reliabilities were above 0.70 except for the CCA subscale, which was 0.61.

Nurses perceived themselves as having a moderate/high level of overall cultural competence ($M = 5.1$, SD 0.67) and a high level of self-reported cultural competence ($M = 4.5$, SD 0.71). Analysis of the CCA subscale scores indicated a high level of cultural awareness and sensitivity ($M = 6.04$, SD 0.5) and a moderate number of CCBs demonstrated ($M = 4.73$, SD 1.1). The mean diversity experience score, which provides an overall index of exposure to diversity, was 9.93 (SD 1.9), indicating a moderate/high exposure to diversity.

TABLE 1. Demographic Characteristics of Study Sample ($n = 120$)

Data	n	%	M	SD	Range
Age	117		45.36	12.19	21–70
Gender					
Female	112	92.6			
Male	9	7.4			
Race or ethnicity					
White	99	81.8			
Black/African American	8	6.6			
Hispanic/Latino	5	4.1			
Asian	9	7.4			
Education					
Diploma	14	11.6			
Associate degree	35	28.9			
Bachelor's degree	51	42.1			
Graduate degree	21	17.4			
Years RN experience			17.01	13.40	0–49
<1	7	5.8			
1–5	32	26.4			
6–10	8	6.6			
>10	74	61.2			
Hours worked per week			35.63	5.8	20–48
24	17	14.2			
32	22	18.3			
36	24	20.0			
40	54	45.0			
>40	3	2.5			
Prior diversity training					
Yes	110	90.9			
No	11	9.1			

Nurses reported experiencing a moderate/high level of total psychological empowerment ($M = 5.42$, SD 0.7). They reported a high sense of meaning ($M = 6.32$, SD 0.06) and competence ($M = 6.10$, SD 0.7) in their work, a moderate/high sense of self-determination ($M = 5.14$, SD 1.2), and a moderate ability to make an impact on organizational outcomes ($M = 4.13$, SD 1.3).

Pearson's product-moment correlation analysis indicated that total cultural competence was not significantly related to total psychological empowerment ($p \geq .05$). Additional analysis of the CCA and PEQ subscale scores demonstrated that the PEQ meaning subscale was significantly correlated with self-reported cultural competence ($r = 0.24$, $p < .01$), CCBs ($r = 0.22$, $p < .05$), and total cultural competence ($r = 0.23$, $p < .05$). The PEQ competence subscale was significantly associated with CCBs ($r = 0.20$, $p < .05$). Correlations between cultural competence (CCA) and psychological empowerment (PEQ) are presented in Table 3.

TABLE 2. Descriptive Statistics for Major Study Variables

Instrument	Mean	Standard Deviation	Score Range	Cronbach Alpha
CCA				
Cultural awareness and sensitivity	6.05	0.47	1–7	0.61
Cultural competence behaviors	4.73	1.08	1–7	0.89
Total cultural competence	5.13	0.67	1–7	0.86
PEQ				
Meaning	6.32	0.64	1–7	0.86
Competence	6.10	0.74	1–7	0.72
Self-determination	5.15	1.16	1–7	0.80
Impact	4.14	1.30	1–7	0.87
Total empowerment	5.43	0.71	1–7	0.84

CCA, Cultural Competence Assessment; PEQ, Psychological Empowerment Questionnaire.

Additional statistical analysis conducted for demographic effects on the major study variables used a lower alpha level of significance of 0.01 due to the number of tests performed. There were no significant relationships between the demographic variables and total cultural competence or total psychological empowerment. There was a significant positive correlation between years working and competence score ($r = 0.34$, $p < .001$), where more years working was associated with higher competence scores.

In addition, there was a significant difference in cultural competence based on years of RN experience ($F(3, 116) = 6.23, p = .001$). The Bonferroni post hoc tests showed nurses with less than 1 year of experience had lower scores than nurses with 5 to 10 years of experience ($p < .001$), and also lower scores than nurses with more than 10 years' experience ($p = .001$). The mean score for nurses with less than 1 year of experience was 3.6 (SD = 1.1), while the mean for nurses with 5 to 10 years of experience was 5.0 (SD = 0), and for nurses with more than 10 years of experience the mean was 4.5 (SD = 0.6).

DISCUSSION

Because each patient has a unique experience of health and illness, all encounters between nurses and patients can be viewed as cross-cultural encounters (Wepa, 2005). Culture, therefore, remains an important organizing constructing guiding nursing practice and in developing nursing knowledge (Dreher & MacNaughton, 2002). Findings from this study provide preliminary evidence of a relationship between cultural competence and dimensions of psychological empowerment. The results are noteworthy given the absence of research on psychological empowerment as a factor that affects the achievement of cultural competence.

In this study, the PEQ meaning subscale correlated significantly with total cultural competence. Meaning occurs when there is a fit between job requirements and an individual's beliefs, values, and behaviors (Spreitzer, 1995); it is a reflection of the individual's intrinsic caring about a task and its purpose (Thomas & Velthouse, 1990). The nurses in this study reported a high sense of meaning, which indicates that they highly value and care about the work they do. The correlation between meaning and total cultural competence suggests that cultural awareness and sensitivity and CCBs are influenced by the nurse's intrinsic caring about their work with patients. Nurses with high perceptions of meaning in their work may be more motivated to become culturally aware and sensitive and develop the knowledge and behaviors required to meet patients' cultural-specific care needs. Having a passion for work that is personally meaningful may enhance the nurse's capacity for what Doorenbos, Schim, Benkert, and Borse (2005) describe as culturally attuned nursing. They describe this as the "complex interplay of sensitivity, knowledge, behaviors, and awareness" (Doorenbos et al., 2005, p. 325) that results in culturally congruent care. A sense of meaning in their work may facilitate the nurse's commitment to the ongoing process of becoming culturally competent.

The PEQ meaning subscale also correlated significantly with the CCBs subscale (CCA). CCBs, which include conducting cultural assessments, respecting cultural customs, and seeking information and resources (Doorenbos et al., 2005), may be more frequently and consistently demonstrated in practice by nurses for whom work is personally meaningful and important. Similar to the relationship with total cultural competence, meaning may be a mechanism through which nurses develop the attitudes, knowledge, and skills that contribute to CCBs. Meaning has been described as the driver of empowerment that energizes individuals about their work (Kizilos, Nason, & Spreitzer, 1997). Nurses who experience psychological empowerment through a high sense of meaning may be more motivated to minimize barriers to care, such as communication difficulties, and incorporate cultural preferences into care planning.

The third significant correlation with the PEQ meaning subscale was self-reported cultural competence, which reflects the nurse's assessment of their competence working with people from different cultures. The nurses in this study described themselves as having a high level of cultural competence. Given that 91% of the nurses participated in prior diversity training and reported a moderate/high level of exposure to diversity, the favorable self-assessment of cultural competence is not surprising. The correlation between meaning and self-reported cultural competence, similar to total cultural competence and CCBs, reinforces the role that caring deeply about work may have on nurses' perceptions and behaviors. Although the use of self-evaluation measures is problematic in many ways (e.g., they do not include directly observable behavior and the patient does not participate in the evaluation process), it is a practical approach to obtaining information that can provide insight into behaviors. Thus, the

TABLE 3. Correlations Between Cultural Competence (CCA) and Psychological Empowerment (PEQ)

	CCA Total	Cultural Awareness and Sensitivity	Cultural Competence Behaviors	Self-Reported Cultural Competence
PEQ total	0.12	-0.09	0.15	0.16
Meaning	0.23*	0.08	0.22*	0.24**
Competence	0.17	-0.06	0.20*	0.15
Self-determination	-0.04	-0.14	-0.01	0.05
Impact	0.09	-0.08	0.11	0.10

*$p < .05$.

**$p < .01$.

nurse's perception of her own cultural competence may be a credible indicator of CCBs. Favorable self-assessment of cultural competence may possibly reflect a social desire for cultural expertise, although neither the overall CCA nor its subscales have shown correlation with social desirability as measured by the Marlowe–Crowne Social Desirability Scale (S. M. Schim, personal communication, November 7, 2011).

In addition to experiencing psychological empowerment through a high sense of meaning, the nurses in this study also reported a high sense of competence. Competence, or self-efficacy, is related to the belief in one's ability to perform work activities with skill (Spreitzer, 1995). The results of this study demonstrated a significant correlation between the PEQ competence subscale and CCBs. Nurses who are self-assured about their professional skills may be more confident in their abilities to provide individualized care to all patients, regardless of cultural background. This sense of competence may result in the demonstration of culturally competent behaviors. This finding supports Dreher and MacNaughton's (2002) contention that cultural competence is fundamentally the same as nursing competence, because it reflects the nurse's ability to be equally therapeutic with all patients. Previous research (Kizilos et al., 1997) has identified a significant relationship between competence and work effectiveness, suggesting that nurses who experience psychological empowerment through a sense of competence may be more effective in meeting their patient's cultural care needs. These nurses may demonstrate more innovative behaviors when implementing culturally appropriate interventions, consistent with Knol and van Linge's (2009) finding that psychological empowerment is a predictor of innovative behavior.

A significant positive correlation between years of RN experience and PEQ competence scores was found in this study, as well as a significant difference between years of RN experience and self-reported cultural competence. Nurses with more years of experience had higher competence scores and higher self-reported cultural competence. Self-confidence and competence in professional nursing practice develop over time through experiential learning and skill acquisition (Benner, 2001). As a result, nurses with more years of experience may perceive themselves as more competent in their clinical practice. Similarly, competence in providing cultural-specific care develops over time, partly as a result of learning from previous cross-cultural encounters (Schim, 2005). Nurses with more years of experience perceive themselves as having greater mastery of the skills required to provide care to patients from a broad range of cultural backgrounds, and therefore assess themselves as having higher levels of cultural competence.

The results of this study did not support a significant correlation between total cultural competence and total psychological empowerment. While this finding was not significant with respect to the overall construct of psychological empowerment, empirical evidence suggests that each of its four dimensions contribute to different outcomes (Kizilos et al., 1997). Just as meaning and competence have been shown to demonstrate differential relationships with work effectiveness, work satisfaction, and job-strain (Kizilos et al., 1997), meaning and competence in this study demonstrated differential relationships with total cultural competence and its dimensions. The meaning and competence dimensions of psychological empowerment may be more important to the manifestation of cultural competence than the other dimensions of psychological empowerment (self-determination and impact).

LIMITATIONS

Several limitations were related to the study design and sampling methodology. The cross-sectional nature of the design, nonprobability convenience sampling strategy, and small sample size ($n = 120$) limit generalizations to a greater population of nurses. Since participation in the study was voluntary, nurses who completed the questionnaires may not have been a representative sample. Furthermore, the majority of the study participants were white females with a mean age of 45.4. While this sample may have reflected the demographics of the nursing population in the United States, it would be important to know the relationship between the study variables in other ethnic and racial groups of nurses, and in nurses who may have been socialized in another culture (e.g., immigrant nurses).

Additional study limitations include self-reporting of cultural competence and psychological empowerment rather than direct observation of behaviors. The CAS subscale's weak alpha reliability coefficient (0.61) may have also made it difficult to find significant relationships with the CAS. Finally, there may have been other variables influencing the findings that were not accounted for.

CONCLUSION AND IMPLICATIONS FOR FUTURE RESEARCH

This is the first study to examine the relationship between cultural competence and psychological empowerment among acute care nurses. Major findings suggest that the ability to provide culturally competent care may be related to the nurse's experience of psychological empowerment through a sense of meaning and competence in work. These results contribute to a growing body of empirical knowledge regarding factors that influence culturally competent practice. Further research is required to determine if study findings are similar in hospitals in different regions of the United States and with different demographics in nurses and patient populations. While the sample size was adequate to detect statistically significant differences, increasing the sample size and including nurses from other specialties would enhance generalization. It would also be important for future research to investigate the effect of nurses' socialization in another country on the relationship between cultural competence and psychological empowerment. Additional knowledge may be gained from conducting an intervention study that includes a continuing education session on cultural competence, and a pretest–posttest design to evaluate the effect on cultural competence.

REFERENCES

Avolio, B. J., Zhu, W., Koh, W., & Bhatia, P. (2004). Transformational leadership and organizational commitment: Mediating role of psychological empowerment and moderating role of structural distance. *Journal of Organizational Behavior, 25,* 951–968. doi:10.1002/job.283

Benner, P. (2001). *From novice to expert: Excellence and power in clinical nursing practice* (Commemorative ed.). Upper Saddle River, NJ: Prentice Hall.

Burns, N., & Grove, S. K. (2009). *The practice of nursing research: Conduct, critique, and utilization* (6th ed.). St. Louis: Elsevier Saunders.

Campinha-Bacote, J. (1999). A model and instrument for addressing cultural competence in health care. *Journal of Nursing Education, 38*(5), 203–206.

DeCicco, J., Laschinger, H., & Kerr, M. (2006). Perceptions of empowerment and respect: Effect on nurses' organizational commitment in nursing homes. *Journal of Gerontological Nursing, 32*(5), 49–57.

Doorenbos, A. Z., Schim, S. M., Benkert, R., & Borse, N. N. (2005). Psychometric evaluation of the cultural competence assessment instrument among health care providers. *Nursing Research, 54*(5), 324–331. doi:10.1097/00006199-200509000-00006

Dreher, M., & MacNaughton, N. (2002). Cultural competence in nursing: Foundation or fallacy? *Nursing Outlook, 50*(5), 181–186. doi: 10.1067/mno.2002.125800

Faulkner, J., & Laschinger, H. (2008). The effects of structural and psychological empowerment on perceived respect in acute care nurses. *Journal of Nursing Management, 16*(2), 214–221. doi:10.1111/j.1365-2834.2007.00781.x

Hochwalder, J. (2007). The psychosocial work environment and burnout among Swedish registered and assistant nurses: The main, mediating, and moderating role of empowerment. *Nursing and Health Sciences, 9,* 205–211. doi:10.1111/j.1442-2018.2007.00323.x

Jirwe, M., Gerrish, K., & Emami, A. (2006). The theoretical framework of cultural competence. *Journal of Multicultural Nursing & Health, 12*(3), 6–16.

Kanter, R. M. (1993). *Men and women of the corporation.* New York: Basic Books.

Knol, J., & van Linge, R. (2009). Innovative behavior: The effect of structural and psychological empowerment on nurses. *Journal of Advanced Nursing, 65*(2), 359–370. doi:10.1111/j.1365-2648.2008.04876.x

Laschinger, H. K., Finegan, J., Shamian, J., & Wilk, P. (2004). A longitudinal analysis of the impact of workplace empowerment on work satisfaction. *Journal of Organizational Behavior, 25,* 527–545. doi:10.1002/job.256

Laschinger, H. K., Gilbert, S., Smith, L., & Leslie, K. (2010). Towards a comprehensive theory of nurse/patient empowerment: Applying Kanter's empowerment theory to patient care. *Journal of Nursing Management, 18,* 4–13. doi:10.1111/j.1365-2834.2009.01046.x

Laschinger, H. K., & Wong, C. (1999). Staff nurse empowerment and collective accountability: Effect on perceived productivity and self-rated work effectiveness. *Nursing Economics, 17*(6), 308–316.

Leggat, S. G., Bartram, T., Casimir, G., & Stanton, P. (2010). Nurse perceptions of the quality of patient care: Confirming the importance of empowerment and job satisfaction. *Health Care Management Review, 35*(4), 355–364. doi:10.1097/HMR.0b013e3181e4ec55

Purdy, N., Laschinger, H. K., Finegan, J., Kerr, M., & Olivera, F. (2010). Effects of work environments on nurse and patient outcomes. *Journal of Nursing Management, 18,* 901–913. doi:10.1111/j.1365-2834.2010.01172.x

Salman, A., McCabe, D., Easter, T., Callahan, B., Gold-stein, D., Smith, T. D., … Fitzpatrick, J. J. (2007). Cultural competence among staff nurses who participated in a family-centered geriatric care program. *Journal for Nurses in Staff Development, 23*(3), 103–111. doi:10.1097/01.NND.0000277179.40206.be

Schim, S. M. (2005). A picture on the front of the box. *Journal of Professional Nursing, 21*(5), 255–256. doi:10.1016/j.profnurs.2005.08.001

Schim, S. M., & Miller, J. E. (1999). *Cultural competence program core components.* Detroit, MI: Henry Ford Health System/Oakland University Center for Academic Nursing. Available from s.schim@wayne.edu

Schim, S. M., Doorenbos, A., Benkert, R., & Miller, J. (2007). Culturally congruent care: Putting the puzzle together. *Journal of Transcultural Nursing, 18*(2), 103–110. doi:10.1177/1043659606298613

Schim, S. M., Doorenbos, A. Z., & Borse, N. N. (2005). Cultural competence among Ontario and Michigan healthcare providers. *Journal of Nursing Scholarship, 37*(4), 354–360. doi:10.1111/j.1547-5069.2005.00061.x

Schim, S. M., Doorenbos, A. Z., & Borse, N. N. (2006). Cultural competence among hospice nurses. *Journal of Hospice and Palliative Nursing, 8*(5), 302–307. doi:10.1097/00129191-200609000-00016

Schim, S. M., Doorenbos, A., Miller, J., & Benkert, R. (2003). Development of a cultural competence assessment instrument. *Journal of Nursing Measurement, 11*(1), 29–40. doi:10.1891/jnum.11.1.29.52062

Spreitzer, G. M. (1995). Psychological empowerment in the workplace: Dimensions, measurement, and validation. *Academy of Management Journal, 38*(5), 1442–1465. doi:10.2307/256865

Spreitzer, G. M., Kizilos, M. A., & Nason, S. W. (1997). A dimensional analysis of the relationship between psychological empowerment and effectiveness, satisfaction, and strain. *Journal of Management, 23*(5), 679704. doi:10.1177/014920639702300504

Taylor, R. A., & Alfred, M. V. (2010). Nurses' perceptions of the organizational supports needed for the delivery of culturally competent care. *Western Journal of Nursing Research, 32*(5), 591–609. doi:10.1177/0193945909354999

Thomas, K., & Velthouse, B. (1990). Cognitive elements of empowerment: An "interpretive" model of intrinsic task motivation. *Academy of Management Review, 15*(4), 666–681. doi:10.5465/AMR.1990.4310926

U. S. Census Bureau. (2010). *United States population projections: 2000 to 2050.* Retrieved from http://www.census.gov/population/www.projections/2009projections.html

Wepa, D. (Ed.). (2005). *Cultural Safety in Aotearoa New Zealand.* Auckland: Pearson Education.

CULTURAL COMPETENCE AND PSYCHOLOGICAL EMPOWERMENT AMONG ACUTE CARE NURSES

Critique by *Emerson E. Ea and Salena A. Gilles*

OVERALL SUMMARY

As the patient population in U.S. acute care facilities, and indeed throughout the health care system, becomes more diverse and multicultural there is a need for nurses and other health professionals to develop cultural sensitivity and competence. Health beliefs, practices, and expectations vary among those from different cultural groups. The researchers linked psychological empowerment to cultural competence among nurses working in one hospital in the northeast, and found that these nurses had a high level of cultural competence and were moderately psychologically empowered. Although there was not the expected relationship between cultural competence and psychological empowerment, there were important relationships identified in the results. Most important, the authors provide a very comprehensive review of the prior research related to these variables and link their study to the prior research. This serves to advance the science so that future research can build on what is currently known. This work is particularly important in advancing our understanding of cultural competence. Overall, the research was very logically and clearly presented.

TITLE

Does the title include the key concepts/variables/phenomenon of interest?

The title of the article, "Cultural Competence and Psychological Empowerment Among Acute Care Nurses," accurately captures the focus of this article, and provides the readers a quick overview of what will be discussed in the article.

Is it concise (12 words or less) and professionally stated?

The title is concise at nine words and is professionally stated.

RESEARCHER(S) CREDIBILITY

Educational credentials?

The educational credentials for all authors are listed as well as a brief description of their current employment and their research and/or practice interests.

Prior methodological research experience of the authors (i.e., methodological expertise)?

Based on the information about the authors, there is no direct way to determine their methodological expertise. The information about the authors suggests that these authors have both methodological expertise and context experience as evidenced by their educational and practice background.

Subject matter content experience (prior research on the subject matter)?

A literature search indicates that the second author has content expertise in cultural aspects of care and that the last author has content expertise in empowerment. The first author has content expertise related to nurses practicing in acute care.

ABSTRACT

Does it clearly and concisely summarize the main features of the report (problem, methods, results, and conclusions)?

The abstract of the article provides the reader the significance of the study and its purpose, which was to describe the relationship between cultural competence and psychological empowerment among acute care nurses in an urban hospital in southern Connecticut. The abstract also included the theoretical framework of the study but did not include a summary of the methods used in the study, the results, and conclusions.

Does or does not include references?

As appropriate, the abstract does not include references.

Is it concise (150–250 words or less)?

The abstract is concise at less than 150 words.

Does it entice you to read the rest of the article (interesting)?

The abstract provides enough information to entice the readers to continue to read the rest of the article.

INTRODUCTION/PROBLEM

Is the research problem or phenomenon of interest clearly stated?

The problem statement is clear. There are two major variables of interest in the study—cultural competence and psychological empowerment. At the end of this section, the authors stated the purpose of the study, which was to determine the relationship between cultural and psychological empowerment. At the beginning of this section, the authors emphasized the important role of nurses in providing culturally congruent care in influencing patient outcomes. This was followed by a discussion of the role of empowerment in making autonomous decisions among professional nurses.

Is it succinct?

The authors succinctly discussed each of these variables and linked these variables at the end of the introduction.

Does it answer the "so what" question?

The authors link the two main variables at the end of the introduction and thus answer the "so what" question.

RESEARCH AIMS/OBJECTIVES

Is the research aim/objective clearly stated?

The purpose of the study is clearly written. The reader is presented with information that builds from the two major variables of the study: cultural competence and psychological empowerment.

Is it concisely written?

> The introduction is concise.

Does it follow logically from the research problem/phenomenon of interest?

> There is a logical flow of information in the beginning section of the article that concluded with stating the purpose of the study.

SIGNIFICANCE

Is the significance to nursing and health care clearly written?

> The authors indicate that it is important for nurses to be cognizant of the differences in cultural beliefs among patients and thus the need for nurses to provide culturally competent care. They also identify the need for understanding the changes in the cultural complexity of the U.S. population.

Does the significance follow from the research aim/objective?

> The significance of the study to nursing and health care is not directly stated. The authors do identify the lack of prior research linking the study variables, but do not directly tie this to their argument regarding the significance of understandings of culture to the study aims.

BACKGROUND

Is there an explicit description of a theoretical perspective or conceptual framework? If not, is it implied?

> Included in the introduction is a discussion of the theoretical framework used in the study. The study used the Cultural Competence Model, which describes cultural competence as made up of four interconnected constructs that include (a) cultural diversity, (b) cultural awareness, (c) cultural sensitivity, and (d) cultural competence behaviors (CCBs). The authors presented a figure in the article of a jigsaw puzzle made up of the four components of cultural competence that clearly demonstrated how these constructs are interrelated.

Are there clear theoretical/conceptual definitions of the concepts?

> Each of the constructs—cultural competence, and psychological empowerment—was clearly defined by the authors.

LITERATURE REVIEW

Primary sources only?

> Only primary sources were cited in the literature review.

Current (within the past how many years)?

> Aside from the classic articles that were cited, the literature review is current and includes references within 10 years of the publication date of the article.

Is the search strategy included?

> The search strategy was not presented.

Is literature relevancy to the research aims/objectives?

> The literature review is directly relevant to the study purpose. A comprehensive literature review for each of the main study variables—cultural competence, and

psychological empowerment—is included. The authors separately described cultural competence and psychological empowerment in the literature review. The studies included in the literature review on cultural competence described relevant research that explored cultural competence among nurses. The authors were able to synthesize those factors that have been shown to relate to cultural competence among nurses. The section on psychological empowerment also presented results of relevant and mostly up-to-date studies that investigated this construct among nurses. The authors provided a clear summary at the end of this section for each of the variables of interest.

Is it chronologically presented (old to current)?

The authors did not present the studies chronologically (old to current). Rather, the authors presented the results of the studies based on synthesized ideas or categories. For example, the section on psychological empowerment discussed the studies that relate to psychological empowerment such as perception of job satisfaction, innovative behavior, and its mediating effect on nurses' perception of burn-out and organizational commitment.

Is it comprehensive? If not, is sufficient background literature provided?

The literature review is very comprehensive and provides a thorough assessment of the state of the science in the areas of study.

RATIONALE FOR THE STUDY

Is there a gap in the literature that this study will fill (will it extend prior knowledge)? Is the rationale clearly stated?

The authors identify the gap in the literature and state that there were no prior studies of the relationship between cultural competence and psychological empowerment, the main variables in this study. The gap in the literature is clearly stated as the authors indicate there are no prior studies linking the two main variables.

Is this a follow-up or replication study?

No, this is an original study linking the two main variables: cultural competence and psychological empowerment.

RESEARCH QUESTION(S) AND/OR HYPOTHESES

Are these explicitly and clearly stated?

There were no research questions explicitly stated but the main research question is implied from the statement of the study purpose.

Do they include the variables/phenomena of interest?

The purpose statement to describe the relationship between cultural competence and psychological empowerment includes the two main variables of interest.

Do they follow from the research aim/objective?

There were no specific research questions stated, but the research aim is clear.

METHODS
Research Design/Paradigm
Is the research design clearly stated?

The design was clearly stated and was appropriate for addressing the research objective, as it allowed the authors to gain more information regarding the area of study, while examining the relationships between the variables.

Is there consistency between the research design and paradigm?

In the introduction of the study, the authors emphasized the importance of nurses being knowledgeable about the diverse health beliefs and practices of their patients, as they are the major provider of direct health care services. Based on what is currently known about the topic, the use of a descriptive design is appropriate.

Is this the best choice of design to address the research problem/phenomenon of interest?

Use of a quantitative descriptive correlational design was the best choice to examine the relationship between cultural competence and psychological empowerment.

Is there rigor in the design?

The quantitative descriptive design provides the necessary rigor for addressing the relationship between the main study variables.

SETTING
Is the setting clearly described?

The setting is clearly stated. Including the geographic location of the hospital, type or unit, and the number of beds.

What biases are introduced as a result of selecting this particular setting?

The findings of this study cannot be generalized to other areas of clinical practice among nurses. The study also was conducted in an urban location, which further limits the generalizability of study findings.

SAMPLING PLAN AND SAMPLE
Is the sampling plan clearly identified?

The sampling plan is clearly identified as a nonprobability convenience sampling strategy.

Does it represent the population of interest?

The sampling plan included only nurses working in the acute care hospital selected for the study and thus represents the population of interest.

Is the sampling plan consistent with the research aim/objective?

The sampling plan is consistent with the research objective to determine the relationship between cultural competence and psychological empowerment among acute care nurses. Inclusion and exclusion criteria were clearly identified.

Is the sample size sufficient (e.g., power analysis or data saturation)?

> A power analysis was used to determine the sample size, necessitating a minimum of 83 participants to detect statistically significant differences. A final sample size of 120 nurses was obtained.

VARIABLES

Are variables clearly identified?
Are variables operationally defined and consistent with theoretical concepts?
Are independent and dependent variables identified, if applicable?

> The variables, cultural competence and psychological empowerment, were clearly identified, operationally defined, and consistent with the theoretical framework used in the study—Cultural Competence Model. Background variables, including questions about age, gender, prior cultural diversity training, self-identified race or ethnicity, and level of education, hours worked per week, and years of nursing experience, were also included. Because this was a descriptive study, there were no independent and dependent variables identified by the authors.

METHOD OF DATA COLLECTION

What are the methods of data collection?

> Survey questionnaires were given to nurse managers, who informed their staff where the questionnaires were located on the units. Consent to participate in the study was indicated by completing and returning the questionnaire.

Are validity and reliability clearly addressed for prior research and current study, if applicable?
Do the measures/instruments address the underlying theoretical concepts or phenomenon of interest?

> The two instruments used in the study were the Cultural Competence Assessment (CCA) and the Psychological Empowerment Questionnaire (PEQ). The two subscales of the CCA included cultural awareness and sensitivity and CCB. The PEQ measured four constructs, including meaning, competence, self-determination, and impact. The validity and reliability of the two instruments used in the study were clearly addressed. The authors cited results of several studies that pertain to validity and reliability of the instruments used in study. These instruments addressed the underlying theoretical concepts developed in the Cultural Competence Model, which discusses the four constructs of provider-level competence.

Were human rights protected?
Are other ethical issues identified?

> Institutional review board and human rights committee approval was obtained prior to conducting the study. There were no other ethical issues that needed to be addressed in this study.

Is the data-collection method appropriate for the research design?

> The research protocol was clear, described in sufficient detail, and appropriate for the research design.

Is there bias in the data collection?

> Study variables were self-reported, which could introduce bias in the results.

What is the fidelity of intervention addressed, if applicable?

> Not applicable.

DATA ANALYSIS

Are data analysis techniques described (e.g., statistical tests, methodology for qualitative analysis)?

Statistical Program for Social Sciences (SPSS) software was used to analyze the data. The detail that the authors presented regarding the analyses was useful, appropriate, and comprehensive. The researchers present the Cronbach alphas for the total score and subscale scores of cultural competence and psychological empowerment. In order to characterize the study sample, descriptive statistics were computed. To answer the research question, a Pearson's product–moment correlation was computed to determine the relationship between the two major study variables.

Does the analysis answer the research question?
Is it appropriate?

The main analysis was a Pearson correlation between the two main study variables: cultural competence and psychological empowerment. This analysis was appropriate to answer the research question implied in the study. Additional analyses were undertaken to determine the effects of background variables on the major study variables.

Is the analysis comprehensive? Are themes identified?

The analyses were comprehensive and presented in detail.

Is there bias in the analysis (trustworthiness? credibility?)?

The researchers report on multiple analyses related to demographic variables and to control for bias report setting the significance level at $p < .01$ for these additional analyses.

RESULTS

Are sample characteristics described and fully reported?

The sample characteristics, including gender, age, race, hours worked per week, college degree, and participation in cultural diversity training, were described and fully reported in detail in tables, and summary in text.

Are findings presented related to research aim/objective?

The findings are related to the implied research objective to determine the relationship between cultural competence and psychological empowerment. The authors reported that there was not a statistically significant relationship between these two main study variables, yet there were statistically significant relationships between several subscale scores. Additional analyses revealed that there were no significant relationships between the demographic variables and total cultural competence and total psychological empowerment with one exception. There was a significant difference in cultural competence based on years of RN experience; those with more experience had higher levels of cultural competence.

Are all outcome variables addressed, if applicable?

All outcome variables are presented, including subscale scores on the cultural competence measure.

Are results clearly presented in text and/or tables/figures?

The researchers utilized tables to display the demographic characteristics of the study sample, as well as the descriptive statistics for the major study variables. The information was presented clearly and the significance of the results was reported.

The Cronbach alphas for all of the subscales for both measures are also reported in a comprehensive table.

Is significance of results reported, if applicable?

Significance levels of all results are presented.

DISCUSSION OF RESULTS
Do the authors link the findings to previous research studies?

The authors provide a very detailed discussion of their results in relation to previous research on both cultural competence and psychological empowerment.

Are the conclusions comprehensive, yet within the data?

The authors' statements regarding study results do not go beyond the data but are presented as tentative interpretations that should be further explored.

Do the authors interpret the results in the discussion?

The authors interpret the results in great detail in the Discussion section of the paper. This is particularly important in light of the lack of statistical significance between total scores on the two main variables, which was the major focus of the study. The significant findings related to subscale scores are described in detail in the Discussion section. Of particular interest are the significant relationships between the "meaning" subscale scores on the psychological empowerment scale and the positive relationship to total cultural competence, the subscale of CCBs, and the subscale of self-reported cultural competence. The authors interpret these findings in relation to the literature on empowerment.

Are the findings generalizable or transferable?

The authors address the questions of lack of generalizability and transferability of the findings in the Limitations section of the paper.

LIMITATIONS
Identified? Accurate? Inclusive?

The limitations of the study were identified, including the use of self-evaluation methods as opposed to directly observed behaviors, and the influence of other variables not accounted for in this study. In addition, there was only a 20% nurse response rate, limiting generalizations to a greater population of nurses. There was a lack of diversity in study participants, with the majority of the study participants being White females with a mean age of 45.4 years, not allowing for the assessment of the relationship between the study variables in other ethnic and racial groups of nurses. In considering the internal reliability of the instruments used, the Cronbach alpha coefficient for the total CCA and PEQ suggested strong reliability (>.84) but the CCA subscale was <.7, which the authors admit may have made it difficult to find significant relationships with the cultural awareness and sensitivity.

IMPLICATIONS
Are there implications for practice, education, research?

The authors identified the lack of research on psychological empowerment as a factor that can affect the achievement of cultural competence and that there is little empirical research that demonstrates the effectiveness of cultural competence training and education in improving clinical outcomes. Yet they did not specifically address the implications of the research findings for practice or education. However, they did make several recommendations for future research.

Are there implications for clinical significance?

The clinical significance of the study is not explicitly addressed by the authors. Yet it is implied that there is a need for more cultural competence among nurses. The introduction to the study is focused on the need for culturally competent nurses, particularly with the changes in population demographics.

RECOMMENDATIONS
Recommendations for future study/study replication?

Because the convenience sampling strategy did not yield a sample that was diverse and representative of the population of interest, the authors agree that further studies are required in similar settings in different regions with diverse nurse and patient populations. In addition, investigating the impact of nurses' socialization in another country on the study variables is recommended as a potential area for future research. Lastly, future research via an intervention study with education on cultural competence may be beneficial.

CONCLUSION
Is it succinct and does it tie everything together?

The conclusion is succinct and ties everything together. Implications for nursing research are presented in the conclusion. The researchers acknowledge that this is the first study to examine the relationship between cultural competence and psychological empowerment among acute care nurses, but also recognize that, based on the additional analyses, the results contribute to the current growing body of knowledge investigating factors that influence cultural competence.

PALAUANS WHO CHEW BETEL NUT: SOCIAL IMPACT OF ORAL DISEASE

3

M. T. Quinn Griffin RN, MSN, PhD, FAAN, ANEF
Associate Professor
Frances Payne Bolton School of Nursing, Case Western Reserve University,
Cleveland, Ohio

M. Mott DNP, APRN, CNS
Instructor (retired), Las Vegas, Nevada

P. M. Burrell PhD, APRN, APMHCNS-BC, CNE
Professor, College of Nursing and Health Sciences, Hawaii Pacific University, Kaneohe, Hawaii

J. J. Fitzpatrick RN, PhD, MBA, FAAN
Elizabeth Brooks Ford Professor, Frances Payne Bolton School of Nursing, Case Western Reserve
University, Cleveland, Ohio

Background: Chewing betel nut is a tradition extending from Southeast Asia to the Pacific. Globally, betel nut is the fourth main psychotropic substance containing a stimulant, arecoline, that has a similar effect to nicotine. In Palau, there is broad acceptance of betel nut chewing. One of the largest immigrant groups in Hawaii is the Palauans. Chewing betel nut has significant social implications that make it difficult for those who engage in this practice to separate potential oral disease from the social importance. However, little is known about the social impact of oral disease from chewing betel nut on Palauans in Hawaii.

Aim: The study aimed to describe the perceptions of betel-chewing Palauans in Hawaii regarding betel nut and to determine the social impact of oral disease among these individuals.

Methods: Descriptive study conducted on the island of Oahu, Hawaii with 30 adult Palauans. Data were collected using the Oral Health Impact Profile-14 to measure perceptions of social impact of oral disease on well-being. Demographic and general health information was collected.

Results: Participants perceived little negative social impact of oral disease on well-being.

Discussion: Families, peers, and society exert a strong influence on the decision to chew betel nut, a known carcinogen. Participants in this study showed little concern on the impact of betel nut chewing on their oral health. They continue the habit in spite of the awareness of potential for oral disease.

Quinn Griffin M. T., Mott M., Burrell P. M., & Fitzpatrick J. J. (2014). Palauans who chew betel nut: Social impact of oral disease. *International Nursing Review, 61,* 148–155. doi:10.1111/inr.12082. Reprinted with permission from John Wiley and Sons © 2014 International Council of Nurses.

Implications for nursing and health policy: Nurses face challenges in educating Palauans about the negative aspects of bethel nut, particularly those related to oral health especially when they do not perceive problems. Nurses must be involved in the development of health policies to design and implement strategies to promote behavioral change, and to ensure clinical services that are culturally sensitive to bethel nut chewers.

KEY WORDS: betel nut, Hawaii, oral health, Palua, social impact

Funding: No funding received for this study.

INTRODUCTION

The ancient custom of chewing betel nut and betel leaf is a tradition practiced by several hundred million people in much of the areas from Southeast Asia to the Pacific (Parsell 2005). The betel nut, the fruit of the palm *Areca catechu* Linnaeus, is often used in the form of a *betel quid*—a mixture of tobacco, betel leaves, lime and flavorings such as fennel seed. The quid is placed between the cheek and the gum and frequently left in the mouth for hours or overnight. In Palau, the betel nut's skin is chewed along with lime, leaf, and tobacco, and the juice is not swallowed but spat out. Betel nut is the fourth main psychoactive substance in the world (Rajan et al. 2007). It contains a stimulant, arecoline, an alkaloid comparable with nicotine in its stimulating, mildly intoxicating effect. Rajan et al. (2007) reported that 96% of participants in their study stated that chewing betel nut made them feel good, relaxed, elated, or high. Betel chewing is addictive and as other additive substances it increases the availability of dopamine in the "pleasure" area of the mesolimbic system in the brain.

BETEL CHEWING IN PALAU

There is a broad acceptance of betel nut and tobacco use within all sectors of the population in Palau (Republic of Palau, Ministry of Health, Bureau of Public Health, Division of Oral Health 2006). Older and younger generations alike enjoy the use of betel nut. In Palau, 63% of middle school and 75% of high school students have chewed betel nut, and most chewed it with tobacco (World Health Organization [WHO] 2012). Students of Palauan origin were significantly more likely to have tried betel nut than students of other ethnic backgrounds. Even with the knowledge that betel nut use can cause serious health problems, the Tobacco Control Program does not strongly discourage betel nut use but advocates for chewers to use betel nut without tobacco (Republic of Palau, Ministry of Health, Bureau of Public Health, Division of Oral Health 2006).

This study was designed to (a) describe the perceptions of betel-chewing Palauans in Hawaii regarding betel nut, and to (b) determine the social impact of oral disease among these individuals.

BACKGROUND

The literature review utilized the search engines MEDLINE, PubMed, BioMed, MDConsult, and Google from 1994 to 2013 using the keywords betel nut, oral health, oral cancer, and Oral Health Impact Profile (OHIP). The literature was searched for references on prevalence of betel nut use, oral health among persons who chew betel nut and the social impact of betel nut use.

BETEL NUT CHEWING

After caffeine, alcohol, and nicotine, betel nut is the fourth most commonly used substance of abuse in the world (Gupta & Ray 2004). Different countries have different ways of preparing betel quid with a great variety of ingredients. The use of commercially prepared betel nut is a lucrative industry bringing in the equivalent of several hundred million U.S. dollars per year (Gupta & Ray 2004). In light of recent migration of Micronesians to Hawaii, Pobutsky and Neri (2012) examined the sociocultural significance of betel nut use among Micronesians. Because of the large influx of Micronesian migrants in Hawaii over the past decade, there has been interest recently in Hawaii about the link to oral cancers by betel nut chewing. There is increasing evidence that Chuukese and other Marshallese in Hawaii have taken up chewing betel nut as a form of ethnic regional identity. Social pressures due to migrant status may contribute to betel nut use.

Betel nut chewing has been shown to directly affect oral health. The impact of oral health on a person's quality of life reflects complex cultural values, social norms, beliefs, and tradition. In many cultures, teeth stained red, black, or patterned indicate marriageability or coming of age. Yet in other cultures, particularly in the younger age groups, the coloration of teeth and missing teeth may lead to embarrassment and self-consciousness limiting social interaction and communication among betel nut chewers (Oakley et al. 2005).

BETEL NUT AND ORAL HEALTH

The adverse oral health effects associated with betel nut use had been well documented. Several researchers have linked betel nut chewing to the development of oral mucosal lesions, oral leukoplakia, oral precancer and cancer, periodontal disease, as well as submucous fibrosis, which has a high rate of malignant transformation and is extremely debilitating with no known cure (Avon 2004; Parsell 2005; Shiu & Chen 2004). Lee et al. (2005) further implicated betel nut chewing to the development of esophageal cancer. While chewing betel nut is a widely practiced form of recreational drug use in Bangladesh, Cambodia, Guam, India, Malaysia, Palau, Papua New Guinea, and Thailand, it is also the leading cause of oral cancer in those areas (Jeng et al. 2001). Betel nut chewing is implicated in oral leukoplakia and submucous fibrosis (Lee et al. 2003). Lee and colleagues (2003) used a gender age-matched case control study in southern Taiwan to explore the association between betel quid chewing on oral leukoplakia and submucous fibrosis. There was a preponderance of younger patients with oral submucous fibrosis and older patients with oral leukoplakia with betel quid chewing as a major cause.

SOCIAL IMPACT OF ORAL HEALTH ISSUES

Gerreth (2006) in a study with 85 Hindu subjects assessed evidence of betel nut chewing and the degree of abrasive changes in teeth. A total of 71.76% of the patients were habitual betel chewers. Abrasive changes were more severe in men than women and increased with age. Gerreth concluded the abrasive changes were linked to the duration of betel chewing. Chatrchaiwiwatana (2006) used two large datasets from Thailand to study the relationship between betel quid chewing and oral diseases. Interestingly, the results indicated that betel quid chewing was linked to a reduction in dental caries. However, bethel quid chewing was related to increased periodontitis and the likelihood of increasing tooth loss. Abrasive changes, periodontitis and tooth loss may all contribute to reduced feelings of well-being, poorer health, and feelings of embarrassment in social situations because of poor dental health.

SUMMARY

Betel nut is the fourth most commonly used substance of abuse in the world. The literature reviewed showed that chewing betel nut was linked to the development of oral health problems, including oral precancer and cancer, periodontal disease, gum disease and addiction. There were no prior studies of perception of oral health issues among betel nut chewers among Palauans in Hawaii.

METHODS

The study was conducted on the island of Oahu in Hawaii. The study was conducted during a meeting of the Ngerchumebai Young Palauans Association (NYPA), a social organization of Palauans with approximately 150 members. The primary investigator met with the president of the NYPA to discuss this study and obtain permission to approach the potential participants.

POPULATION

According to the US Census Bureau's American Community Survey (U.S. Census Bureau 2011), in 2011, the foreign share of the population was 17.9%, an increase from 14.7% in 1990 (U.S. Census Bureau 2000). One of the largest groups arriving is the Micronesians, as well as Palauans and Marshallese. They come to Hawaii for medical care under the Compact of Free Association (COFA). Under the terms of COFA, citizens of the Republic of Palau are able to have access to health services in the United States (Compact of Free Association 1986). Because of poor health outcomes in the COFA region, many Palauans come to Hawaii for medical treatments including treatment for oral cancer related to chewing betel nut (Riklon et al., 2010). Palauans were chosen for this study as little is known about chewing betel nut and the social impact of oral disease on Palauans in Hawaii.

SAMPLE

The sample was drawn from Palauan adults who attended the NYPA social gathering. Following discussions with the president of the NYPA, a convenience sample was deemed the best approach for this study due to difficulties identifying Palauans who chew bethel nut. Although use of a convenience sample does not allow generalization of results to the wider research population, a nonprobability, nonrandom sampling where subjects are selected based on their convenient accessibility was chosen for this pilot so that baseline information could be collected and then used to guide further studies in this area. The inclusion criteria were native Palauan adults (18 years or older) who were betel nut chewers and who were able to speak and read English. They had to be willing to spend at least 1 hour with the investigator to complete the questionnaire.

INSTRUMENTS

Demographic and background information was obtained through the use of a 6-item demographic sheet and a 12-question health survey focused on betel nut use and its impact on the participants' health and well-being. This instrument was developed by the researcher and it included the following items: Who introduced them to betel nut? Do they chew with/without tobacco? Number of daily/weekly chews? and Who in family chews? All items and the scoring used are displayed in Table 1.

The OHIP-14 measuring people's perceptions of the social impact of oral disorders on their well-being was developed in Australia (Slade 1997). The original OHIP contains 49 questions (Slade & Spencer 1994). A shortened version (OHIP-14) of OHIP-49 has been developed (Slade 1997) and is used in settings where use of the longer instrument is inappropriate. The OHIP has been widely used in studies of people with different cultural backgrounds. Researchers have used the OHIP in Finland (Harju et al. 2002), Sri Lanka (Ekanayake & Perera 2003), Hungary (Szentpetery et al. 2006), and Australia (Slade 1997). The OHIP-14 has excellent reliability in different cultural samples, for example, with an older Japanese sample the Cronbach's alpha was 0.95 (Ikebe et al. 2004). In Finland, the Cronbach's coefficient alpha was 0.93 (Harju et al. 2002). In a Sri Lanka study, the Cronbach's alpha for the translated Sinhalese scale was 0.93 (Ekanayake & Perera 2003), and in Hungary, Szentpetery and colleagues (2006) reported Cronbach's alpha values between 0.71 and 0.96.

The items on the OHIP-14 are Likert type with five response choices ranging from 0 for "never" to 4 for "fairly often" for each item. The scale has a range of 0 to 56 with higher scores indicating reduction in oral-related quality of life (Slade 1997). The items are related to perceptions of problems or discomforts with the mouth and teeth on nutrition, social interactions, and reduction in life satisfaction (Slade 1997). There is no Palauan version of the OHIP-14; however, all the Palauans in this study spoke, read and wrote English. All instruments were administered in English. The licensee for OHIP-14, BioMed Central, Ltd. (Springer Science+Business, London, UK) permitted open access and verbatim copying and redistribution in all media for any purpose. This permission was printed on all copies OHIP-14 used in this study.

PROCEDURE

Permission to conduct this study was obtained from the institutional review board (IRB) at Case Western Reserve University, Cleveland, Ohio, along with permission from the President of the NYPA. A waiver of written consent was obtained from the IRB. Prior to giving the potential participant the survey, the researcher checked that each of the potential participants met the inclusion criteria. A paper survey was provided to each eligible study participant. To allow for privacy and confidentiality, surveys were completed in a quiet private area at the NYPA social gathering. Study participants completed the background data sheet and the OHIP-14 instrument, and returned the completed survey to the researcher. Completing the questionnaires indicated the participants' consent to be part of the study. The researcher placed each completed survey in a locked box that she kept with her at

TABLE 1. SAMPLE CHARACTERISTICS

Frequency Counts for Selected Variables (*N* = 30)			
Variable	*Category*	*N*	*%*
Marital status	Single	15	50.0
	Married	15	50.0
Education level	High school graduate	10	33.3
	Completed 2 years of college	11	36.7
	Completed 4 years of college	6	20.0
	Advanced degree	3	10.0
Occupation	Construction	1	3.3
	Tourism	2	6.7
	Business	1	3.3
	Professional	3	10.0
	Unemployed	4	13.3
	Others	19	63.3
Results			
Who introduced to betel nut?	Mother	2	6.7
	Mother, father, sister	1	3.3
	Mother, family members, friends	1	3.3
	Father	2	6.7
	Sister	1	3.3
	Sister, family members, friends	1	3.3
	Family members, friends	22	73.3
Chew with tobacco	Yes	23	77.0
	No	7	23.3
Chew without tobacco	Yes	10	33.3
	No	20	66.7
Number of daily chews	Once a day	2	6.7
	Twice a day	1	3.3
	Three times a day	4	13.3
	Four times a day	10	33.3
	Other	11	36.7
Number of weekly chews	Once a week	2	6.7
	Twice a week	1	3.3
	Three times a week	3	10.0
	Four times a week	9	30.0
	Other	15	50.0
Who in family chews?	Mother	3	10.0
	Mother, father	2	6.7
	Mother, father, brother	2	6.7

(continued)

TABLE 1. SAMPLE CHARACTERISTICS (*continued*)

Frequency Counts for Selected Variables (*N* = 30)			
Variable	*Category*	*N*	*%*
	Mother, father, brother, sister	4	13.3
	Mother, father, sister	1	3.3
	Mother, brother	1	3.3
	Father, brother, sister	2	6.7
	Brother	4	13.3
	Brother, sister	1	3.3
	Sister	3	10.0
	Other	5	16.7
Children who chew	Yes	2	6.7
	No	28	93.3
Who introduced children to betel nut?	Other	30	100
Any teeth problems in past year?	Yes	5	16.7
	No	25	83.
Any mouth sores in past year?	Yes	5	16.7
	No	25	83.3
Any difficulty swallowing in past year?	Yes	3	10.0
	No	27	90.0
Did you see the doctor for any of your health problems?	Yes	13	43.3
	No	17	56.7

all times. Participants received $5.00 at the completion of the questionnaires as a token of appreciation for their participation.

RESULTS

The sample included 15 male (50%) and 15 female (50%) native Palauans who were 18 years old and older. Participants chewed betel nut from once a day (6.7%) to more than four times a day (36.7%). Sample characteristics are included in Table 1.

Bethel Nut Usage

The main results of 12 items related to betel nut usage are reported in this section. Detailed results are in Table 1. When asked "who introduced you to bethel nut?" participants revealed that immediate family members were involved with only a small percentage of participants, specifically, mothers (*n* = 3, 10%), fathers (*n* = 3, 10%), and sisters (*n* = 2, 6%). The majority of participants reported that other family members (aunts, uncles) and friends exerted the most influence with regard to their introduction to bethel nut. Combined, these groups represented 22 participants, 73.3%.

Participants were asked four questions related to their experience of chewing betel nut. The majority (*n* = 23, 77%) of the participants reported chewing betel nut with tobacco. However, when asked if they chewed without tobacco, a total of 10 (33.3%) reported that they did while 20 (66.7%) did not chew without tobacco. The number of daily chews of betel nut ranged from once a day (6.7%, $n = 2$) to more than four times a day for 11 (36.7%) respondents. When asked to indicate the number of weekly chews of betel nut, half ($n = 15$, 50%) stated that they chewed betel nut more than four times a week.

There were three questions related to betel nut chewing within the family. Respondents were asked one question related to family members chewing betel nut. Responses to this question ranged from one family member ($n = 10$, 33.3%) to more than three family members ($n = 4$, 13.3%). There were two questions related to children chewing betel nut. A small percentage (6.7%, $n = 2$) of respondents had children who chewed betel nut, whereas 93.3% ($n = 28$) reported that their children did not chew betel nut. The 6.7% who stated that their children chewed betel nut claimed that it was other family members (aunts, uncles) and friends and not the immediate family who introduced the children to betel nut.

ORAL HEALTH RESULTS

Results related to physiological impact of oral disease

Four questions related to physiological impact of oral disease were asked. Study participants were asked if they have had trouble pronouncing any words because of problems with their teeth, mouth, or dentures. The majority (93.3%, $n = 28$) of the respondents reported that they have never experienced any trouble. When asked about experiencing painful aching in their mouth, a total of 73.3% ($n = 22$) stated that they never had a painful mouth. The third question was related to difficulty doing their usual jobs because of problems with their teeth, mouth, or dentures. The majority (86.7%, $n = 26$) of the respondents stated that they never had this problem. The final question was related to being totally unable to function because of problems with teeth, mouth, or dentures. Again, the majority (86.7%, $n = 26$) of the respondents reported that they never had any problems in this regard. Detailed results are in Table 2.

Results related to psychological impact of oral disease

There were six questions related to psychological impact of chewing betel nut. Study participants were asked if they have felt self-conscious because of problems with their teeth, mouth, or dentures. The majority of respondents (60%, $n = 18$) indicated that they never experienced this problem. When asked about feeling tense because of problems with their teeth, mouth, or dentures, a total of 23 (76.7%) respondents reported that they never felt tense in relation to oral problems. The third question was related to difficulty relaxing because of problems with their teeth, mouth or dentures. For this question, the majority (83.3%, $n = 25$) of the respondents indicated that they never had difficulty relaxing in relation to issues with oral health. Study participants were asked if they have been a bit embarrassed because of problems with their teeth, mouth, or dentures. A total of 73.3% ($n = 22$) stated that this was never the case. Responses to a question related to being irritable with other people because of problems with their teeth, mouth or dentures revealed that the majority (76.7%, $n = 23$) were never a bit irritable with others due to oral health problems. The sixth question asked the study participants if they felt that life in general was less satisfying because of problems with their teeth, mouth, or dentures. Almost all

TABLE 2. SOCIAL IMPACT OF ORAL DISEASE (*N* = 30)

Variable	Category	*n*	%
Physiological impact			
Trouble pronouncing words	Never	28	93.3
	Hardly ever	2	6.7
Painful mouth	Never	22	73.3
	Hardly ever	7	23.3
	Occasionally	1	3.3
Difficulty doing usual jobs	Never	26	76.7
	Hardly ever	3	10.0
	Occasionally	1	3.3
Totally unable to function	Never	26	86.7
	Hardly ever	2	6.7
	Occasionally	2	6.7
Psychological impact			
Felt self-conscious	Never	18	60.0
	Hardly ever	7	23.3
	Occasionally	4	13.3
	Very often	1	3.3
Felt tense	Never	23	76.7
	Hardly ever	6	20.0
	Occasionally	1	3.3
Difficult to relax	Never	25	83.3
	Hardly ever	4	13.3
	Occasionally	1	3.3
A bit embarrassed	Never	22	73.3
	Hardly ever	5	16.7
	Occasionally	2	6.7
	Very often	1	3.3
A bit irritable with other people	Never	23	76.7
	Hardly ever	6	20.0
	Occasionally	1	3.3
Nutritional impact			
Sense of taste has worsened	Never	26	86.7
	Hardly ever	3	10.0
	Occasionally	1	3.3
Discomfort when eating	Never	22	73.3
	Hardly ever	5	16.7
	Occasionally	2	6.7
	Very often	1	3.3

(continued)

TABLE 2. SOCIAL IMPACT OF ORAL DISEASE (*N* = 30) (*continued*)

Variable	Category	*n*	%
Diet been unsatisfactory	Never	26	86.7
	Hardly ever	3	10.0
	Very often	1	3.3
Interruption of meals	Never	23	76.7
	Hardly ever	6	20.0
	Very often	1	3.3

(93.3%, *n* = 28) of the respondents reported that they never felt like this. Detailed results are in Table 2.

Results related to nutritional impact of oral disease

There were four questions addressing the nutritional impact of oral health problems. Study participants were asked if they felt that their sense of taste has worsened because of problems with their teeth, mouth, or dentures. Over three-quarters (86.7%, *n* = 26) reported that they never experienced changes in their sense of taste due to problems with teeth, mouth, or dentures. Reponses to the question related to discomfort when eating due to problems with teeth, mouth, or dentures revealed that 73.3% (*n* = 22) never found it uncomfortable to eat any foods because of oral health problems. Almost all (86.7%, *n* = 26) of the respondents did not agree that their diet had been unsatisfactory because of problems with their teeth, mouth, or dentures. The final question in this section asked about interruption of meals because of problems with the teeth, mouth, or dentures. Over three-quarters of the respondents (76.7%, *n* = 23) stated that this never happened. Detailed results are in Table 2.

DISCUSSION

Families, peers and society exert a strong influence on the decision to chew betel nut, a known carcinogen. The use of betel nut is woven into the culture and society of Palauans. The participants in this study showed little concern on the impact of betel nut chewing on their oral health. They continue the habit in spite of the awareness of potential for oral disease. Few participants in this study reported oral health issues or feeling that their oral health had a negative social impact on their lives. Only a small percentage of the participants experienced embarrassment, had to interrupt meals, experienced discomfort and had dissatisfaction with their diet because of problems with their teeth, mouth, or dentures. These findings related to impact on their lifestyle are supported in the literature. Family and social influence in chewing betel nut are evident in studies by Pobutsky and Neri (2012) and Oakley et al. (2005). In this study, it was interesting to note that 28 of the 30 participants reported that their children did not chew betel nut, and the two who had children chewing betel nut claimed that it was other family members who introduced the children to betel nut. These findings may indicate that there may be some information available encouraging children not to chew bethel nut, and also letting this population know that children should be discouraged from chewing. These findings warrant further investigation as building on this information along with developing strategies to promote behavioral change may help decrease the health effects of betel nut chewing and improve the health of Palauans.

Also, family influence was apparent in the answer to the question, "Who introduced you to betel nut?" Close family members and friends exerted the most influence. Interestingly, no participant mentioned a brother as introducing them to betel nut chewing but they specifically mentioned a sister. Further investigation may reveal cultural rationales for this finding.

There are challenges for health care providers and nurses in particular in educating Palauans about the negative aspects of bethel nut, particularly those related to oral health especially when they do not perceive problems. Also, the Palauans in this study had no intentions of giving up their habit of chewing betel nut. Nurses are caring for patients throughout the life span and are ideally placed to provide health education related to betel nut chewing and the implications for ill health. Nurses can identify betel nut chewers by incorporating questions related to chewing in their patient health assessment. Once these patients are identified, nurses can develop strategies with each patient to promote behavioral change.

However, betel nut chewing is a major issue and its eradication needs to be tackled at a state level in Hawaii. Multidisciplinary teams of health care providers including nurses along with the policy makers must work together to develop state policies to educate the people about the dangers of betel nut chewing. This education needs to be implemented at all education levels. Use of social media and tailored health messages for younger age groups is needed. Perhaps the development of a teenage betel nut quit program similar to the tobacco cessation programs is needed. Oakley et al. (2005) stated that dental aesthetics was a consideration for young people when making decisions related to chewing. Capitalizing on this information may help to reduce chewing in younger age groups. Health policies to develop and implement strategies to promote behavioral change are needed. Partnerships and alliances with Palauans and other Micronesians, and health departments, hospitals, and community clinics will make an impact in reaching the populations at risk of the health problems related to betel nut chewing. Health policies must be developed to ensure there are clinical services that are culturally sensitive to *bethel* nut chewers. Nurses must be involved in the development of these services. When planning these services, education will be needed for nurses about betel nut and the health issues involved.

LIMITATIONS

The small convenience sample who participated in the study was limited to Palauans who live in Hawaii and who chew betel nuts. Their perceptions of the social impact of oral disease on their well-being may not be representative of Palauans living in Hawaii, or those afflicted with oral cancer as a result of chewing betel nut. A larger study is needed with a power analysis in order to obtain the required sample size to investigate relationships among variables.

RECOMMENDATIONS FOR FUTURE RESEARCH

A sample of Palauans with oral cancer may present a different perception of the social impact of chewing betel nut. Also, it is recommended that a more comprehensive study be undertaken among this group of Palauans so that we might better understand the cultural and social components of chewing betel nut, and the meaning that this has within this cultural group. Studies with powered samples are required to investigate relationships among variables of interest in this population. Comparison studies with samples of betel nut chewers in Palau and Hawaii could be conducted also. In this study, there was no independent assessment of dental and oral health. Such an assessment would have provided objective data in addition to the participants' perceptions of their oral health issues. It may be that some of these participants have some oral disease but had adapted their lifestyle and diet to reduce the impact of the problem. Future studies could add such objective data and perhaps questions related to dental care and visits to the dentist.

CONCLUSION

The participants in this study did not feel that their habit of chewing betel nut impacted their lives or their oral health. They continued to work, earn a living, take care of their families and socialize. As with any habit or addiction, like cigarette smoking, drinking alcohol, or using illicit drugs, it is important for health professionals to first recognize the problem, and then to assist the individuals and the communities to understand the health consequences of their behavior. Although this study was conducted in Hawaii, the results have international implications as betel chewing is common in most Asian and Pacific countries (Pobutsky & Neri 2012). Methods of chewing may differ between the countries but many of the health issues are the same. Therefore, there is an urgency to investigate bethel nut chewing further and to develop national and international health policies to reduce health issues related to betel nut chewing.

CONFLICT OF INTEREST

The authors have no conflict of interest.

AUTHOR CONTRIBUTIONS

MM, PMB, MTQG, and JJF: Conceptualized and designed the study. MTQG, MM, PMB, and JJF: Drafted the manuscript.

REFERENCES

Avon, S.L. (2004) Oral mucosal lesions associated with use of quid. *Journal of the Canadian Dental Association*, **70** (4), 244–248.

Chatrchaiwiwatana, S. (2006) Dental caries and periodontitis associated with betel quid chewing: analysis of two data sets. *Journal of the Medical Association of Thailand*, **89** (7), 1004–1011.

Compact of Free Association (COFA) (1986) Republic of Palau.

Ekanayake, L. & Perera, I. (2003) Validation of a Sinhalese translation of the Oral Health Impact Profile-14 for use with older adults. *Gerodontology*, **20** (2), 95–99.

Gerreth, K. (2006) Tooth wear in Hindu betel nut chewers. *Przeglad Lekarski*, **63** (10), 882–886.

Gupta, P.C. & Ray, C.S. (2004) Epidemiology of betel quid usage. *Annals, Academy of Medicine, Singapore*, **33** (4 Suppl), 31s–36s.

Harju, P., Lahti, S. & Hausen, H. (2002) *Oral Health Impact among Adult Finns – A Pilot Study*. Available at: http://iadr.confex.com/iadr/2002SanDiego/techprogram/abstract_13025.htm (accessed 1 July 2013).

Ikebe, K., et al (2004) Application of short-form oral health impact profile on elderly Japanese. *Gerodontology*, **21** (3), 167–176.

Jeng, J.H., Chang, M.C. & Hahn, L.J. (2001) Role of areca nut in betel quid-associated chemical carcinogenesis: current awareness and future perspectives. *Oral Oncology*, **37** (6), 477–492.

Lee, C.H., et al. (2003) The precancer risk of betel quid chewing, tobacco use and alcohol consumption in oral leukoplakia and oral submucous fibrosis in southern Taiwan. *British Journal of Cancer*, **88** (3), 366–372.

Lee, J.M., et al. (2005) Safrole-DNA adducts in tissues from esophageal cancer patients: clues to areca-related esophageal carcinogenesis. *Mutation Research*, **565** (2), 121–128.

Oakley, E., Demaine, L. & Warnakulasuriya, S. (2005) Areca (betel) nut chewing habit among high-school children in the Commonwealth of the Northern Mariana Islands (Micronesia). *Bulletin of the World Health Organization*, **83** (9), 656–660.

Parsell, D. (2005) Palm-nut problem: Asian chewing habit linked to oral cancer. *Science News*, **167** (3), 43–44. doi: 10.2307/4015878.

Pobutsky, A.M. & Neri, E.I. (2012) Betel nut chewing in Hawaii: is it becoming a public health problem? Historical and socio-cultural considerations. *Hawaii Journal of Medicine & Public Health*, **71** (1), 23–26.

Rajan, G., Ramesh, S. & Sankaralingam, S. (2007) Areca nut use in rural Tamil Nadu: a growing threat. *Indian Journal of Medical Sciences*, **61** (6), 332–337.

Republic of Palau, Ministry of Health, Bureau of Public Health, Division of Oral Health (2006) *Oral Health in Palau Disease Burden and Plan*. RPMH, Bureau of Public Health, Division of Oral Health. Koror, Palau.

Riklon, S., Alik, W., Hixon, A. & Palafox, N.A. (2010) The 'compact impact' in Hawaii: focus on health care. *Hawaii Medical Journal*, **6** (Suppl 3), 7–12.

Shiu, M.N. & Chen, T.H. (2004) Impact of betel quid, tobacco and alcohol on three-stage disease natural history of oral leukoplakia and cancer: implication for prevention of oral cancer. *European Journal of Cancer Prevention*, **13** (1), 39–45.

Slade, G.D. (1997) Derivation and validation of a short-form oral health impact profile. *Community Dental Oral Edidemiology*, **25** (4), 284–290.

Slade, G.D. & Spencer, A.J. (1994) Development and evaluation of the Oral Health Impact Profile. *Community Dental Health*, **11** (1), 3–11.

Szentpetery, A., et al. (2006) The Hungarian version of the oral health impact profile. *European Journal of Oral Sciences*, **114** (3), 197–203.

U.S. Census Bureau (2000) *The Foreign-Born Population*. US Department of Commerce, Washington, DC.

U.S. Census Bureau (2011) *American Community Survey (1–Year Estimates)*. US Department of Commerce, Washington, DC.

World Health Organization (WHO) (2012) *New Report Reveals High Prevalence of Betel, Tobacco Chewing in Western Pacific*. Available at: http://www.wpro.who.int/mediacentre/news/2012/20120323/en/ (accessed 31 January 2013).

PALUANS WHO CHEW BETEL NUT: SOCIAL IMPACT OF ORAL DISEASE

Critique by *Anne Folte Fish*

OVERALL SUMMARY

The authors conducted a small, clinically meaningful, descriptive, and well-executed study in a unique population in Hawaii. They present a compelling case for further study of the social impact of oral disease from chewing betel nut, an addictive psychotropic substance that is culturally rooted in ancient traditions. Clearly there are major national and international health-related policy implications. A fact that was somewhat surprising was that betel quids are commercially prepared and a lucrative industry, representing a significant barrier to policy change.

TITLE

Does the title include the key concepts/variables/phenomenon of interest?

The title is highly instructive. It includes the population, the issue, and the specific phenomenon of interest. Immediately the reader can easily see the health care issue to be investigated. The title may also bring to mind, for some readers, pictures in *National Geographic* of indigenous peoples with red mouths.

Is it concise (12 words or less) and professionally stated?

The title is concise at less than 12 words and is professionally stated.

RESEARCHER(S) CREDIBILITY

Educational credentials?

The credentials of the primary author are PhD, RN, FAAN, ANEF (Academy of Nursing Education). She is a professor of nursing at a university that is a globally recognized leader in nursing education and research. The other authors are also doctorally prepared nursing faculty, with the exception of the second author, who is a retired instructor.

Prior methodological research experience of the authors (i.e., methodological expertise)?

A literature search reveals that collectively, the authors have extensive prior methodological research experience in conducting quantitative studies on a wide variety of phenomena of interest.

Subject matter content experience (prior research on the subject matter)?

Dr. Quinn has a long history of scholarship and transcultural, methodological, and content expertise related to this study, specifically about social issues, health beliefs, and health behaviors. Dr. Burrell also has relevant research experience with a cultural focus.

ABSTRACT (BACKGROUND)
Does it include the key components (objective/aim, background/rationale, methods, results, and conclusion)?

> The background information includes the key components plus implications. The message in the opening paragraph is clear: Betel nut is a known carcinogen.

Does or does not include references?

> The abstract appropriately does not include references.

Is it concise (150–250 words or less)?

> The abstract is concise, but longer than the criteria of 150 to 250 (a total of 297 words).

Does it entice you to read the rest of the article (interesting)?

> The abstract is interesting because of its focus on a societal norm that has real health consequences.

INTRODUCTION/PROBLEM
Is the research problem or phenomenon of interest clearly stated?

> The authors clearly describe the prevalence of betel nut chewing in Hawaii, particularly among Palauans, and its adverse effects on oral health, including the development of cancer. Strong cultural acceptance and societal implications of chewing betel nut contribute to its continued practice.

Is it succinct?

> The problem is succinctly summarized in the Summary section of the introduction.

Does it answer the "so what" question?

> The introduction answers in a direct way the "so what" question. The socially accepted habit of betel nut chewing has serious health implications.

RESEARCH AIMS/OBJECTIVES
Is the research aim/objective clearly stated?

> The research aim is clearly stated in the last paragraph of the introduction: to describe Hawaiian Palauans' perceptions of betel nut chewing and determine the social impact of oral disease.

Is it concisely written?

> The research aim is concisely written.

Does it follow logically from the research problem/phenomenon of interest?

> The aim flows logically from the previously identified research problem/phenomenon of interest.

SIGNIFICANCE
Is the significance to nursing and health care clearly written?

> The significance to nursing is not explicitly stated but health care implications are clearly described. The authors refer to the global prevalence and acceptance of betel nut chewing, its addictive qualities, and adverse effects on oral health.

Does the significance follow from the research aim/objective?

> The significance flows from the research aim/objective.

BACKGROUND
Is there an explicit description of a theoretical perspective or conceptual framework? If not, is it implied?

> A pathophysiological framework embedded in a sociocultural framework is implied.

Are there clear theoretical/conceptual definitions of the concepts?

> The authors explain betel quid, a common form of betel chewing, and provide specific examples of oral disease.

LITERATURE REVIEW
Primary sources only?

> All sources were primary sources.

Current (within the past how many years)?

> Dates of sources ranged from 1986 to 2013. Older sources are included if they represent hallmark or landmark papers about the topic or if little is known about the phenomenon of interest. If possible, more recent literature (within 2–3 years of publication) should be included.

Is the search strategy included?

> The article describes the search strategy used.

Is literature relevant to the research aims/objectives?

> Strong lines of evidence are presented regarding betel nut use and oral pathology, all relevant to the research aims.

Is it chronologically presented (old to current)?

> The research was not presented chronologically but rather began with background on betel nut chewing, betel nut and oral health, and the social impact of oral health issues. This organization assists the reader to first understand cultural customs that contribute to betel nut chewing followed by the social and health consequences.

Is it comprehensive? If not, is sufficient background literature provided?

> The section on the literature review is extensive and interesting, and provides sufficient background information. The summary succinctly reinforces the high global use of betel nut and the resulting oral health issues.

RATIONALE FOR THE STUDY
Is there a gap in the literature that this study will fill (will it extend prior knowledge)? Is the rationale clearly stated?

> The clearly stated research aim reflects the gap in the literature that is be filled.

Is this a follow-up or replication study?

> This is a unique, first-of-a-kind study on this topic in this population in Hawaii.

RESEARCH QUESTION(S) AND/OR HYPOTHESES
Are these explicitly and clearly stated?

> Although research questions were not stated, they can be easily inferred from the study aim/purpose.

Do they include the variables/phenomenon of interest?

> Variables of interest were included: perceptions of betel nut chewing in the study population and social impact of oral disease.

Do they follow from the research aim/objective?

> The variables follow from the research aim.

METHODS
Research Design/Paradigm
Is the research design clearly stated?

> The research design is clearly stated in the abstract, but not in the text, as a quantitative descriptive design.

Is there consistency between the research design and paradigm?

> This quantitative research design is consistent with the positivist approach to using statistics and drawing inferences from the data

Is this the best choice of design to address the research problem/phenomenon of interest?

> The descriptive design is the best choice of design for the issue studied, particularly because there have been no previous studies investigating this phenomenon of interest.

Is there rigor in the design?

> The presentation of the methods section is well organized, reflecting that rigor is likely high within this descriptive approach.

SETTING
Is the setting clearly described?

> The study was conducted on Oahu, Hawaii, during a meeting of a sociocultural organization, the Ngerchumebai Young Palauans Association (NYPA). More detail was provided in the Methods section as to why that setting was chosen.

What biases are introduced as a result of selecting this particular setting?

> Bias is related to the single site and study results might vary in other settings.

SAMPLING PLAN AND SAMPLE
Is the sampling plan clearly identified?

> A small convenience sample ($n = 30$) was identified. Nonrandom sampling is often used in nursing research especially when using descriptive designs.

Does it represent the population of interest?

> The sample represented the population of interest on Oahu in Hawaii.

Is the sampling plan consistent with the research aim/objective?

> This sampling method is consistent with the research aim/objective of describing perceptions of betel nut chewing among Palauans in Hawaii and investigating the social impact of oral disease.

Is the sample size sufficient (e.g., power analysis or data saturation)?

> The authors do not describe the use of power analysis and acknowledge that the small sample size limits generalization of study findings.

VARIABLES

Are variables clearly identified?

> The outcome variables are clearly identified in the research aim; however, the study also includes a statement about the lack of an objective measure of the oral pathologies they state result from the betel nut chewing.

Are variables operationally defined and consistent with theoretical concepts?

> The operational definitions are described in the Instruments section and include the use of a researcher-developed health survey as well as the Oral Health Impact Profile (OHIP-14). A reader unfamiliar with the latter acronym would need to use additional resources to learn that it stands for OHIP.

Are independent and dependent variables identified, if applicable?

> In studies, the independent and dependent variables are rarely named as such, but the article is clear about the dependent variables measured in this descriptive study. The study's outcome variables are sample characteristics in Table 1 and the social impact variables in Table 2.

METHOD OF DATA COLLECTION

What are the methods of data collection?

> Data-collection methods are straightforward and described in the Procedure section. During a meeting of the NYPA, study participants completed a demographic sheet and two surveys and returned them to the primary author.

Are validity and reliability clearly addressed for prior research and current study, if applicable?

> Reliability of the OHIP instrument reported in other studies was acceptable. Internal reliability and validity were not addressed. The 12-question health survey was researcher developed. There was no content validity reported, therefore, reliability and validity testing is required in future studies. The questions seem in line with the concepts in the study.

Do the measures/instruments address the underlying theoretical concepts or phenomenon of interest?

> The measures/instruments address the phenomenon of interest, such as perceptions of betel nut chewing and social impact of oral disease in this particular population.

Were human rights protected?

> Protection of human subjects was stated by describing permissions obtained from institutional review boards and the president of the NYPA. Privacy and confidentiality were also addressed. Participants' completion of surveys implied consent.

Are other ethical issues identified?

No other ethical issues were identified. Participants received $5.00 for completing questionnaires; however, the sum is too nominal to be considered coercive.

Is the data-collection method appropriate for research design?

Obtaining data from questionnaires is appropriate for a descriptive research design.

Is there bias in data collection?

The use of a self-report questionnaire, common in descriptive research, introduces an element of bias in the data that can affect the validity of findings.

What is the fidelity of intervention addressed, if applicable?

In the absence of an intervention this is not applicable.

DATA ANALYSIS

Are data analysis techniques described (e.g., statistical tests, methodology for qualitative analysis)?

From a review of the results it is clear that the authors utilized simple descriptive statistics, that is, mean and percentage, to summarize the sample and measures.

Does the analysis answer the research question?

The data analysis does answer the underlying questions about perceptions of betel nut chewing and social impact of oral disease in this population.

Is it appropriate?

The use of descriptive statistics is appropriate for providing a simple summary of quantitative data.

Is the analysis comprehensive? Are themes identified?

The data analysis was sufficiently comprehensive to provide the reader with an understanding of the participants' perception of betel nut chewing and the social impact of oral disease.

Is there bias in the analysis (trustworthiness? credibility?)?

While there does not appear to be overt bias in the data analysis, the use of self-report data introduces an element of bias that can influence the validity of findings.

RESULTS

Are sample characteristics described and fully reported?

The sample characteristics are described and displayed in Table 1.

Are findings presented related to research aim/objective?

Study findings on perceptions of betel nut chewing and its social impact on oral health are described in the article's Results section.

Are all outcome variables addressed, if applicable?

The outcome variables of interest are addressed in the Results section and presented in tables.

Are results clearly presented in text and/or tables/figures?

> The authors displayed participant sample characteristics in Table 1 and the social impact of oral disease in Table 2.

Is significance of results reported, if applicable?

> Because the authors did not hypothesize about comparisons between or within groups of individuals, significance is not applicable.

DISCUSSION OF RESULTS

Do the authors link the findings to previous research studies?

> The authors link their findings to two previous studies that reported strong family and social influence on an individual's decision to chew betel nut. Given the lack of prior studies in this population on the phenomenon of interest, referencing only two other studies is acceptable.

Are the conclusions comprehensive, yet within the data?

> The discussion of results is comprehensive but the authors do not go beyond what was found.

Do the authors interpret the results in the discussion?

> Results are interpreted in the article's discussion section. The authors describe the study participants' intention to continue betel nut chewing because of minimal concerns about health or negative social impact. Of note is that the vast majority of participants' children did not chew betel nut, offering promise for behavior change in younger Palauans.

Are the findings generalizable or transferable?

> The authors state that the perceptions of the study participants may not be representative of Palauans living in Hawaii.

LIMITATIONS

Identified? Accurate? Inclusive?

> The limitation paragraph is well written, accurate, and inclusive. The authors identify the small convenience sample and lack of power analysis as limitations. Additional limitations are conducting the research during one gathering of a social organization as well as the use of self-report for dental and oral health rather than an independent, objective assessment.

IMPLICATIONS

Are there implications for practice, education, research?
Are there implications for clinical significance?

> The implications are for practice, education, policy, and research, all of which are highly clinically significant. Nurses are challenged to educate and facilitate behavior change in Palauans who chew betel nut, given they do not perceive problems with this deeply embedded cultural tradition. Nurses are called on to participate in policy development that ensures the availability of culturally sensitive services addressing the health needs of betel nut chewers.

RECOMMENDATIONS
Recommendations for future study/study replication?

Future studies are recommended utilizing betel nut chewers who already have oral cancer. Also, the authors recommend comparing nut chewers in Hawaii and Palau, and obtaining independent assessments of oral health. Future studies can determine whether betel nut chewers adapt their lifestyle and diet to reduce the impact of their oral problems. Research on dental care practices and dental visits is also warranted.

CONCLUSION
Is it succinct and does it tie everything together?

The succinct conclusions tie the following ideas together: the lack of impact found regarding betel nut chewing on oral health, need for people addicted to recognize the health consequences, and the urgency of understanding the phenomenon to further develop national and international health policies related to betel nut chewing.

A RANDOMISED CLINICAL TRIAL OF THE EFFECTIVENESS OF HOME-BASED HEALTH CARE WITH TELEMONITORING IN PATIENTS WITH COPD

4

Janet E. McDowell
Department of Respiratory Medicine, Lagan Valley Hospital,
Northern Ireland, UK

Sally McClean
School of Computing and Information Engineering, University of Ulster, Northern Ireland, UK

Francis FitzGibbon
School of Engineering, University of Ulster, Northern Ireland, UK

Stephen Tate
Department of Respiratory Medicine, Lagan Valley Hospital, Northern Ireland, UK

SUMMARY

We studied the effect of telemonitoring in addition to usual care (TUC) compared to usual care (UC) alone in patients with chronic obstructive pulmonary disease (COPD). A total of 110 patients with moderate to severe COPD were recruited from a specialist respiratory service in Northern Ireland. Patients had at least two of: emergency department admissions, hospital admissions, or emergency general practitioner (GP) contacts in the 12 months before the study. Exclusion criteria were patients who had any respiratory disorder other than COPD, or were cognitively unable to learn the process of monitoring. Patients were randomized to receive 6 months of home TUC, or 6 months of UC. The primary outcome measure was disease-specific quality of life, as measured by the St. George's Respiratory Questionnaire for COPD patients (SGRQ-C). Of 100 patients completing the study, 48 patients were randomized to telemonitoring and 52 patients were randomized to the control group. The SGRQ-C scores improved significantly in the intervention group compared to UC ($p = .001$). The Hospital Anxiety and Depression Scale (HADS) anxiety score was significantly higher in the telehealth group compared to the UC group ($p = .01$). There were significantly more contacts with the Community Respiratory Team (CRT) in the telemonitoring group compared to the control group ($p = .029$). There were no significant between-group differences in EQ-5D scores, HADS depression scores, GP activity, emergency department visits, hospital

McDowell, J. E., McClean, S., FitzGibbon, F., Tate, S. (2015). A randomised clinical trial of the effectiveness of home-based health care with telemonitoring in patients with COPD. *Journal of Telemedicine and Telecare*, 21(2), 80–87. doi:10.1177/1357633X14566575. Reprinted by Permission of SAGE Publications, Ltd.

admissions, or exacerbations. The total cost to the health service of the intervention over the 6-month study period was £2039, giving an estimated incremental cost-effectiveness ratio (ICER) of £203,900. In selected patients with COPD, telemonitoring was effective in improving health-related quality of life and anxiety, but was not a cost-effective intervention.

INTRODUCTION

Chronic obstructive pulmonary disease (COPD) is a major burden on health care systems worldwide.[1] In the United Kingdom, COPD accounts for 1.4 million consultations with general practitioners (GPs) and over 1 million hospital bed-days annually.[2] This represents a cost to the health service of approximately £982 million per year[2] (£1 = 1.3 Euro or US$1.6).

Exacerbations of COPD are associated with increased hospital admissions and costs, reduced social contact, increased anxiety, and reduced health-related quality of life.[2-4] The management of patients with COPD includes well-established interventions such as pulmonary rehabilitation, inhaled therapies, and smoking cessation which can reduce rates of exacerbation and improve health-related quality of life.[2, 5-7] However, it is now recognized that COPD is a multisystem disorder and patients often suffer from additional comorbidities, including anxiety and depression, cardiovascular disease, and osteoporosis, which significantly increase their health care requirements. This realization has led to attempts to develop integrated care strategies, including the use of telemedicine, which may allow more comprehensive and effective overall management of these patients.

Telemonitoring may allow early intervention for acute exacerbations of COPD and thereby improve quality of life. Four recent systematic reviews of telemonitoring in patients with COPD provide conflicting evidence for its value in improving health status and reducing health care interventions.[8-11] The studies on which the reviews were based were typically underpowered and applied different models of monitoring, making comparisons difficult. All four reviews recommended better quality research.

The primary objective of the present study was to assess the effect of telemonitoring in patients with COPD of moderate to severe disease severity; the primary outcome was health-related quality of life. The secondary objectives were to assess the effect of telemonitoring on health care utilization, exacerbations, satisfaction, and cost-effectiveness.

METHODS

The study was a two-center, randomized controlled clinical trial. Patients were recruited between August 2009 and January 2010 from a specialist respiratory service in Northern Ireland. The study was approved by the appropriate ethics committee. Written informed consent was given by all patients.

The inclusion criteria were a diagnosis of moderate to severe COPD (GOLD stage 2 or 3), and at least two of: emergency department admissions, hospital admissions, or emergency GP contacts in the 12 months before the study. The exclusion criteria were any respiratory disorder other than COPD, and patients cognitively unable to learn the process of monitoring.

Patients were randomized to receive usual care (UC) or telemonitoring in addition to usual care (TUC). Patients were randomized using a concealed, computer-generated randomization procedure prepared by a researcher with no clinical involvement in the trial. Details of the allocated group were placed in sequentially numbered envelopes and opened consecutively on receiving informed patient consent.

Patients in the UC group received a standardized home-based program of specialist respiratory assessment and monitoring provided by the local Community Respiratory Team (CRT) and GP. The program was developed from department of health guidelines.[12] The CRT physiotherapist and nurse offered each patient at least two home visits within 2 weeks of receiving the referral. During these visits, the patient received disease-specific education, including recognition of the signs and symptoms of exacerbation; advice on smoking cessation, if necessary; review of self-management techniques and CRT contact details for future use. If patients experienced an exacerbation of their condition, they contacted the CRT or their GP and a decision was made about whether they could be managed at home by the CRT or required hospitalization. During evenings, weekends, and bank holidays, patients were advised to use the out-of-hours GP service or the hospital emergency department. If hospital admission was required, the community team worked closely with the hospital team to support early discharge. Patients managed at home during an exacerbation were monitored closely by the CRT until stable. In addition, all patients were offered pulmonary rehabilitation or access to a weekly maintenance exercise class.

Patients in the TUC group received the standardized home-based program of care as described previously and, in addition, a home telehealth system (HomMed, Honeywell, USA) was provided by Home Telehealth Ltd (HTL) for a period of 6 months. The telecommunications device was connected directly to the patient's home telephone line by an HTL technician. The monitoring process is shown in Figure 1. The system was preloaded with personal information, including monitoring start time, clinical observations (blood pressure, heart rate, oxygen saturations), and questions relating to symptoms (difficulty in breathing, cough, sputum, tiredness). The HTL technician instructed the patient on use of the equipment and observed the patient self-monitoring. The monitoring session lasted for approximately 10 minutes during which the patient would attach a finger probe and blood pressure cuff and respond "yes" or "no" to the set questions. Patients received a courtesy call from the CRT within 24 hours of monitor installation and a further demonstration from the technician was requested if necessary.

Patients monitored their clinical observations and answered questions relating to symptoms each morning at the agreed time for 5 continuous days. The daily data were transmitted via the telephone line to a server and downloaded by HTL. A trend report was sent to the CRT by email and normal limits were set for each clinical observation using the 5-day report for guidance. Patients then monitored their clinical observations and questions relating to symptoms each morning at the agreed time for a period of 6 months, with daily data transmitted and downloaded by HTL. A dedicated HTL nurse reviewed the daily data within 10 minutes of its arrival and compared it to the set normal limits. An alert indicated that one or more of the patient's clinical observations was outside the set normal limits or the patient had answered "yes" to a question relating to their symptoms. Following an alert, the HTL nurse contacted the patient to obtain additional information, advised the

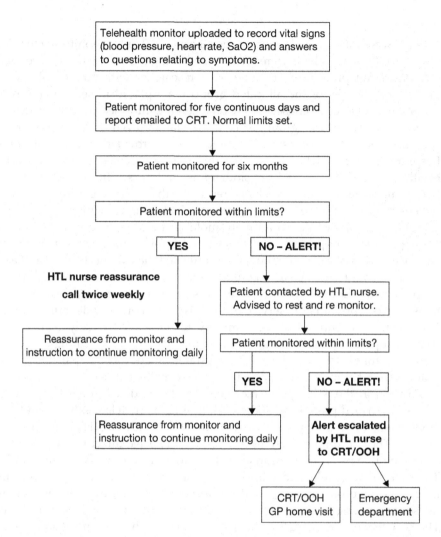

FIGURE 1. Telemonitoring system.

CRT, community respiratory team; HTL, home telehealth limited; OOH GP, out of hours general practitioner.

patient to sit down and relax for 30 minutes and to repeat the monitoring. The second set of results was reviewed and if these were within normal limits, the HTL nurse contacted the patient and provided reassurance. If the second set of results remained outside the limits, the alert was escalated to the CRT. The CRT decided whether a home visit or an emergency department admission was required.

If an alert occurred at the weekend, and needed to be escalated, the HTL nurse contacted the out-of-hours GP who took appropriate action and provided a report for the CRT documenting the outcome of the escalation. If patients were monitored within normal limits for 3 to 4 days and no alerts were created, the HTL nurse contacted the patient to ensure that they were not experiencing any difficulties with their respiratory condition that had not been detected by the monitor.

Outcomes

The primary outcome was quality of life, as measured by the St George's Respiratory Questionnaire for COPD patients (SGRQ-C).[13] Secondary outcomes were the EuroQol five-dimension questionnaire (EQ-5D) score; anxiety and depression, as measured by a change in the Hospital Anxiety and Depression Scale (HADS); health care utilization; number of exacerbations; satisfaction and cost-effectiveness.

SGRQ-C scores, EQ-5D scores, EQ-5D scores supplemented by a visual analog scale (EQ-VAS) and HADS scores were assessed for all patients at baseline and again at 6 months. Data on health care utilization and exacerbations of COPD was collected retrospectively for all patients at the end of the 6-month study period from hospital coding, GP records, and CRT records. GP contacts were included only if the consultation was for respiratory causes. Exacerbations of COPD were defined as the rapid and sustained worsening of sputum production and dyspnoea.[14] Cost-effectiveness analysis was based on the change in the EQ-VAS score in the TUC group and the cost of the intervention during the 6-month study period. Details on the cost of the intervention were provided by HTL. Details on CRT costings were provided by the Finance Department of the hospital. The change in EQ-VAS score was used to calculate the quality-adjusted life year (QALY) gain/loss accrued and the cost of the intervention was used to estimate the incremental cost-effectiveness ratio (ICER). An ICER of less than £20,000 was considered cost-effective.[15]

Patients in the TUC group were asked to indicate their response to the following questions (agree/disagree/don't know): telemonitoring helped me feel more in control of my health on a day-to-day basis; if I had the opportunity to use telemonitoring again, I would do so. Finally, patients in the TUC group were asked to report any difficulties experienced with the monitoring equipment.

Sample Size

The sample size was determined using data provided by Koff et al.[16] Calculation showed that 50 patients per group would be necessary to detect an 8.0-unit improvement in the SGRQ with an SD of 15 at the 5% significance level. To allow for 10% dropout, 55 patients were randomized to each group.

Data Analysis

Statistical analyses were performed using a standard package (PASW version 18, Predictive Analytics Software). No formal statistical tests were applied to baseline characteristics. The change in SGRQ-C scores, EQ-5D scores, and HADS scores was compared using analysis of covariance (ANCOVA) between the two groups and followed the intention to treat principle. Six-month health care utilization and exacerbations were compared using unpaired two sample t-tests between the two groups. The exception was GP out-of-hours activity which had a highly skewed distribution, so a nonparametric Mann–Whitney test was used instead. QALY analysis was used to estimate cost-effectiveness.

RESULTS

A total of 110 patients (58% female) were randomized with 100 patients completing the study. The progress of patients through the study and the reasons for withdrawal are shown in Figure 2. Five patients died (two in the TUC group and three in the UC group) and five patients in the TUC group withdrew from the trial because the monitoring process was stressful ($n = 3$) or time-consuming ($n = 2$). One GP surgery would not release information on patient-GP contacts (two patients in the UC group).

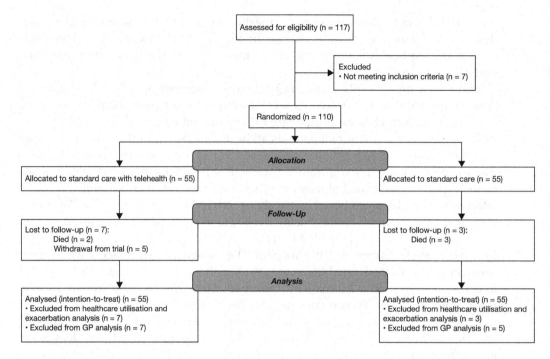

FIGURE 2. Flow of participants through the trial.

Baseline Data

The demographics and baseline characteristics of the groups were similar (Table 1), including SGRQ-C and EQ-5D scores (Table 2). The baseline HADS scores indicated mild anxiety and depression in both groups, and the baseline SGRQ-C total score indicated poor health status in both groups. The baseline EQ-5D and EQ-VAS scores were lower than would be expected in patients with moderate to severe disease severity, again indicating poor health status.

Quality of Life

The total SGRQ-C scores recorded at 6 months improved in the TUC group compared to the UC group (mean 61.1 vs. 66.8), with a significant between-group difference (p = .001) (Table 3). This between-group improvement exceeded the minimum clinically important difference of at least four units. The component SGRQ scores recorded at 6 months changed as follows: the symptoms score improved in the TUC group compared to the UC group (mean 71.5 vs. 79.0), with a significant between-group difference (p = .002). The activity score improved in the TUC group compared to the UC group (mean 77.8 vs. 82.8), with a significant between-group difference (p = .003). The impact score improved in the TUC group compared to the UC group (mean 47.7 vs. 53.0), with a significant between-group difference (p = .03) (Table 3).

The total EQ-5D scores recorded at 6 months declined in the TUC and improved in the UC group (mean 0.57 vs. 0.49), with a nonsignificant between-group difference (p = .08) (Table 4). The EQ-VAS scores recorded at 6 months declined in the TUC group and improved in the UC group (mean 48.8 vs. 46.6), but the between-group difference was not significant (p = .50) (Table 4).

TABLE 1. Characteristics of the Two Groups at Baseline. The Values Shown Are the Mean (SD)

	Telemonitoring With Usual Care (*n* = 55)	Usual Care (*n* = 55)
Age, years	69.8 (7.1)	70.2 (7.4)
Females, %	58.2	54.5
Current smokers, %	38.2	32.7
Smoking history, pack years	49.4 (25.4)	43.0 (19.9)
Living alone, %	23.6	32.7
FEV1, % predicted	45.5 (13.7)	43.4 (11.3)
FVC, % predicted	71.7 (15.5)	70.4 (17.3)
BODE index	5.7 (1.8)	5.4 (2.1)
Long-term oxygen therapy, %	27.3	25.5
Ambulatory oxygen therapy, %	40.0	32.7
Influenza vaccination, %	98.2	90.9
Current pulmonary rehabilitation	18.2	16.4
EQ-5D score	0.49 (0.35)	0.52 (0.30)
EQ VAS	50.1 (18.0)	45.5 (23.1)
HADS anxiety score	8.3 (5.2)	7.9 (4.3)
HADS depression score	6.8 (3.8)	7.9 (3.9)
Emergency department visits[a]	1.02 (0.9)	1.42 (1.3)
Hospitalizations[a]	0.82 (0.9)	1.05 (0.9)
Hospital length of stay, days[a]	5.67 (8.7)	6.38 (7.3)
Urgent GP contacts[a]	5.98 (4.1)	6.11 (3.8)
Previous exacerbations[a]	4.29 (2.2)	4.75 (2.4)

[a]In previous year.

Anxiety and Depression

The HADS anxiety scores recorded at 6 months improved in the TUC group compared to the UC group (mean 7.15 vs. 8.81), with a significant between-group difference (*p* = .01) (Table 4). This between-group improvement exceeded the minimum clinically

TABLE 2. Baseline SGRQ-C Scores. The Values Shown Are the Mean (SD)

	Telemonitoring With Usual Care (*n* = 55)	Usual Care (*n* = 55)
SGRQ-C total score	63.6 (15.9)	64.2 (14.5)
SGRQ-C components		
Symptoms	75.1 (15.1)	75.3 (17.6)
Activity	79.7 (19.7)	80.9 (17.4)
Impact	50.1 (18.2)	50.5 (17.8)

TABLE 3. Changes in Disease-Specific Health-Related Quality of Life. The Values Shown Are the Mean (SD)

	Telemonitoring With Usual Care (*n* = 55)	Usual Care (*n* = 55)	Mean Difference (95% CI)	*p*-Value[a]
SGRQ-C total score	61.1 (17.0)	66.8 (15.0)	5.75 (2.32 to 9.18)	.001
SGRQ-C components				
Symptoms	71.5 (17.3)	79.0 (15.9)	7.42 (2.77 to 12.07)	.002
Activity	77.8 (21.0)	82.8 (16.3)	5.01 (1.79 to 8.23)	.003
Impact	47.7 (19.3)	53.0 (18.8)	5.24 (0.49 to 9.99)	.031

[a]Two-sided *p*-value for between-group difference.

important difference of at least 1.32 units. The HADS depression scores recorded at 6 months improved in the TUC group compared to the UC group (mean 6.87 vs. 7.50), but the between-group difference was not significant (*p* = .29) (Table 4).

Health Care Utilization and Exacerbations

Analysis of health care utilization and exacerbations was carried out on 48 patients in the TUC group and 52 patients in the UC group. At 6 months, there was a higher number of emergency department visits, hospitalizations, and longer length of hospital stay in the UC group compared to the TUC group, but the differences were not significant (*p* = .40, *p* = .42, *p* = .59, respectively) (Table 5). At 6 months, there was a significantly higher number of CRT contacts in the TUC group compared with the UC group (mean difference 3.2 contacts, *p* = .029) (Table 4). No significant differences were observed in study period exacerbations between the two groups (*p* = .22) (Table 5).

Analysis of GP contacts was carried out on 48 patients in the TUC group and 50 patients in the UC group. At 6 months, there was a significantly higher number of GP contacts in the UC group than the TUC group (mean difference 1.3 contacts, *p* = .003) and a significantly higher number of out-of-hours GP contacts in the TUC group compared with the UC group (mean difference 0.45 contacts, *p* = .015) (Table 6). There were no significant differences between the groups in combined GP and GP out-of-hours contacts (mean difference 0.90 contacts, *p* = .079) (Table 6).

TABLE 4. Changes in Generic Health-Related Quality of Life, Anxiety and Depression. The Values Shown Are the Mean (SD)

	Telemonitoring With Usual Care (*n* = 55)	Usual Care (*n* = 55)	Mean Difference (95% CI)	*p*-Value[a]
EQ-5D score	0.57 (0.32)	0.49 (0.33)	0.08 (−0.01 to 0.18)	.08
EQ-VAS	48.8 (17.6)	46.6 (18.8)	2.18 (−4.25 to 8.61)	.50
HADS anxiety score	7.15 (4.50)	8.81 (4.20)	1.66 (0.37 to 2.95)	.01
HADS depression score	6.87 (3.67)	7.50 (3.92)	0.63 (−0.55 to 1.81)	.29

[a]Two-sided *p*-value for between-group difference.

TABLE 5. Summary

	Telemonitoring With Usual Care (*n* = 48)	Usual Care (*n* = 52)	Mean Difference (95% CI)	*p*-Value[a]
Emergency department visits	0.60 (0.9)	0.79 (1.3)	0.19 (−0.25 to 0.63)	.40
COPD total hospitalizations	0.50 (0.9)	0.65 (1.0)	0.15 (−0.22 to 0.53)	.42
COPD total length of stay, days	3.4 (7.7)	4.3 (8.5)	0.87 (−2.36 to 4.10)	.59
CRT total contacts	10.1 (7.8)	6.9 (7.0)	3.2 (0.33 to 6.15)	.029
Total exacerbations	2.35 (1.8)	2.81 (1.9)	0.45 (−0.28 to 1.19)	.22

[a]Two-sided *p*-value for between-group difference.

Satisfaction

Patient satisfaction in the TUC group was high: 84% of patients agreed with the statement that "telemonitoring helped me feel more in control of my health on a day to day basis"; 81% of patients agreed with the statement that "if I had the opportunity to use telemonitoring again I would do so" and only 17% of patients experienced difficulties with the equipment.

Cost-Effectiveness

The between-group difference in quality of life was 2.18 units. If perfect life is represented by 1 unit, this improvement in the EQ-VAS score is equivalent to 0.02 units. The cost of telemonitoring per patient was estimated at £10.12 per day, or £1847 per patient over the 6-month study period. CRT contacts increased by 3.2 in the TUC group, as calculated from overall yearly costs. This is approximately £192 per patient over the 6-month study period. The observed improvement in EQ-VAS score (0.02) over the 6-month study period (0.5 years) represents 0.01 QALYs. The total cost to the health service of the intervention over the 6-month study period was £1847 + £192 = £2039. This gives an estimated ICER of £2039 / 0.01 / = £203,900.

DISCUSSION

The present study demonstrates that telemonitoring and a standard home-based program of care is associated with improved quality of life and reduced anxiety,

TABLE 6. Summary of GP Contacts During the 6-Month Study Period. The Values Shown Are the Mean (SD)

	Telemonitoring With Usual Care (*n* = 48)	Usual Care (*n* = 50)	Mean Difference (95% CI)	*p*-Value[a]
Total daytime GP contacts	1.25 (1.7)	2.57 (2.5)	1.32 (0.54 to 2.04)	.003[a]
Total out-of-hours GP contacts	0.69 (1.1)	0.24 (0.7)	0.45 (0.10 to 0.81)	.015[a]
Total GP contacts	1.94 (2.22)	2.84 (2.8)	0.90 (−0.11 to 1.91)	.079

[a]Two-sided *p*-value for between-group difference.

compared to a standard home-based program of care alone in patients with moderate to severe COPD and a history of frequent health care utilization. The observed improvements were accompanied by significantly increased contacts with the specialist community team. There were no significant effects of telehealth on depression, number of emergency department visits, hospitalizations, GP activity, or exacerbations over a 6-month period. Telehealth in this setting was not a cost-effective intervention.

Limitations

The study had certain limitations. The primary outcome assessors were not blind to treatment allocation. However, questionnaires were administered according to published guidelines to reduce bias. It was not possible to use blinding of participants due to the type of intervention. We did not conduct further poststudy analysis of quality of life, anxiety, and depression to determine whether the improvements were maintained after telemonitoring ceased. Telehealth in the present study was not cost-effective. However, the findings may not be generalizable to other COPD populations.

Interpretation

We observed an improvement in SGRQ-C scores (5.75 units) similar to that found in a systematic review of studies investigating pulmonary rehabilitation (6.11 units).[17] Similar findings were reported in a study conducted by Koff et al. who applied a home-based model of care in addition to telemonitoring compared to no intervention over a 3-month period and reported that SGRQ improved by 10.3 in the intervention group compared to 0.6 in the control group.[16]

In contrast, two recent randomized controlled trials reported that telemonitoring did not confer a significant benefit on health-related quality of life.[18, 19] Our study differed from previous trials as patients received regular reassurance calls from the HTL nurse (at least one call every 4 days) in addition to the increased contacts with the specialist community team. The study was conducted over a particularly severe winter during which many patients became isolated in their homes. It is possible that the reassurance provided through these regular contacts reduced anxiety and increased confidence, enabling patients to feel more in control of their symptoms and more able to carry out activities of daily living. This is reflected in the enhanced quality of life and also suggested by the satisfaction questionnaire, with 84% of patients feeling more in control of their health with telemonitoring. Since reduced quality of life and increased anxiety remain a major problem in patients with COPD, telemonitoring and/or increased specialist health care contacts may be useful in the care of these patients. A small number of patients found the monitoring process to be stressful or time-consuming, and therefore it may not be a suitable intervention for all patients with COPD.

The present study, in agreement with previous studies, showed no significant effect of telemonitoring on hospital activity and exacerbations.[18,20] In our trial, telemonitoring was associated with a significant increase in workload for the specialist community team and the out-of-hours GP service, but there was no significant reduction in hospital activity. The trial, however, was not powered to definitively analyze health care utilization. A future, longer study would be required to determine whether the changes in quality of life observed in our study were associated with any changes in hospital activity. Only one previous randomized controlled trial has shown significantly reduced hospitalizations, reduced exacerbations, and reduced urgent GP contacts with telemonitoring compared to no intervention. That study was conducted over a 12-month period in a heterogeneous group of patients with chronic respiratory failure and only included a subgroup of patients with COPD (240 patients, 101 with COPD).[21] It did not include a typical COPD population, as all were on long-term oxygen therapy and/or noninvasive ventilation, and the telehealth system itself recorded only oxygen saturations.

In conclusion, the present study demonstrates that, in selected patients with COPD, telemonitoring is effective in improving health-related quality of life and anxiety but is not a cost-effective intervention.

ACKNOWLEDGMENTS

The authors thank the patients who participated in the trial, the Lisburn Community Respiratory Team and the Downpatrick Community Respiratory Team. They also thank Barbara Hanna, Gail McKeown, Hilary Sloan, Jenna Chaviel, Jennifer Howard, Elaine Jackson, Claire Gault, Aileen Mulhall, Hugh Harrison, and Rosemary McCoubrey. The study was funded by a grant from the European Centre for Connected Health. The researchers were independent from the funders.

REFERENCES

1. Rabe KF, Hurd S, Anzueto A, et al. Global strategy for the diagnosis, management, and prevention of chronic obstructive pulmonary disease: GOLD executive summary. *Am J Respir Crit Care Med* 2007;**176**:532–55.

2. National Clinical Guideline Centre. Chronic obstructive pulmonary disease: management of chronic obstructive pulmonary disease in adults in primary and secondary care. See http://guidance.nice .org.uk/CG101/Guidance/pdf/English (last checked 18 July 2014).

3. Andersson F, Borg S, Jansson SA, et al. The costs of exacerbations in chronic obstructive pulmonary disease (COPD). *Respir Med* 2002;**96**:700–8.

4. Seemungal TA, Donaldson GC, Paul EA, Bestall JC, Jeffries DJ, Wedzicha JA. Effect of exacerbation on quality of life in patients with chronic obstructive pulmonary disease. *Am J Respir Crit Care Med* 1998;**157**:1418–22.

5. Calverley PM, Anderson JA, Celli B, et al. Salmeterol and fluticasone propionate and survival in chronic obstructive pulmonary disease. *N Engl J Med* 2007;**356**:775–89.

6. Kanner RE, Connett JE, Williams DE, Buist AS. Effects of randomized assignment to a smoking cessation intervention and changes in smoking habits on respiratory symptoms in smokers with early chronic obstructive pulmonary disease: the Lung Health Study. *Am J Med* 1999;**106**:410–6.

7. Papadopoulos G, Vardavas CI, Limperi M, Linardis A, Georgoudis G, Behrakis P. Smoking cessation can improve quality of life among COPD patients: validation of the clinical COPD questionnaire into Greek. *BMC Pulm Med* 2011;**11**:13.

8. Bartoli L, Zanaboni P, Masella C, Ursini N. Systematic review of telemedicine services for patients affected by chronic obstructive pulmonary disease (COPD). *Telemed J E Health* 2009;**15**:877–83.

9. Polisena J, Tran K, Cimon K, et al. Home telehealth for chronic obstructive pulmonary disease: a systematic review and meta-analysis. *J Telemed Telecare* 2010;**16**:120–7.

10. Bolton CE, Waters CS, Peirce S, et al. Insufficient evidence of benefit: a systematic review of home telemonitoring for COPD. *J Eval Clin Pract* 2011;**17**:1216–22.

11. McLean S, Nurmatov U, Liu JL, Pagliari C, Car J, Sheikh A. Telehealthcare for chronic obstructive pulmonary disease. *Cochrane Database Syst Rev* 2011;**7**:CD007718.

12. Department of Health, Social Services and Public Safety in Northern Ireland. A healthier future: a strategic framework for respiratory conditions. See http://www.dhsspsni.gov .uk/pcd_-_respiratory_framework.pdf (last checked 18 July 2014).

13. Meguro M, Barley EA, Spencer S, Jones PW. Development and validation of an improved, COPD-specific version of the St. George Respiratory Questionnaire. *Chest* 2007;**132**:456–63.

14. Burge S, Wedzicha JA. COPD exacerbations: definitions and classifications. *Eur Respir J Suppl* 2003;**41**:46s–53s.

15. National Institute for Health and Clinical Excellence. Guide to the methods of technology appraisal. See http://www.nice.org.uk/article/PMG9/chapter/Foreword (last checked 24 November 2014).

16. Koff PB, Jones RH, Cashman JM, Voelkel NF, Vandivier RW. Proactive integrated care improves quality of life in patients with COPD. *Eur Respir J* 2009;**33**:1031–8.

17. Lacasse Y, Goldstein R, Lasserson TJ, Martin S. Pulmonary rehabilitation for chronic obstructive pulmonary disease. *Cochrane Database Syst Rev* 2006;**4**:CD003793.

18. Pinnock H, Hanley J, McCloughan L, et al. Effectiveness of telemonitoring integrated into existing clinical services on hospital admission for exacerbation of chronic obstructive pulmonary disease: researcher blind, multicentre, randomised controlled trial. *BMJ* 2013;**347**:f6070.

19. Lewis KE, Annandale JA, Warm DL, Hurlin C, Lewis MJ, Lewis L. Home telemonitoring and quality of life in stable, optimised chronic obstructive pulmonary disease. *J Telemed Telecare* 2010;**16**:253–9.

20. Lewis KE, Annandale JA, Warm DL, et al. Does home telemonitoring after pulmonary rehabilitation reduce health-care use in optimized COPD? A pilot randomized trial. *COPD* 2010;**7**:44–50.

21. Vitacca M, Bianchi L, Guerra A, et al. Tele-assistance in chronic respiratory failure patients: a randomised clinical trial. *Eur Respir J* 2009;**33**:411–8.

A RANDOMISED CLINICAL TRIAL OF THE EFFECTIVENESS OF HOME-BASED HEALTH CARE WITH TELEMONITORING IN PATIENTS WITH COPD

Critique by *Rebecca Witten Grizzle*

OVERALL SUMMARY

Telemonitoring programs are increasingly used to manage the care of individuals with a chronic disease in their home environment. This randomized controlled trial (RCT) was designed to assess the effect of telemonitoring on health-related quality of life (QOL) in individuals with chronic obstructive pulmonary disease (COPD), which is characterized by frequent exacerbations and hospitalization. Study findings reinforce the key role of the telehealth nurse's reassurance of individuals' self-care abilities, which may improve QOL.

TITLE

Does the title include the key concepts/variables/phenomenon of interest?

The title describes the research design, setting, patient population, and intervention in a clear manner.

Is it concise (12 words or less) and professionally stated?

Although professionally stated, it is not concise at 18 words long. The authors could have shortened the title to *RCT of Home-Based Care With Telemonitoring of COPD Patients* given that the term *effectiveness* is implied and RCT is a well-known acronym for randomized controlled trial.

RESEARCHER(S) CREDIBILITY

Educational credentials?

The researchers' credentials are not listed in the first page of the article, only their respective work affiliations. It is assumed that the first and fourth authors are pulmonologists, as they work for the Department of Respiratory Medicine at Lagan Valley Hospital in Northern Ireland. The second and third authors are professors at the University of Ulster.

Prior methodological research experience of the authors (i.e., methodological expertise)?

The second author is the primary author of a systematic review of telehealth care for COPD, but it is not clear if any of the authors have methodological expertise in planning and conducting RCTs as primary researchers.

Subject matter content experience (prior research on the subject matter)?

Overall, they have the clinical and technical subject matter expertise to conduct research in this field. However, because of the researchers' desire for a comprehensive program impacting psychosocial outcomes, the addition of research team members from nursing and/or health psychology would have strengthened this aspect of the study.

ABSTRACT (SUMMARY)
Does it include the key components (objective/aim, background/rationale, methods, results, and conclusion)?

This unstructured abstract contains the overall purpose of the study, but background or rationale is not provided. The methods are presented in detail, along with a summary of relevant findings and conclusion. The abstract contains acronyms such as HADS, EQ-5D, and ICER, which are not defined and require the reader to search the article for further understanding.

Does or does not include references?

The abstract appropriately does not include references.

Is it concise (150–250 words or less)?

It is slightly long at 270 words.

Does it entice you to read the rest of the article (interesting)?

A reader with particular interest in telemonitoring and COPD may be curious to find out why the intervention increased anxiety levels and which of the "selected patients" could possibly benefit as alluded to in the abstract. However, those with less interest may pass on reading the remainder of the article due to the lack of cost-effectiveness and no significant differences between groups on key outcomes.

INTRODUCTION/PROBLEM
Is the research problem or phenomenon of interest clearly stated?

The clinical and societal burden of COPD and its associated comorbidities is stated.

Is it succinct?

The research problem is stated clearly and concisely.

Does it answer the "so what" question?

The authors point to the need for integrated and comprehensive management, such as using telehealth strategies, to improve health outcomes, including QOL. COPD seems to be a significant health problem that is worthy of study.

RESEARCH AIMS/OBJECTIVES
Is the research aim/objective clearly stated?

The authors state the primary and secondary objectives of the study in the last paragraph of the introduction. The main aim is to determine the effectiveness of telemonitoring on health-related QOL. The secondary aims are to test the impact of the intervention on patient satisfaction, health services utilization, and costs.

Is it concisely written?

The research objectives are written succinctly.

Does it follow logically from the research problem/phenomenon of interest?

The primary and secondary objectives of the study flow directly from the stated research problem.

SIGNIFICANCE
Is the significance to nursing and health care clearly written?

The significance to health care professionals is implied as patient outcomes, such as QOL and health care utilization, have important implications for nurses, particularly those in home health care. The costs to society are made clear, particularly given that health care in Ireland is provided by the government. Not only do exacerbations of COPD cause a burden to the health care system, but individuals are affected physically and psychologically.

Does the significance follow from the research aim/objective?

The significance to health care professionals flows from the stated research objectives.

BACKGROUND
Is there an explicit description of a theoretical perspective or conceptual framework? If not, is it implied?

There is no conceptual or theoretical framework that guided the intervention study. One can assume that the researchers use a biomedical framework with biopsychosocial aspects, given the assessment of vital signs, symptoms, anxiety, depression, and QOL. To strengthen the study, the researchers could have based the telemonitoring intervention on patient self-management concepts or a transitional care model.

Are there clear theoretical/conceptual definitions of the concepts?

The author did not explicitly define any key concepts, such as health-related QOL.

LITERATURE REVIEW
Primary sources only?

There was no separate Literature Review section, possibly due to journal space restraints; however, 11 works are briefly cited in the Introduction section. Five articles are primary sources, with relevant variables of QOL, treatment, costs, and smoking cessation interventions.

Current (within the past how many years)?

Six articles are older than 5 years (1998–2009), and only five articles are within 5 years of the study's 2015 publication date.

Is the search strategy included?

No search strategy was identified.

Is literature relevant to the research aims/objectives?

Although the research aim is to determine the effectiveness of the telemonitoring intervention, the literature review did not include any relevant RCTs. However, four of the articles are systematic reviews, representing a higher level of evidence. Two articles are clinical guidelines or expert opinions, which is considered a lower level of evidence.

Is it chronologically presented (old to current)?

The literature review is not presented chronologically.

Is it comprehensive? If not, is sufficient background literature provided?

Literature is comprehensive enough to justify the rationale for conducting the study.

RATIONALE FOR THE STUDY

Is there a gap in the literature that this study will fill (will it extend prior knowledge)? Is the rationale clearly stated?

The authors note that there are conflicting findings on the effectiveness of telemonitoring among COPD patients in four systematic reviews of these interventions. Recommendations are for higher quality studies with adequate power. To meet the gap in research knowledge, they used standardized outcome measurements addressing the psychosocial aspects of the disease, as well as health care utilization and costs.

Is this a follow-up or replication study?

This is not a follow-up or replication study.

RESEARCH QUESTION(S) AND/OR HYPOTHESES

Are these explicitly and clearly stated?

No research questions or hypotheses are explicitly stated. It is assumed that the researchers hypothesize that telemonitoring with usual care is more effective in improving the stated health care outcomes than with usual care alone.

Do they include the variables/phenomenon of interest?

Based on the primary and secondary objectives, it can be inferred that health-related QOL, health care utilization, COPD exacerbations, patient satisfaction, and cost-effectiveness are the outcome variables of interest.

Do they follow from the research aim/objective?

The presumed hypothesis flows logically from the research objectives.

METHODS

Research Design/Paradigm

Is the research design clearly stated?

The research design, a dual-center RCT, is clearly stated in the Methods section and alluded to in the title.

Is there consistency between the research design and paradigm?

Because the researchers were comparing two interventions, a quantitative analysis approach from the positivist paradigm is appropriate.

Is this the best choice of design to address the research problem/phenomenon of interest?

RCTs are considered the most rigorous quantitative research design on the evidence-based practice (EBP) hierarchy.

Is there rigor in the design?

This study contained elements for a good RCT, such as intention-to-treat analyses. Rigor would be improved if patients were randomly sampled and their general practitioners were blinded to their assignment to intervention or usual care groups.

SETTING
Is the setting clearly described?

The setting was identified as two health centers with pulmonary specialist services in Northern Ireland, but they are not described beyond that.

What biases are introduced as a result of selecting this particular setting?

Given that this part of Ireland has government-sponsored health care, selection bias can be introduced by the use of a nonrandom sample in this type of setting. Also, there may be a threat of *compensatory rivalry of the no-treatment group*. Health care providers who know that their patients are in the usual care group (and not in the intervention group), may give these patients better care to avoid unfavorable comparisons.

SAMPLING PLAN AND SAMPLE
Is the sampling plan clearly identified?

The sampling plan is not identified, but is assumed to be a nonrandom sampling method, such as using convenience or consecutive samples.

Does it represent the population of interest?

Patients meeting the inclusion criteria of moderate to severe COPD and recent emergency or hospital admission were invited to participate. Patients were excluded if they were cognitively unable to learn the technology or had other pulmonary comorbidities, which is consistent with the aims of determining whether telemonitoring is effective with COPD patients.

Is the sampling plan consistent with the research aim/objective?

Although random sampling is ideal for an RCT, a nonrandom sampling strategy is still appropriate method for determining the effectiveness of a clinical intervention.

Is the sample size sufficient (e.g., power analysis or data saturation)?

Sample size requirements were calculated using a 0.05 level of significance, but the power level was not specified. The required sample size was 50 patients per group, and the researchers oversampled by 10% due to anticipated dropouts. There were 110 patients who were randomized to intervention conditions, and 10 participants were eventually lost to follow-up, so the sample size was adequate.

VARIABLES
Are variables clearly identified?

Health-related QOL is identified as the primary outcome variable of interest. Secondary outcomes are identified as health care utilization, exacerbations, cost-effectiveness, and patient satisfaction with telemonitoring.

Are variables operationally defined and consistent with theoretical concepts?

The QOL variable was operationally defined as the score on St. Georges' Respiratory Questionnaire for COPD patients (SGRQ-C), which is subdivided into symptoms, activity, and impact scores. Another QOL variable was the score on the EuroQol five-dimension questionnaire (EQ-5D) and the associated visual analog scale (EQ-VAS). It is not clear what five aspects of living comprise the EQ-5D scale. Anxiety and depression symptoms were measured by the Hospital Anxiety and Depression Scale

(HADS). This measure has been used with patients in community settings, but it is unclear whether it measures state or trait anxiety levels. It is also unclear whether a higher score on any of these scales indicates a higher level of the construct. Because there were no conceptual definitions identified, it is difficult to determine whether the measurements are consistent.

Are independent and dependent variables identified, if applicable?

Although not explicitly identified, the independent variable is easily inferred as telemonitoring and the primary dependent variable is health-related QOL. Additional dependent variables include health care utilization, exacerbations, cost-effectiveness, and patient satisfaction.

METHOD OF DATA COLLECTION

What are the methods of data collection?

QOL and anxiety and depression data were collected by surveys, but it was unclear whether they were self-administered or researcher-administered scales. Quality of data collected can vary depending on the health literacy level of the patient and/or the data collector training.

Are validity and reliability clearly addressed for prior research and current study, if applicable?

Validity and reliability of the measurements were not discussed, and readers are left to explore the literature to determine appropriateness. The home telehealth system was identified, but calibration of sphygmomanometers or pulse oximeter probes was not mentioned.

Do the measures/instruments address the underlying theoretical concepts or phenomenon of interest?

The research instruments that measure anxiety, depression, and QOL appear to address the underlying concept of QOL related to living with COPD.

Were human rights protected?

Human rights of research participants were vaguely discussed with the mention of written informed consent and ethics committee approval.

Are other ethical issues identified?

It was not clear how researchers avoided coercive methods to recruit participants, given patients' dependence on government-sponsored care and their potential status as members of vulnerable populations, such as elderly or severely ill persons.

Is the data-collection method appropriate for research design?

Data was collected at baseline and 6 months, which is consistent with a pretest–posttest intervention design. However, given the variable disease course among patients, surveys could have been administered within a week of an exacerbation. The usual care and telemonitoring protocols were described in good detail.

Is there bias in data collection?

The only systematic bias in data-collection methods was that patients without access to a home telephone line could not participate (i.e., impoverished patients or those who only use mobile phones).

What is the fidelity of intervention addressed, if applicable?

The authors did not discuss a manipulation check to determine whether he intervention was delivered and received as intended, such as a follow-up call to patient to ensure that triage decisions were understood. It is unclear whether the monitoring alerts were followed up consistently.

DATA ANALYSIS

Are data analysis techniques described (e.g., statistical tests, methodology for qualitative analysis)?

Data analysis methods were well described. Using a standard statistical software package, outcome measures were compared between the two groups using analysis of variance (ANOVA) after the intention-to-treat principle was applied.

Does the analysis answer the research question?

The analyses address the research objectives. However, statistical analyses were not done to measure whether there were significant differences between groups prior to the intervention. The authors stated that groups were similar in terms of demographics and baseline characteristics, but acknowledged that they did not apply any statistical analyses to this baseline data.

Is it appropriate?

Instead of examining the change in the usual care or intervention group mean from its baseline to determine the relative effectiveness in that group, the researchers compared the groups to each other only at the end of the study. This may not yield accurate findings if the groups were not equally matched or equivalent on baseline levels of the variables, despite the groups being assigned by a computer-generated randomization procedure.

Is the analysis comprehensive? Are themes identified?

Apart from not addressing the differences between groups at baseline, the data analyses appear to be comprehensive.

Is there bias in the analysis (trustworthiness? credibility?)?

There do not appear to be explicit biases in the analyses.

RESULTS

Are sample characteristics described and fully reported?

Table 1 displays the sample's baseline characteristics by group, and groups appear to be different in clinically significant ways, such as in smoking history and oxygen use. The percentage differences in the majority of baseline characteristics are large enough to potentially affect outcomes.

Are findings presented related to research aim/objective?

The findings related to the research objectives are presented in an organized narrative format by each outcome variable using the subheadings: *baseline data, QOL, anxiety and depression, health care utilization and exacerbations, satisfaction*, and *cost-effectiveness*. There are six tables that summarize baseline and follow-up data. However, because the researchers only compare the mean differences in scores between the groups and not the change in a group from baseline, it is difficult to interpret the results.

In addition, it is unclear whether lower QOL scores, including symptoms, activity, and impact subscores, indicate poorer health, and whether higher scores mean a higher level of QOL, as one would expect. Typically, a reader would expect a lower level of a score to indicate a lower level of the construct being measured. Presenting study findings in the opposite format makes interpretation difficult and can be especially confusing for a novice reader of research as it is counterintuitive.

The anxiety or depression scores were also difficult to interpret. The authors wrote that the HADS depression scores at follow-up were improved with telemonitoring, compared to usual care (6.87 vs. 7.50). But the baseline HADS depression score was 6.8 for the telemonitoring group, and 7.9 for the usual care group, indicating that depression scores remained almost the same for both groups.

Are all outcome variables addressed, if applicable?

All outcome variables of interest are addressed in both the text and in tables.

Are results clearly presented in text and/or tables/figures?

The authors use a variety of tables to display demographic characteristics and results related to the outcome variables.

Is significance of results reported, if applicable?

Significant study findings are presented but without comparing each group's change from the respective baseline it is difficult to interpret the results.

DISCUSSION OF RESULTS

Do the authors link the findings to previous research studies?

The authors placed their findings in the context of a previous study of home-based care with monitoring and a systematic review of pulmonary rehabilitation that supported improvements in patients' QOL. However, these findings differ from two more recent RCTs that did not significantly impact QOL with the use of telemonitoring. The authors conclude that their intervention was likely more successful in reducing anxiety and improving QOL because it included more frequent reassurance calls from the telehealth nurse and more frequent contacts with the pulmonary specialists than recent studies. They note that this clinical trial was performed during a particularly severe winter that prevented patients from leaving their homes. They suggest that the additional reassurance and support were helpful in reducing patient anxiety and improving confidence.

Are the conclusions comprehensive, yet within the data?

The discussion of study findings is comprehensive but the authors' conclusions, although interesting, may be going beyond the data, as the purpose of the study was not to test the effectiveness of nursing reassurance and patient empowerment. More frequent visits with the specialists did not result in lower hospitalization utilization, and as a result the intervention was not found to be cost-effective, consistent with findings from several other RCTs of this nature.

Do the authors interpret the results in the discussion?

The authors interpret study findings in the interpretation section of the article.

Are the findings generalizable or transferable?

There is no explicit discussion of the generalizability of study findings.

LIMITATIONS
Identified? Accurate? Inclusive?

The researchers state that the main limitations of the study are the lack of blinding to treatment conditions, the limited generalizability to other populations of COPD patients, and the inability to conduct follow-up assessment of QOL, anxiety, and depression after telemonitoring ended. It is not clear why the authors listed the lack of follow-up as a limitation, as this was not conducted as a longitudinal study beyond 6 months. The first two limitations are accurate in that the data collectors and treating physicians were not blinded to assignment to intervention or control groups. Thus, this could have introduced the threat to internal validity of *compensatory rivalry of the no-treatment group*. The threat to external validity is the limited generalizability, in that these findings may not be extended to patients beyond Northern Ireland or to countries without universal health care.

IMPLICATIONS
Are there implications for practice, education, research?
Are there implications for clinical significance?

The authors did not outline specific implications for clinical practice or education, given the lack of cost-effectiveness. However, there may be some implications for future research studies in this area. Considering the key role of the telehealth nurse and the need for an underlying conceptual framework, future studies should investigate the role of the nurse in promoting patient self-efficacy and patient self-management of COPD at home.

RECOMMENDATIONS
Recommendations for future study/study replication?

The only recommendation is to conduct a longer study in the future that is powered to be able to more carefully analyze health care utilization trends and determine whether QOL is associated with changes in hospital usage.

CONCLUSION
Is it succinct and does it tie everything together?

The conclusion is stated concisely in the last sentence and tie together all of the components of the study. The telemonitoring intervention is successful in improving QOL and reducing anxiety, but is not cost-effective.

USING TEXT REMINDER TO IMPROVE CHILDHOOD IMMUNIZATION ADHERENCE IN THE PHILIPPINES

5

Mary Joy Garcia-Dia, DNP, MA, RN
New York University Rory Meyers College of Nursing and Nursing
Informatics Center for Professional Nursing Practice
New York–Presbyterian Hospital
New York, New York

Joyce J. Fitzpatrick, PhD, MBA, RN, FAAN
Frances Payne Bolton School of Nursing
Case Western Reserve University
Cleveland, Ohio

Elizabeth A. Madigan, PhD, RN, FAAN
Frances Payne Bolton School of Nursing
Case Western Reserve University
Cleveland, Ohio

John W. Peabody, MD, PhD, FACP
QURE Healthcare and University of California
San Francisco
and University of California
Los Angeles, California

ABSTRACT

A comparative descriptive study was conducted to determine the effectiveness of text messages with pictures compared with plain text messages or verbal reminders in improving measles, mumps, and rubella (MMR) immunization compliance in the rural areas of the Philippines. We found that text messaging with or without pictures is a feasible and useful tool in MMR immunization compliance for childhood immunization. Texting with pictures ($n = 23$), however, was no more effective than plain text messaging ($n = 19$) or verbal reminder ($n = 17$) in improving MMR immunization compliance. Compared with parents who received verbal reminders alone, either type of text reminders was linked to parents bringing their child for MMR immunization on a timelier basis, as defined by the difference between the scheduled visit (SV) and the actual visit,

Garcia-Dia, M. J., Fitzpatrick, J. J., Madigan, E. A., & Peabody, J. W. (2017). Using text reminder to improve childhood immunization adherence in the Philippines. *CIN: Computers, Informatics, Nursing*, *35*(4), 212–218. Retrieved from http://journals.lww.com/cinjournal/Abstract/2017/04000/Using_Text_Reminder_to_Improve_Childhood.7.aspx although this was not statistically significant. Mobile technology that uses text reminders for immunization can potentially improve the communication process between parent, the public health nurse, and health care provider. Future studies can explore the application of plain text messages or text messages with pictures to improve compliance more broadly for maternal and child health care especially in rural areas of developing countries and may be a helpful tool for health promotion for this population.

KEY WORDS: global health, immunization, mobile technology, public health, text messaging

Between 2013 and 2014, the Centers for Disease Control determined that measles outbreaks in the United States primarily originated in other countries (Philippines, Turkey, Vietnam, Italy, Germany, and the Netherlands) infecting unimmunized populations or individuals whose immunizations were not up-to-date.[1,2] In 2015, measles, mumps, rubella (MMR) started to fall below the 95% target needed for herd immunity, which is cause for alarm.[3]

The attitude and acceptance of parents, both in developing countries and wealthier nations, are the single biggest limiting factor with vaccine deployment.[4-6] The majority of parents view MMR as benign and are unaware that these diseases often lead to long-term sequelae and can kill 1% to 5% of infected individuals.[7] This health literacy gap points to a fundamental need for more effective communication between parents and public health officials.

The criticality of adhering strictly to scheduled immunization may not be fully understood by parents at the time of their consultation because of low health literacy and language barriers. These communication barriers can lead to immunization delays, undervaccination, and missed vaccination.[8] Other barriers include socioeconomic status, inadequate access, time constraints, high out-of-pocket cost and low reimbursements for vaccine administration, misconceptions of parents about the severity of vaccine-preventable diseases, current safety of vaccines, and fragility of vaccine supply.[9] Nurses could, however, work with parents in achieving their child's full health potential by implementing mobile technology and utilizing text messaging in promoting timely vaccination.

SIGNIFICANCE

Research studies done in the United States have demonstrated parents' acceptance of using text message reminders for communicating appointments.[10-12] Compared with other technology or application, mobile phones require minimal infrastructure setup particularly in developing countries. Parents worldwide can quickly learn how to receive and send text messages with the phone's simple function and intuitive navigation. According to the International Telecommunications Union in 2010, there were 5 billion wireless subscribers, with 90% having access to mobile networks, 80% of which are in rural areas, with 4.2 trillion text messages sent.[13] More recently, providers or clinicians have the option to combine text message with pictures potentially further facilitating their communication with the parents.[14]

In developing countries, appointment reminders for immunization could potentially leverage widespread cell phone coverage to increase compliance with vaccine visits. Among developing countries, the Philippines, with a population of 101,696,333 (2016), has 100 million mobile subscribers and 2 billion texts sent daily.[15,16] The Philippines might be an ideal country to use text messaging to increase immunization compliance, particularly in rural areas where health literacy remains low, poverty and lower education are problematic, and community health workers conduct house calls to remind parents of immunization visits.[17] The combination of health communication and text messaging, including the possibility of augmenting them with pictures, could stimulate a meaningful response to declining and delayed immunizations.[18]

MATERIALS AND METHODS
Design and Research Questions

The study is a comparative descriptive analysis of two intervention groups (plain text message and text message with pictures) and a control group (verbal reminder/usual care) to determine if these interventions are more effective than verbal reminders in improving the parents' adherence to immunization schedules and/or the timeliness of bringing the child for immunization. The research questions were as follows:

1. Is text messaging with or without pictures superior to verbal reminders (usual care) in improving MMR adherence?

2. Will text messaging result in more timely immunization compared with usual care?

3. Is text messaging with pictures superior to plain text message alone in improving MMR adherence?

4. Are parents more satisfied in receiving text message with pictures compared with plain text message alone?

Operational Definition

Research Questions 1, 2, and 3: To determine which intervention is superior, the study used immunization and the timeliness of the immunization as its dependent variable. Timeliness of vaccine administration is determined by the difference in the number of days between scheduled date of appointment visit and actual date of visit that the child was brought in for immunization.

Research Question 4: Parents' satisfaction in receiving immunization reminders is evaluated through a Usability Questionnaire with a 5-point Likert scale.

PROCEDURE

Of the seven recommended vaccines that children need to receive before the age of 2 years, MMR was selected as the focus of the study. As per the World Health Organization (WHO)[19] recommendations (2009), children should have one dose of MMR between 12 and 15 months of age. The Philippines had implemented WHO's recommendation through the Expanded Program on Immunization. Specifically, in the municipality of Bago City, Lag-Asan, and Poblacion, barangay health teams conduct house visits to remind parents of their child's MMR immunization schedule. Despite this program, from 2013 to 2014, of the 5,281 children scheduled for MMR immunization, only 3,352 children completed their MMR shots. Thus, there was an opportunity to increase adherence and send timely reminders with MMR shots through text messaging. To comply with institutional review board (IRB) requirements, a letter of intent was submitted to the office of the mayor, and a letter of cooperation was obtained from the chief health officer in charge of the Bago City health center. Locally, the University of the Philippines School of Economics' IRB approved the research study in addition to Case Western Reserve University's IRB approval.

Inclusion criteria were parents with a minimum of sixth-grade education and with a child (or children) between the ages 12 and 24 months needing MMR immunization. Parents who had children who missed their MMR vaccination after 15 months of age were excluded. A chart review was then conducted at the community health center to determine eligibility for the study based on the inclusion/exclusion criteria. A convenience sample size of 75 parents was obtained based on an expression of interest during a recruitment session. After obtaining written, informed consent and providing HIPAA [Health Insurance Portability and Accountability Act notification forms (both of which were translated in Tagalog), participants were asked to pick a number randomly from a box. Parents who had an odd number were assigned to plain text message only, and those who have an even number were assigned to text message with pictures. From the chart review, the control group was randomly selected based on children who had MMR immunization due from December 2014 to February 2015. All participants were requested to fill out the sociodemographic questionnaire.

Operationally, the researcher explained the study's purpose, duration (3 months), and the rules in using the mobile phone (for research purpose and not for personal use). As part of the study, a prepaid phone card and a GSM (global system for mobiles) cell phone (Torque DTV5, Torque Mobile, The Philippines) capable of receiving text messages with pictures were then provided to minimize any participation or functional biases. The local PHN sent a text reminder once 7 to 10 days prior to the scheduled appointment date. The text message sent to the parents in their local dialect was direct and purposely simple: "Bago City Health Clinic: Palihug dala kay (ngalan sang bata) para sa iya MMR sa (petsa)" (English translation: Bago City Health Clinic: Please bring [name of child] for MMR on [date]"). After the message was received, participants were requested to acknowledge receipt of message by return text. After their child's vaccination, parents were requested to fill out the usability (satisfaction) questionnaire. Participants who brought their child past the scheduled appointment date were asked to fill out the reason for delay questionnaire. The participation rate was 100% for the two intervention groups at the end of the study.

INSTRUMENTS

We performed a manual chart review of paper medical records to collect data on the date of the immunization visit and as a guide on when to send the immunization reminders to the two interventions and the control groups. The scheduled immunization date was compared against the actual date of when the participant brought his/her child for vaccination to determine adherence. A survey questionnaire was distributed to determine participants' level of satisfaction with receiving/sending text messages.[20] Higher scores indicated greater satisfaction and agreement in using text messaging for immunization reminders, with 5 indicating highest score (strongly agree) and 1 indicating lowest score (strongly disagree). Parents who brought their child after the scheduled date for immunization were requested to fill out an additional survey to determine reasons for the delay, which were categorized into the following:

1. Environmental reasons: work schedule conflict, no transportation money, child was sick, no babysitter for other children, distance and time to travel, other reasons ("I forgot")

2. Technological reasons: low battery, no charge, electrical outage, low coverage (low bar), and broken phone, other reasons

DATA ANALYSIS

All data collected were entered into a statistical software package, IBM SPSS Statistics version 20 (IBM, Armonk, NY) and reviewed for consistency. We performed frequency distributions to describe the percentage of responses of each of the demographic questions (age, educational level, number of children). To account for the small sample size and the nonnormal distribution of the data, we used three nonparametric tests: Mann–Whitney U test and Wilcoxon rank sum test for two independent variables to compare the sums of the rankings of the intervention group and Kruskal–Wallis H test to determine if a difference exists in the distribution of values between the intervention and control groups.

RESULTS
Sample Characteristics

All of the parent participants were female; the average age was 30.4 years. They were predominately high school graduates (68%), with the rest either college graduates (16%), had some level of college (10.7%), or elementary graduates (5.3%). The mean number of children per family was 2.4; 45.3% of the participants had one child, 28% had two children, 12% had three children, 9.3% had four children, and 5.4% had 5 to 6 children. Per the inclusion criteria, the participants' children ranged in age from 12 to 14 months (December 2013–February 2014).

Descriptive Statistics

To determine whether text messaging in Groups 1 and 2 was superior to the control group who received only verbal reminder during the home visit for their MMR immunization rates (Research Questions 1 and 2), we performed a Kruskal–Wallis test. We found that there was no significant difference in the groups ($H_2 = 5.316$, $p > .05$, with 2 degrees of freedom), indicating that the immunization rates did not differ significantly from each other (Figure 1).

When we compared timelines among the three groups, we found that text message reminders for MMR immunization were timelier in either text (i.e., the intervention) groups compared with the verbal reminders. We noted that 20% of parents from the control group brought their child back for MMR after 90 days compared with 4% from the text group (19 days). However, the result showed no statistical difference ($H2 = 5.262$, $p > .05$) (Figure 2). Based on the difference (average number of days), Group 1 parents (plain text) brought their child within 1 (0.96) day, and Group 2

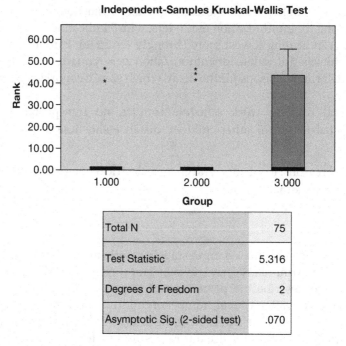

Independent-Samples Kruskal-Wallis Test

Total N	75
Test Statistic	5.316
Degrees of Freedom	2
Asymptotic Sig. (2-sided test)	.070

1.The test statistic is adjusted for ties.
2.Multiple comparisons are not performed because the overall test does not show significant differences across samples.

FIGURE 1. Parents' rank based on their adherence to the scheduled immunization visit: intervention and control groups.

parents (text with pictures) within 2 to 3 (2.72) days, whereas the Group 3 parents (verbal reminders) brought their child 20 to 21 (20.64) days later.

We examined whether text with pictures was superior to text message alone (Research Question 3) using the Mann–Whitney U test. The ranking result showed no significant difference ($U = 363, p > .05$). Using the actual visit date, we determined whether the parents' adherence to the scheduled date in bringing their child for immunization among those parents who received text message alone (mean rank of 23.48) differed from that of parents who received text message with pictures (mean rank of 27.52). Using the Wilcoxon rank sum test, we observed that there was no significant difference in the results of the rank ($W = 0.980, p > .05; Z = -0.025$) (Table 1).

We compared the difference in the number of days between the scheduled visit and the actual visit that the parents brought the child for immunization (Table 2). We found no significant difference in timeliness between the intervention groups.

The Usability Questionnaire (user satisfaction survey) was used to determine the parents' satisfaction in using text messaging (Research Question 4). Group 1 parents (plain text) were 92% ($n = 23$) satisfied with the study using text message, whereas 8% ($n = 2$) responded neutrally. Group 2 (text with pictures) were 96% ($n = 24$) satisfied, with only 4% ($n = 1$) not satisfied. Parents who received and read plain text messages 100% agreed that it was easy. For Group 2, 80% of the parents who received and read text message with pictures agreed that it was easy, whereas 20% disagreed. When asked if it was easy to send text messages, 100% of the parents from Group 1 agreed.

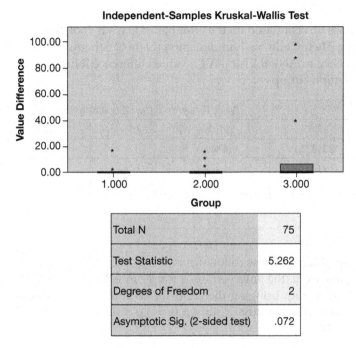

Independent-Samples Kruskal-Wallis Test

Total N	75
Test Statistic	5.262
Degrees of Freedom	2
Asymptotic Sig. (2-sided test)	.072

1.The test statistic is adjusted for ties.
2.Multiple comparisons are not performed because the overall test does not show significant differences across samples.

FIGURE 2. Timelines of visit based on the number of days it took for the parents to bring their child for immunization (date of scheduled visit [SV] minus date of actual visit [AV] = value difference [number of days]): intervention and control groups.

Eighty percent of Group 2 parents agreed that it was easy to send text messages, 8% ($n = 2$) disagreed, and 12% ($n = 3$) neutrally responded. Further analysis using Kruskal–Wallis test showed no significant difference in the satisfaction between the uses of text alone compared with text with pictures ($H_2 = 0.192, p > .05$), indicating that the groups did not differ significantly from each other with their level of satisfaction in using text messaging for immunization reminders.

TABLE 1. Parents' Ranks Based on Their Adherence With the Scheduled Immunization Visit: Intervention Groups

	Rank				
Group	1	42	43	46	48
1 (Text $n = 25$)	23 (92%)	1 (4%)			1 (4%)
2 (Text with picture $n = 25$)	19 (76%)		3 (12%)	2 (8%)	1 (4%)
Total	42	1	3	2	2

TABLE 2. Timelines of Visit Based on the Number of Days It Took for the Parents to Bring Their Child for Immunization (Date of Scheduled Visit [SV] Minus Date of Actual Visit [AV] = Value Difference [Number of Days]): Intervention Groups

Group	Value Difference in Days (Scheduled Visit)				
	0d	5d	7d	14d	19d
1 (Text n = 25)	23 (92%)	1 (4%)			1 (4%)
2 (Text with picture n = 25)	19 (76%)		3 (12%)	2 (8%)	1 (4%)
Total	42	1	3	2	2

For those children whose follow-up visit was delayed, the survey results showed seven parents from the intervention groups mostly cited environmental factors prevented them from bringing the child for immunization: work schedule conflict ($n = 1$), no babysitter for other children ($n = 1$), child was sick ($n = 3$), and other ("I forgot") ($n = 2$).

DISCUSSION

This study is one of the first to evaluate the effectiveness of plain text messages compared with text messages with pictures in determining adherence rates and timeliness to the immunization schedule for MMR. We found that text messaging was well received, but that there was no marginal benefit from adding pictures to the text messages. We also found that the texting intervention groups were satisfied in using text messages for immunization reminders, and the intervention suggests easy adoption of mobile technology with no training required.

We wondered why there was no marginal benefit from texting with pictures versus plain texting and did a post–data collection interview. Public health nurses found that text with picture took longer to upload. Parents provided the same feedback describing instances when the picture never fully loaded. It is possible that there may be a marginal benefit of adding pictures, but we were unable to observe this because of these technical problems related to the time uploading or downloading pictures. Pictures are aimed at those challenged with literacy and low education. However, our study population was well educated, with as many as 27% of the population having a college education, and all but four in 20 had graduated from high school, mitigating some advantages pictures were expected to confer.

A study by Ahlers-Schmidt et al.[21] utilized a user-centered design to evaluate participants' level of comprehension in receiving and replying to a text message sent to their personal phone. The participants ranked the text messages based on how critical the information was and their intention to act on it. The outcome of the study showed that short, specific text content could result in higher comprehension, making it likely parents would schedule their child for immunization.

A study in Kenya, using text reminders, evaluated whether SMS reminders improved diphtheria, pertussis (whooping cough), and tetanus (DPT) vaccine compliance when done along with cash incentive to parents of children who required immunizations[22] This study showed that it is feasible to set up an integrated mobile phone-based system to both remind and incentivize parents to immunize their children.

LIMITATIONS

The sample size was relatively small masking statistical differences, for example, in the timeliness of immunizations. We also did not extend the follow-up for more than 3 months. Thus, while directionally positive text messaging appeared to increase immunization rates and timeliness, the small sample size likely left the study underpowered. This study used a convenience sample and a nonrandom cohort for the control group, limiting the causal inferences that could be made. The study focused only on MMR vaccine schedule and did not include other vaccines such as DPT, where multiple doses of vaccine (three doses) need to be administered within a tighter timeframe (0–6 months of age). The investigator-supplied phones may not reflect the use of text-capable phones that are privately owned or afforded. The study was limited by technical challenges that appear to have impacted the ability to transmit or download the pictures uncovered after data collection. Lastly, we did not address the question of affordability or the incentives of purchasing the phone and the cost of cellular connectivity. Notwithstanding, this study shows that familiarity with cell phones is widespread even in the poorest settings.

RECOMMENDATIONS

The use of text reminders is already well suited for urban communities and, with appropriate infrastructure, could be implemented in rural areas in developing countries. Government agencies can partner with nonprofit organizations and mobile companies to expand telecommunication coverage and provision of cellular phones to health centers as an auxiliary to standard practice. Expanding the use of text messaging in rural areas may help local health centers streamline the immunization process and set up an automated, safer workflow for community health workers. This could potentially eliminate weekly house visits and long travel hours. If effective, texting holds the promise of saving time and money versus a traditional home visit, although this needs to be verified in future studies.

The use of cell phones has become a primary tool for personal communication in developing countries. The idea of extending a cell phone's function beyond personal and business use in managing one's health does not require additional training and can easily be adopted. However, targeted parents who receive specific health alerts or reminders can potentially ignore the message and fail to respond or act on it. Evaluating parental or individual response over time due to financial constraints or potential reminder fatigue will help researchers find the appropriate balance in sending text reminders based on content, criticality, and frequency.

CONCLUSION

As countries around the world shift its goals from Millennium Development Goal 4: Reducing Childhood Mortality to Sustainable Development Goal 3: Good Health and Well-Being, the underlying challenges of immunization programs with lack of coverage, missed vaccination, undervaccination, and delayed visits leading to catch-up vaccine schedules continue to exist particularly in Europe and Asia.[23,24] This study showed that text messaging by itself can reduce immunization delays and improve parents' adherence to scheduled visits compared with traditional reminders. The use of mobile technology as an intervention through text reminders can likely increase satisfaction and improve the communication process between patients and health care providers particularly in rural and geographically disadvantaged population. Local government can partner with health agencies by providing funds, incentive mechanisms, and policies to decrease health disparities and digital divide in areas with inadequate network and telecommunication infrastructure. Future studies can explore the application of plain text messages or text messages with pictures to improve compliance for maternal and child health care especially in rural areas of developing countries and may be a helpful tool for health promotion for this population.

ACKNOWLEDGMENTS

The authors thank Dr. Ferdinand Ramon Mayoga and Stella Marie Celis, RN, PHN from Bago City Health Center, and Dr. Ramon Clarete from the University of the Philippines for their collaboration and support during the research implementation.

REFERENCES

1. Center for Disease Control and Prevention. National state and local area vaccination coverage among children aged 19–35 months—United States, 2012. *Morb Mortal Wkly Rep* 2013;62: 36.
2. Centers for Disease Control and Prevention. *Measles Cases and Outbreaks.* 2015. http://www.cdc.gov/measles/cases-outbreaks.html. Accessed October 1, 2015.
3. Parry L. Number of children given MMR jab falls for the first time in seven years and coverage is lowest in London. Daily Mail, 2015. http://www.dailymail.co.uk/health/article-3246062/Number-children-given-MMR-jabFALLS-time-seven-years-coverage-lowest-London.html. Accessed February 21, 2016.
4. Opel DJ, Manglone-Smith R, Taylor JA, et al. Development of a survey to identify vaccine-hesitant parents: the parent attitudes about childhood vaccines survey. *Hum Vaccines.* 2011;7: 419–425.
5. Luthy KE, Beckstrand RL, Peterson NE. Parental hesitation as a factor in delayed child immunization. *J Pediatr Care.* 2009;26: 388–394.
6. Center for Disease Control and Prevention. *Immunization Strategies for Healthcare Practices and Providers.* 2015. https://www.cdc.gov/vaccines/pubs/pinkbook/downloads/strat.pdf. Accessed July 14, 2016.
7. Harris KM, Hughbanks-Wheaton DK, Johnson R, et al. Parental refusal or delay of childhood immunization: implications for nursing and health education. *Teach Learn Nurs.* 2007;2: 127–132.
8. Guerra FA. Delayed immunization has potentially serious health consequences. *Pediatr Drugs.* 2007;9: 143–148.
9. Gardner P, Pickering LK, Orenstein WA, et al. Guidelines for quality standards for immunization. *Clin Infect Dis.* 2002;35: 503–511.
10. Peck JL, Stanton M, Reynolds GES. Smartphone preventive health care: parental use of an immunization reminder system. *J Pediatr Health Care.* 2014;28: 35–42.
11. Stockwell MS, Kharbanda EO, Martinez EA, et al. Text 4 Health: impact of text message reminder-recalls for pediatric and adolescent immunizations. *Am J Public Health.* 2012;102: 15–21.
12. Vann J, Szilagyi P. Patient reminder and recall systems to improve immunization rates [review]. *Cochrane Collab.* 2009;1: 1–69.
13. International Communication Union. *ITU Sees 5 Billion Subscriptions Globally in 2010 Online.* 2010. http://www.itu.int/newsroom/press_releases/2010/06.html. Accessed June 1, 2014.
14. Leroy G, Endicott JE, Kauchak D, et al. User evaluation of the effects of a text simplification algorithm using term familiarity on perception, understanding, learning, and information retention. *J Med Internet Res.* 2013;15: 144.

15. Philippines—mobile communications, forecast, broadcasting market: Synopsis. 2015. http://www.budde.com.au/Research/Philippines-MobileCommunications-Forecasts-and-Broadcasting-Market.html. Accessed March 12, 2015.

16. Philippines population (live). 2016. http://www.worldometers.info/worldpopulation/philippines-population/. Accessed February 21, 2016.

17. UNICEF. At a glance: Philippines. 2013. http://www.unicef.org/infobycountry/philippines_statistics.html. Accessed December 22, 2015.

18. Kheir N, Awaisu A, Radoui A, et al. Development and evaluation of pictograms on medication labels for patients with limited literacy skills in a culturally diverse multiethnic population. *Res Soc Admin Pharm.* 2014;10: 720–730.

19. World Health Organization. *The Coverage Estimates and Estimation of Number of Children Vaccinated or Not Vaccinated: WHO/UNICEF Coverage Estimates 2012 Revision.* 2013. http://apps.who.int/immunization_monitoring/globalsummary/timeseries/tswucoveragebcg.html. Accessed June 1, 2014.

20. Dick JJ, Nundy S, Solomon MC, et al. Feasibility and usability of a text message-based program for diabetes self-management in an urban African-American population. *J Diabetes Sci Technol.* 2011;5: 1246–1254.

21. Ahlers-Schmidt CR, Hart T, Chesser A, et al. Using human factors techniques to design text message reminders for childhood immunization. *Health Educ Behav.* 2012;3: 538–543.

22. Wakadha H, Chandir S, Were EJ, et al. The feasibility of using mobile-phone based SMS reminders and conditional cash transfers to improve timely immunization in rural Kenya. *Vaccine.* 2012;31: 987–993.

23. World Health Organization. *State of the World's Vaccines and Immunization.* 2009. http://www.unicef.org/media/files/SOWVI_full_report_english_LR1.pdf. Accessed June 1, 2014.

24. The Millennium Development Goals Report. 2014. http://www.un.org/millenniumgoals/2014%20MDG%20report/MDG%202014%20English%20web.pdf. Accessed June 1, 2014.

USING TEXT REMINDER TO IMPROVE CHILDHOOD IMMUNIZATION ADHERENCE IN THE PHILIPPINES

Critique by *Margaret A. Harris and Karen Bauce*

OVERALL SUMMARY

The use of mobile technology to improve adherence to timely childhood immunization for measles, mumps, and rubella (MMR) in rural areas of the Philippines is described in this quantitative study that compares the effectiveness of two different types of text reminders. The authors used a combination of manual chart review and questionnaire to obtain data from parent participants, and the results are well described. Although the study findings were not statistically significant, the authors suggest that the global popularity of cell phones can be leveraged for health promotion in rural areas of developing countries. This research study may be particularly relevant to nurses with an interest in global health promotion and the strategic application of mobile technology.

TITLE

Does the title include the key concepts/variables/phenomenon of interest?

The title includes the key concepts of the study but refers generally to childhood immunization adherence rather than specifying adherence and timeliness of MMR immunization.

Is it concise (12 words or less) and professionally stated?

Simultaneously, it is concise and comprehensive.

RESEARCHER(S) CREDIBILITY

Educational credentials?

All four authors have doctoral preparation (DNP, PhD, and MD).

Prior methodological research experience of the authors (i.e., methodological expertise)?

An Internet search indicates that each author has significant methodological experience in conducting quantitative research, including intervention studies.

Subject matter content expertise (prior research on the subject matter)?

The same Internet search revealed that all four authors have published extensively in areas such as community/home health care, health care systems, child health outcomes, and global health policy. Dr. Peabody has also conducted other research in the Philippines. Collectively, these authors have diverse expertise in areas essential for this research study.

ABSTRACT
Does it include the key components (objective/aim, background/rationale, methods, results, and conclusion)?

The journal's author guidelines pertaining to the abstract are generic and require only a summary of the major issue, problem, or topic as well as study findings and conclusions. The major issue or problem is not described. The abstract begins with the design of the study and moves directly into results. The abstract finishes with a conclusion and directions for future research.

Does or does not include references?

Appropriately, the abstract does not include citations.

Is it concise (150–250 words or less)?

The abstract is concisely written and within the recommended word count.

Does it entice you to read the rest of the article (interesting)?

Although the abstract describes statistically insignificant results, readers with a strong interest in the use of mobile technology to promote health would be compelled to read the rest of the article.

INTRODUCTION/PROBLEM
Is the research problem or phenomenon of interest clearly stated?

The introduction explains the trends of lower thresholds of herd immunity and dangers of the current trajectories of under-immunization for MMR, especially in six specified countries. One of these six countries is the Philippines, where the study is conducted. The introduction also cites parents' attitudes toward immunizations and communication as barriers to achieving proper immunization levels.

Is it succinct?

The problem of underimmunization is succinctly described in the introduction.

Does it answer the "so what" question?

The adverse health implications of nonadherence to scheduled MMR immunization are clearly described.

RESEARCH AIMS/OBJECTIVES
Is the research aim/objective clearly stated?

The research objective is clearly stated as determining the effectiveness of two interventions versus a control group in improving parental adherence to vaccination schedules and/or timeliness of vaccination.

Is it concisely written?

The research objective is written concisely.

Does it follow logically from the research problem/phenomenon of interest?

The research objective follows logically from the previously identified problem of MMR under vaccination.

SIGNIFICANCE

Is the significance to nursing and health care clearly written?

This section focused on international telecommunications and mobile networks with specific information regarding mobile subscribers and text usage in the Philippines. This provides the rationale for how the text-messaging project could be effective in this country. Although city-specific rates of MMR immunization are reported later in the Procedures section, immunization rates for the Philippines should be included as part of the significance of the issue. If included, this section would clearly address both the need and feasibility for the study and provide a rationale for conducting the study in the Philippines.

Does the significance follow from the research aim/objective?

The significance of improving declining and delayed MMR immunizations follows logically from the research aim.

BACKGROUND

Is there an explicit description of a theoretical perspective or conceptual framework? If not, it is implicit?

There is no mention of a theoretical perspective or a conceptual framework.

Are there clear theoretical/conceptual definitions of the concepts?

The only definitions provided are operational definitions for timeliness of vaccine administration and parents' satisfaction in the Materials and Methods section.

LITERATURE REVIEW

Primary sources only?

There is no systematic review of relevant literature presented, only a reference to previous research conducted in the United States demonstrating parents' acceptance of using text message reminders for communicating appointments. The previous research cited appears to be from primary sources, based on a cursory review of the reference list.

Current (within the past how many years)?

Information cited in the introduction regarding global immunization rates and telecommunication information cited in the Significance section were all within 7 years of publication.

Is the search strategy included?

A search strategy was not included.

Is literature relevant to the research aims/objectives?

The limited information presented is relevant to the research aim but does not provide the reader with any understanding of how text messaging for health reminders has been implemented in other studies.

Is it chronologically presented (old to current)?

The generic reference to previous studies is not presented chronologically.

Is it comprehensive? If not, is sufficient background literature provided?

The literature review would benefit from substantially more information on text messaging for health reminders. If previous research studies are so limited, the authors should state that.

RATIONALE FOR THE STUDY
Is there a gap in the literature that this study will fill (would it extend prior knowledge)? Is the rationale clearly stated?

> This report does not provide a compelling case derived from literature to support the "need" for the research project or the "gap" in knowledge in this area.

Is this a follow-up or replication study?

> This appears to be an original study as replication is not mentioned.

RESEARCH QUESTION(S) AND/OR HYPOTHESES
Are these explicitly and clearly stated?

> The four research questions are clearly stated under Design and Research Questions.

Do they include the variables/phenomenon of interest?

> The variables of interest, immunization, and timeliness of immunization, are included in the research questions.

Do they follow from the research aim/objectives?

> The research questions flow logically from the research aim of determining the effectiveness of interventions to improve immunization and timeliness of immunization.

METHODS
Research Design/Paradigm
Is the research design clearly stated?

> The design is described in the Materials and Methods section as a comparative descriptive analysis of two intervention groups.

Is there consistency between the research design and paradigm?

> There is consistency between the use of the research design to determine the comparative efficacy of two different interventions and the positivist view of an objective reality that can be known through collection and analysis of quantifiable data.

Is this the best choice of design to address the research problem/phenomenon of interest?

> Considering the limited knowledge of the effectiveness of text reminders for childhood immunizations, this is an appropriate design.

Is there rigor in the design?

> There is rigor in the research design in its use of two different interventions and a control group.

SETTING
Is the setting clearly described?

> The study setting for receiving text reminders was the natural environment of the participants residing within Bago City. In addition, parent participants completed study questionnaires or surveys in the Bago City Health Clinic, where their children were brought for their vaccine.

What biases are introduced as a result of selecting this particular setting?

> The potential effects of the variability of the participants' natural environment are unknown and not addressed by the authors. The authors do not mention what time

of day the texts were sent, only that the public health nurse sent one reminder. The time and circumstances under which parents received the messages could greatly influence the effectiveness of the reminders. In addition, it is unknown whether parents were able to complete study questionnaires at the health clinic in privacy, which may introduce an element of bias in their responses.

SAMPLING PLAN AND SAMPLE
Is the sampling plan clearly identified?

The authors used a nonprobability convenience sampling plan, enrolling 75 parents based on their expressed interest during a recruitment session at the health center. The authors report that the control group was randomly selected from chart review but should specify that a sample of 25 was used for each of the three groups. There is also some confusion created with the inclusion and exclusion criteria. Inclusion criteria consist of parents with a minimum of sixth-grade education with a child between the ages of 12 and 24 months who needs an MMR vaccine. The only exclusion criterion is parents who missed their child's MMR vaccination after 15 months of age. The wide age range of the inclusion criteria does not fit with the exclusion criterion. If parents did not have their child vaccinated by 15 months of age with the MMR, they would not be eligible for the study. Why include parents of children aged 15 to 24 months who still need an MMR?

Does it represent the population of interest?

The population of interest was parents of a child or children within a specified age-range requiring MMR vaccination, yet the study sample consisted of only females, presumably the mothers. It is not clear from the text's use of "parents" if the inclusion of fathers was also desired.

Is the sampling plan consistent with the research aim/objective?

The convenience sampling plan is consistent with the research objective and specifically addresses the four research questions.

Is the sample size sufficient (e.g., power analysis or data saturation)?

There is no power analysis so it is unknown whether the sample size is sufficient to detect statistically significant differences among groups.

VARIABLES
Are variables clearly identified?

The outcome variables of interest are clearly identified in the research questions: immunization, timeliness of the immunization, and satisfaction with text reminders for immunization.

Are variables operationally defined and consistent with theoretical concepts?

In the Instruments section, the authors describe how timeliness of MMR immunization, cause of lateness to an immunization appointment, and parents' satisfaction with receiving text massages for immunization reminders were measured. Adherence to the scheduled immunization visit was measured but is not described, leaving the reader to assume it is a dichotomous variable. Because a theoretical framework is not mentioned, there is no consistency with theoretical concepts to consider.

Are independent and dependent variables identified, if applicable?

In the section Operational Definition, the authors identify dependent variables as immunization, timeliness of the immunization, and parent satisfaction in receiving text reminders for immunization. The independent variable is not explicitly identified but is easily understood to be text messaging.

METHOD OF DATA COLLECTION

What are the methods of data collection?

Immunization status and timeliness of immunization were determined by chart review. Demographic information, parent satisfaction, and reason for delay in vaccination were all collected via survey. Reason for delay of immunization and demographic surveys appears to be investigator-developed as there is no reference to previous studies. Parent satisfaction was measured with a usability questionnaire for which little information is provided. The authors provide a citation that leads the reader to believe that this is the same satisfaction questionnaire used in a previous study regarding text-message feasibility for diabetic self-management; without reading the original article it cannot be determined whether the two are equivalent.

Are validity and reliability clearly addressed for prior research and current study, if applicable?

No reliability or validity is mentioned for the Usability Questionnaire and the number and nature of items are not reported. The appropriate implementation of this scale is indeterminable with the information provided.

Do the measures/instruments address the underlying theoretical concepts or phenomenon of interest?

Aside from the usability scale, all other measures directly address the variables of interest.

Were human rights protected?

Human subjects' protection is fully addressed. Permission was granted from the mayor of the city as well as the chief officer of the health center. Appropriate institutional review board approvals were obtained.

Are other ethical issues identified?

The authors do not indicate whether the demographic questionnaire or the satisfaction and reasons for delay of immunization surveys were anonymous or contained personal identifying information.

Is the data-collection method appropriate for research design?

Data collected were indeed descriptive in nature and provided for comparison between two groups. This is consistent with the stated research design.

Is there bias in data collection?

A certain level of bias is presumed to exist in all data collection. In this study it is indeterminable whether explicit bias occurred in data collection because of the lack of information regarding the time of day that text-message reminders were sent.

What is the fidelity of intervention addressed, if applicable?

To enhance the fidelity of the intervention, cell phones with prepaid phone cards were provided to all parent participants. Text messages were sent in the parent participant's local language and dialect. Although the phones were indicated for text messaging with images, post-hoc data revealed that technology issues occurred with downloading text messages with pictures for some parent participants.

DATA ANALYSIS

Are data analysis techniques described (e.g., statistical tests, methodology for qualitative analysis)?

The data-analysis plan with rationale is well described in its own section in the article.

Does the analysis answer the research question?

Each of the four research questions is specifically addressed with appropriate analysis methods.

Is it appropriate?

Given the small sample size, assumptions of normal distribution, and the level of data collected, nonparametric tests were appropriately performed.

Is the analysis comprehensive? Are themes identified?

The authors provide a detailed, comprehensive discussion of the data analysis.

Is there bias in the analysis (trustworthiness? credibility?)?

Although the authors provide a rationale for their choice of nonparametric statistical tests, the lack of reliability and validity information for the parent satisfaction scale can introduce an element of bias in the analysis.

RESULTS

Are sample characteristics described and fully reported?

Sample characteristics are fully reported. Parents' gender, age, and education are described. Demographic data is stated to include parents' age, educational level, and number of children. However, gender of parent must have been ascertained as the first sample characteristic described in the Results section was gender. The means for child's age and the number of children in the family are also reported.

Are findings presented related to research aim/objective?

Study findings are reported with reference to corresponding research questions. All four research questions are addressed.

Are all outcome variables addressed, if applicable?

All outcome (dependent) variables of interest are addressed in the findings.

Are results clearly presented in text and/or tables/figures?

The major findings from the analyses are presented in the text and in graphic form. Although statistically nonsignificant, Figure 1 depicts the large difference between the control group and the two intervention groups in parents' adherence to the scheduled immunization appointment. This dramatic visual creates a lasting impression on the reader. The results of analyses of differences between the two intervention groups are displayed in chart form, which is appropriate for these nonsignificant results.

Is significance of results reported, if applicable?

No statistically significant results were detected among the variables tested.

DISCUSSION OF RESULTS
Do the authors link the findings to previous research studies?

The authors begin the discussion of results by noting that their study is unique in being the first to investigate the efficacy of different types of text-messaging reminders on parental adherence and timeliness with MMR immunization schedules. Stating this information earlier in the article would have provided the reader with important background context and greater understanding of why the authors only described two previous research studies. The authors do not discuss similarities and differences between these earlier studies and their current study. In addition, the limited literature review makes it difficult for the reader to know how text messaging has been implemented in previous studies as health reminders.

Are the conclusions comprehensive, yet within the data?

The authors do not discuss findings beyond the scope of the design and data of the study.

Do the authors interpret the results in the discussion?

The authors do neglect an opportunity to capitalize on the nonsignificant results and what they could mean in the specific setting in which the study was conducted. The authors make a great case for the use of cell phones and, more specific, text messaging in the Philippines. Although they did not assess the cost of obtaining a cell phone and maintaining service, the authors do establish that participants in this region demonstrated familiarity with cell phone usage without any training. This, coupled with the nonsignificant difference between weekly visits and one text reminder on immunization adherence, is a major finding. The cost of cell usage would have to be compared to the cost of a public health nurse visiting each family each week over time. This could save a great deal of resources with similar or better adherence to the immunization schedule. Although this idea is mentioned in the Recommendations section, it should have been explicated in the discussion, as it is the only finding with significant implications for practice.

Are the findings generalizable or transferable?

Because of the small sample size, generalizability of the findings is quite limited. However, this study did advance the feasibility of cell phone use for health promotion in underdeveloped areas.

LIMITATIONS
Identified? Accurate? Inclusive?

The authors accurately identify the small convenience sample, the 3-month duration of the study, and the unknown cost of the connectivity as limitations of the study. The last one could have, with little effort to ascertain the information, been addressed. This information would have bolstered the discussion as previously mentioned.

IMPLICATIONS
Are there implications for practice, education, research?
Are there implications for clinical significance?

The authors describe the implications for practice in the Recommendations section. They appropriately discuss how expanding telecommunications in rural areas is increasing cell phone usage and the benefits of health management applications are clear. These benefits include better health outcomes with fewer resources required.

RECOMMENDATIONS
Recommendations for future study/study replication?

Future areas of research, cited by the authors, include determining the balance of text-message content volume, criticality, and frequency. This would avoid alert overload and maximize effectiveness of textmessage reminders.

CONCLUSION
Is it succinct and does it tie everything together?

The conclusion begins with a summary of the state of childhood immunization in developing countries, which flows well into the results of the study. The authors then discuss the use of mobile technologies in rural areas and the need for local governments to collaborate with health organizations to establish networks for enhanced communication between patients and health care providers. It closes with a recommendation for future studies. The conclusion ties the critical pieces together to tell an important story in a succinct manner.

NURSE CARING BEHAVIORS FOLLOWING IMPLEMENTATION OF A RELATIONSHIP-CENTERED CARE PROFESSIONAL PRACTICE MODEL

6

Carol A. Porter, DNP, FAAN
Edgar M. Cullman, Sr. Chair of the Department of Nursing Chief Nursing
Officer/Senior Vice President, Associate Dean of Nursing Research and Education, The Mount Sinai
Medical Center, New York, NY, USA

Marisa Cortese, PhD, RN
Senior Manager for Quality, Research and Education, Oncology Services. The Mount Sinai Medical
Center, New York, NY, USA

Maria Vezina, EdD, RN, NEA-BC
Senior Director, Nursing Education, Research and Professional Practice, The Mount Sinai Medical
Center, New York, NY, USA

Joyce J. Fitzpatrick, PhD, MBA, FAAN
Elizabeth Brooks Ford Professor of Nursing, Frances Payne Bolton School of Nursing Case Western
Reserve University, Cleveland OH, USA. Senior Adviser, Center for Nursing Research and Education.
The Mount Sinai Medical Center, New York, NY, USA

ABSTRACT

Background: There has been considerable attention to nurse caring in the literature, and recent attention has been focused on the importance of caring not only to patient outcomes, but also to nurse outcomes such as the importance nurses place on caring within their professional role.

Aims: The purpose of this study was to describe nurses' perceptions o their own caring behaviors 6 months after implementation of a new Relationship-Centered Care Professional Practice Model.

Methodology: A descriptive design was used to survey all 1,500 clinical nurses providing care in a large academic medical center. The Caring Behavior Inventory was used, and background data were collected to describe the sample.

Results: Five hundred thirty-eight nurses completed the survey, for a response rate of 35.9%. Participants had high perceptions of caring behaviors in all of the assessed areas: assurance of human presence, knowledge and skill, respectful deference to others, and positive connectiveness.

Porter, C. A., Cortese, M., Vezina, M., & Fitzpatrick, J. J. (2014). Nurse caring behaviors following implementation of a relationship centered care professional practice model. *International Journal of Caring Sciences*, 7(3), 818–822. Retrieved from http://www.internationaljournalofcaringsciences.org/docs/16.%20FITZPATRICK%20ORIGINAL.pdf

Conclusions: Results of this study are consistent with prior research on nurses' perceptions of caring. As in prior research the more observable aspects of care received the higher ratings. Several factors may have contributed to the results of high scores on caring behaviors, including the implementation of a professional practice model that specifically targeted key components of caring in the provision of direct patient care. Further, throughout the implementation of the professional practice model there was considerable attention paid to continuing education targeted toward aspects of caring, provided both for nurse leaders and clinical nurses.

KEY WORDS: caring, nurses, relationship-centered care, professional practice model

INTRODUCTION

Caring has historically been considered an important part of nursing practice. Theories that contain an explication of the concept of nurse caring have received attention in both the scientific and the professional practice arena within the discipline (Watson, 1988, 2008). While a considerable literature exists comparing nurses' and patients' perceptions of caring behaviors, there is no literature that specifically addresses nurses' perceptions of caring behaviors following implementation of a hospital-wide professional practice model (PPM).

BACKGROUND

Research on nurse caring behaviors has spanned the globe. In a recent review of the research literature from 1987 to 2012 on patients' perceptions of nurse caring, Potter and Fogel (2013) concluded that human needs assistance was an important aspect of nurse caring valued by patients, independent of clinical setting or patient population. These researchers also found that nurses ratings of their caring behaviors were consistently higher than the patients ratings of the nurse caring behavior. The most comprehensive comparison study was of patients and nurses in six different European countries (Papastavron et al., 2011). It is important to note that in prior studies both patients' and nurses' ratings of nurse caring behaviors are high, particularly in the areas of care that are directly observable, for example, performance of skills. Further, there is a beginning focus on the link between nurse caring behaviors and patient satisfaction (Wolf, Miller, & Devine, 2003; Larrabee et al., 2004; Green & Davis, 2005; Wu, Larrabee, & Putnam, 2006).

In prior research nurses place high importance on the expressive aspects of caring, for example, listening to the patient, building trust, and the less observable aspects of care, for example, patient monitoring (O'Connell & Landers, 2008; Tucker, Brandling, & Fox, 2009). Even so, the rankings of these less observable aspects of caring by nurses are not significantly higher than the rankings of the more observable caring behaviors. There is a paucity of research on specific programmatic efforts to enhance nurse caring behaviors among nurses.

PURPOSE OF STUDY

The purpose of the present study was to describe nurses' perceptions of caring 6 months after implementation of a new Relationship-Centered Care (RCC) PPM. The PPM that was introduced was developed as part of an overall effort to improve the patient experience with care in the hospital. The RCC Model included attention to relationships with patients and families, relationships to all members of the care team, relationship to the community served, and care of self. Porter and colleagues have provided a comprehensive description of the components of care that were introduced along with the new PPM (Porter, Vezina, McEvoy, & Fitzpatrick, 2013).

RESEARCH METHODS

A descriptive design was used; the Caring Behavior Inventory (CBI) was used to measure nurses' perceptions of caring behaviors. The 1,500 RNs who were working as clinical nurses (directly engaged in clinical practice on the inpatient care units) were invited to participate. Nurse managers, educators, and advanced practice nurses were excluded.

Signed informed consent was waived but all participants were informed that completion of the questionnaire implied consent. RNs who participated in this study were asked to complete a background data sheet that included participant's age, gender, location of work (campus and unit), years of practice, initial type of nursing education, and highest nursing degree held.

The analysis using SPSS consisted of descriptive statistics for background variables. Means and standard deviations were computed for the CBI total and subscale scores.

CARING BEHAVIOR INVENTORY (CBI-24)

The CBI-24 includes 24 items each measured on a 6-point Likert-type scale based on a conceptual definition of nurse caring as an interactive process that occurs between nurses and patients. The CBI-24 measures perception of the frequency of caring behaviors. Total scores range from 6 to 144; higher mean scores indicate higher frequency of caring behaviors.

The scale has four subscales: Assurance of Human Presence (eight items), Knowledge and Skill (five items), Respectful Deference to Others (six items), and Positive Connectedness (five items). Authorization to use the CBI was obtained.

The CBI-24 has demonstrated convergent validity and good test–retest reliability ($r = 0.82$ for nurses) (Wu et al., 2006). Previous research has indicated high internal consistency with Cronbach alpha ranging from 0.92 to 0.96 (Burtson & Stichler, 2010; Palese et al., 2011; Papastavrou, Efstathiou, & Charalambous, 2012; Wu et al., 2006).

RESULTS

Following implementation of the PPM throughout all of the hospital units, the survey was distributed to the 1500 clinical nurses. Five hundred thirty-eight nurses completed the questionnaire (response rate 35.9%). The sample was representative of the population of nurses working on the units. The majority of the nurses were women ($n = 463$, 86.1%); the mean age of the nurses was 39.5 years. Detailed background characteristics are included in Table 1.

Perceptions of Caring Behaviors

Nurses had high perceptions of caring behaviors. The mean total score was 5.54 (out of a possible total mean score of 6.0). Mean scores for all subscales were also high: the Assurance of Human Presence mean score was 5.56; Knowledge and

TABLE 1. Demographic Information

Variables	Number (%)	(*N* = 538)
Gender:		
Male	68	(12.6)
Female	463	(86.1)
Preferred not to answer	7	(1.3)
Age (mean)	39.5	
Years of Practice/Work:		
<1	20	(3.7)
1–2	43	(8.0)
3–5	83	(15.4)
5–10	100	(18.6)
11–15	38	(7.1)
16–20	41	(7.6)
Over 20	158	(29.4)
Preferred not to answer	55	(10.2)

TABLE 2. Means and Standard Deviations Caring Behavior Subscale Scores

Subscales	Means	(SD)
Assurance of human presence	5.56	(±0.54)
Knowledge and skill	5.66	(±0.50)
Respectful deference to others	5.54	(±0.58)
Positive connectiveness	5.34	(±0.68)
Total score	5.54	(±0.53)

Skill mean score was 5.66; Respectful Deference to Others mean score was 5.54 (± 0.58); and Positive Connectedness mean score was 5.34 (± 0.68). These results are in details included in Table 2.

DISCUSSION

The clinical nurses who participated in this study rated all aspects of caring very high. These results are consistent with prior research using the CBI as well as qualitative studies of nurse caring and nurses' perceptions of caring behaviors assessed with other instruments (Potter & Fogel, 2013).

As in other studies, the more observable aspects of care received the highest ratings, even though all aspects were consistently rated above 5 on a 6-point scale. The high ratings of nurses in the present study exceed the ratings of nurses in prior research (Burtson & Stitchler, 2010; Palese et al., 2011).

There are several factors that might be related to the high caring scores among the nurses in the present sample. With the implementation of the PPM there was considerable emphasis placed on direct caring behaviors of the clinical nursing staff providing care at the bedside. Several continuing education programs were introduced and all nurses were engaged in understanding and applying the components of caring that were inherent in the model of care. Nurse leaders also were engaged in the implementation of the PPM, and were supportive of the changes that were introduced to enhance care provisions. In addition, nurse leaders consistently tracked the implementation of the PPM and the caring behaviors on each unit.

LIMITATIONS

One of the major limitations of the study is the lack of a measure of nurse caring behaviors prior to implementation of the PPM. Thus, it is not known the extent to which changes occurred. Also, no attempt was made to discern relationships to other factors, for example, years of practice experience, as the overall lack of variability of the scores did not permit these analyses.

RECOMMENDATIONS FOR FUTURE RESEARCH

There is a need to more fully understand the dimensions of nurse caring. Further study is recommended to determine the meaning that the individual caring behaviors have for nurses. Also, it is important to ascertain if there are variations in the perceived importance of caring behaviors dependent on the patients receiving care. Also, continued study comparing nurses and patient perceptions of caring behaviors of nurses is recommended as are studies linking nurse caring behaviors to patient outcomes.

IMPLICATIONS FOR PRACTICE

While all of the mean scores for nurses' perceptions of caring behaviors were high, it is important to note that the lowest scores were on the subscale of positive connectedness. The interpersonal relationship that nurses develop with their patients should be at the forefront of the work that they do. It is expected that as we continue to implement the RCC PPM this aspect of nurse caring will become increasingly apparent to both nurses and patients. The core principles of the RCC Model include the therapeutic relationship that is developed with patients and team members.

REFERENCES

Burtson, P. L., & Stichler, J. F. (2010). Nursing work environment and nurse caring: relationship among motivational factors. Journal of Advanced Nursing, 66(8), 1819–1831.

Green, A., & Davis, S. (2005). Toward a predictive model of patient satisfaction with nurse practitioner care. Journal of the American Academy of Nurse Practitioners, 17(4), 139–148.

Larrabee, J. H., Ostrow, C. L., Withrow, M. L., Janney, M. A., Hobbs, G. R., & Burant, C. (2004). Predictors of patient satisfaction with inpatient hospital care. Research in Nursing and Health, 27(4), 254–268.

O'Connell, E., & Landers, M. (2008). The importance of critical care nurses' caring behaviours as perceived by nurses and relative. Intensive and Critical Care Nursing, 24, 349–358. doi:10.1016/j.iccn.2008.04.002

Palese, A., Tomietto, M., Suhonen, R., Efstathiou, G., Tsangari, H., Merkouris, A., et al. (2011). Surgical patient satisfaction as an outcome of nurses' caring behaviors: A descriptive and correlational study in six European countries. Journal of Nursing Scholarship, 43(4), 341–350.

Papastavrou, E., Efstathiou, G., & Charalambous, A. (2011). Nurses' and patients' perceptions of caring behaviors: quantitative systematic review of comparative studies. Journal of Advanced Nursing, 67(6), 1191–1205.

Papastavrou, E., Efstathiou, G., Tsangari, H., Suhonen, R., Leino-Kilpi, H., Patiraki, E., et al. (2012). Patients' and nurses' perceptions of respect and human presence through caring behaviors: A comparative study. Nursing Ethics, 19(3), 369–379.

Porter, C. A., Vezina, M., McEvoy, M., & Fitzpatrick, J. J. (2013). Development and implementation of a professional practice model. Nurse Leader.

Potter, D. R., & Fogel, J. (2013). Nurse caring: A review of the literature. International Journal of Advanced Nursing Studies, 2(1): 40–45.

Tucker, A., Brandling, J., & Fox, P. (2009). Improved record keeping with reading handovers. Nursing Management, 16(8), 30–34.

Watson, J. (1988). New dimensions of human caring theory. Nursing Science Quarterly, 1(4), 175–181.

Watson, J. (Ed.). (2008). Assessing and measuring caring in nursing and health science. Springer Publishing Company.

Wolf, Z. R., Miller, P. A., & Devine, M. (2003). Relationship between nurse caring and patient satisfaction in patients undergoing invasive cardiac procedures. MedSurg Nursing, 12(6), 391–396.

Wu, Y., Larrabee, J. H., & Putman, H. P. (2006). Caring Behaviors Inventory: a reduction of the 42-item instrument. Nursing Research, 55(1), 18–25.

NURSE CARING BEHAVIORS FOLLOWING IMPLEMENTATION OF A RELATIONSHIP-CENTERED CARE PROFESSIONAL PRACTICE MODEL

Critique by *Annette Peacock-Johnson and Patricia Keresztes*

OVERALL SUMMARY

Caring is often considered one of the most central concepts in the practice of nursing and is the foundation of the nurse–patient relationship. Although there is a much prior research describing nurse caring behaviors, this is the first study to describe nurse caring behaviors following implementation of a specific professional practice model. The study was conducted at one academic medical center in the northeast. The large sample of acute care nurses across various specialties adds to our overall knowledge of nurse caring. In this study, as in the prior research, nurses' perceptions of their own caring behaviors were high. The researchers frame their results in relation to both future research and professional practice. As professional practice models are an important explicit expectation of Magnet® hospitals, this study adds to our understanding of this core structural component of nursing care delivery. Although the research would have been strengthened with a pretest–posttest design, overall the findings add to our understanding of nurse caring behavior. The report is clearly and logically presented and follows the overall expectations for research reports.

TITLE

Does the title include the key concepts/variables/ phenomenon of interest?

The title of this research article includes the key concepts of interest, nurse caring behaviors, and the professional practice model (Relationship-Centered Care).

Is it concise (12 words or less) and professionally stated?

The title is 13 words (thus a bit lengthy) but appropriate and professionally stated for the manuscript.

RESEARCHER(S) CREDIBILITY

Educational credentials?

All four authors have doctoral degrees and thus have the educational credentials to conduct the study.

Prior methodological research experience of the authors (i.e., methodological expertise)?

The authors have prior research experience with similar studies and thus have the methodological expertise for this study. The last author has several research publications.

Subject matter content experience (prior research on the subject matter)?

The first three authors hold leadership positions in nursing research and education at the institution where the research was conducted; the fourth author holds an advisory position with the institution. Three of the authors were the authors of another related article focused on the description of the Relationship-Centered Care Professional Practice Model. The positions held by the authors imply that they have expertise in the areas of research and practice.

ABSTRACT

Does it include the key components (objective/aim, background/rationale, methods, results, and conclusions)?

All components of the abstract are described, including the background, aims, methods, results, and conclusions. The background sentence could be improved by being more clear and concise. The aim is clearly stated. The design, instrument, and sample are identified within the methodology description. The results are clearly and succinctly stated. The conclusion is comprehensive and includes the results.

Does it include references?

The abstract does not include references.

Is it concise (150–250 words or less)?

The abstract is concise at 239 words, an appropriate length.

Does it entice you to read the rest of the article (interesting)?

The abstract is interesting and invites individuals, particularly those in nursing practice or management, to read the entire article.

INTRODUCTION/PROBLEM

Is the research problem or phenomenon of interest clearly stated?

The phenomena of nurse caring is clearly stated in the introduction. This includes the concept of nurses' perceptions of caring following implementation of a professional practice model. The phenomena of interest is easily identified from the authors' presentation in this introduction.

Is it succinct?

The introduction is brief. Yet, the authors identify the gap in knowledge from a lack of research focusing on factors that may influence nurse caring behaviors.

Does it answer the "so what" question?

Nurse caring is of particular significance to nursing, as there is much literature on the topic and several theoretical perspectives identifying caring as a fundamental concept for the discipline. Professional practice models also are of current significance particularly in light of the Magnet program focus on integration of professional practice models to guide nursing. The "so what" question is answered in the introduction as the authors identify the importance of understanding nurse caring and also professional practice models.

RESEARCH AIMS/OBJECTIVES

Is the research aim/objective clearly stated?

There is no specific research objective stated in the introduction, rather it is implied by the authors' statement of the absence of research linking perceptions of caring behaviors following implementation of a hospital-wide professional practice model.

Is it concisely written?

The introduction is very concise.

Does it follow logically from the research problem/phenomenon of interest?

Yes, the research problem flows logically from the phenomena of interest. The introduction is very precise and parsimonious. The purpose of the study is clearly defined and concisely written.

SIGNIFICANCE
Is the significance to nursing and health care clearly written?

There is no separate section describing the significance of the study to nursing and health care. Yet, caring is one of the most essential aspects of nursing. Nurse caring behaviors are significant to both nursing and health care.

Does the significance follow from the research aim/objective?

The significance follows directly from the research aims. The research objective clearly identifies nurses' perceptions of caring and the importance of caring as the objective of the study. It is not the intent of the study to explore the significance of nurses' perceptions of caring related to other outcomes or variables such as nurse or patient satisfaction.

BACKGROUND
Is there an explicit description of a theoretical perspective or conceptual framework? If not, is it implied?

No theoretical perspective or conceptual framework is identified for this study; the theoretical perspectives on caring are implied, particularly as the authors cite the classic reference to Watson. Theoretical frameworks on caring have been developed, which include Jean Watson's Theory of Human Caring and the middle range Theory of Caring by Kristen Swanson. Both of these theoretical perspectives are related in their focus on caring as the central concept of nursing science and professional practice. Additionally, a model for relationship-based care (RBC) has been developed to enhance relationships with patients/families/colleagues and self. Although the authors identify the Relationship-Centered Care Professional Practice Model used for this study, they do not provide any description of their conceptual model. Inclusion of a conceptual framework would provide a means to more fully understand and describe the phenomena of interest, thereby advancing the science of nurse caring.

Are there clear theoretical/conceptual definitions of the concepts?

There are no theoretical definitions of the concepts presented until the description of the Caring Behavior Inventory (CBI) instrument. In the Instruments section there is a conceptual definition of caring behaviors presented.

LITERATURE REVIEW
Primary sources only?

Fourteen primary references are cited in the review of literature. Two literature reviews on caring are cited. These reviews provide recent comparisons of nurse caring behaviors from studies using various clinical settings, patient populations, or international sites.

Current (within the past how many years)?

References range from 1 year to 27 years old. The oldest references are classic articles focused on nurse caring such as the Watson reference. Watson's work on caring represents seminal literature and is therefore appropriate for inclusion in the Literature Review section.

Is the search strategy included?

The search strategy was not included.

Is literature relevant to the research aims/objectives?

References are relevant to this study on nurses' perceptions of caring and include articles on the instrument and the professional practice model that were used. The literature review appropriately emphasizes nurse ratings and rankings of their caring behaviors as these are the focus of the current study.

Is it chronologically presented (old to current)?

The literature review is not presented in chronological order but is summarily presented based on findings from the research. The relationship of nursing caring behaviors to patient outcomes is briefly mentioned, but is not the focus of the current study. Although the literature review is not exhaustive, sufficient background is included to provide context for this study.

RATIONALE FOR THE STUDY

Is there a gap in the literature that this study will fill (would it extend prior knowledge)? Is the rationale clearly stated?

Previous research has examined nurses' and patients' perceptions of nurse caring behaviors, including the importance of various caring behaviors, and relationships between nurse caring behaviors and patient satisfaction. A clear gap in knowledge is identified and limited research exists that examines ways to enhance nurse caring behaviors through the implementation of a professional practice model. This study is not a replication study. This study aims to expand what is known by exploring nurses' perceptions of caring when using a professional practice model. The rationale for the study is clearly stated.

RESEARCH QUESTIONS AND/OR HYPOTHESES

Are these explicitly and clearly stated?

The research purpose is explicit and clearly stated: to describe nurses' perceptions of caring six months after implementation of a new Relationship-Centered Care Professional Practice Model. Specific research questions regarding the importance nurses' place on various caring behaviors or the possible relationships between caring behaviors and demographic variables are not stated.

Do they include the variables/phenomena of interest?

The variable of interest, nurses' perceptions of their own caring behaviors, is clearly identified.

Do they follow from the research aim/objective?

> This main variable of interest, nurse caring behaviors, follows from the study purpose statement.

METHODS

Research Design/Paradigm

Is the research design clearly stated?

> The research design is clearly stated as a descriptive design using survey instruments.

Is there consistency between the research design and paradigm?

> The design uses a nonexperimental survey approach that is appropriate to address and describe the phenomenon of nurse caring behaviors.

Is this the best choice of design to address the research problem/phenomenon of interest?

> Yes, for a purely descriptive study such as this one, the choice of design is appropriate.

Is there rigor in the design?

> Rigor could have been enhanced by surveying the nurses prior to the implementation of the professional practice model. The design is postmeasure only.

SETTING

Is the setting clearly described?

> The setting is identified in the abstract as a large academic medical center but is not described in the article.

What biases are introduced as a result of selecting this particular setting?

> All of the authors have an affiliation with the setting of the research study. In addition, three of the four authors also wrote the article describing the professional practice model used in the study. Associations with the professional practice model and the institution used for the study could potentially introduce bias into the study.

SAMPLING PLAN AND SAMPLE

Is the sampling plan clearly identified?

> The sampling plan is clearly identified. In this study, no statistical tests or correlations are undertaken.

Does it represent the population of interest?

> The sample represents the population of interest. It includes 1,500 clinical nurses directly engaged in clinical practice on the inpatient care units in the academic medical center where the research was conducted. Exclusion criteria are described and include those nurses not in direct patient care such as managers, educators, and advanced practice nurses.

Is the sampling plan consistent with the research aim/objective?

> The sampling plan is appropriate for the objective, which is to describe nurse caring behaviors.

Is the sample size sufficient (e.g., power analysis or data saturation)?

> Because the study is only descriptive, a power analysis is not needed.

VARIABLES
Are variables clearly identified?

> The variable of nurse caring behaviors is clearly identified and operationalized by the use of the CBI-24.

Are variables operationally defined and consistent with theoretical concepts?

> There were no explicit theoretical concepts identified. The main variable, nurse caring behaviors, is measured by the CBI-24. There is no explicit operational definition of the main variable but it is implied that the scores on the CBI will be used to define nurse caring behaviors.

Are independent and dependent variables identified, if applicable?

> Ideally, the independent variable is implementation of the Relationship-Centered Care Professional Practice Model; nurses' perceptions of caring is the dependent variable. As the authors noted in the Limitations section, measures of nurse caring were not taken prior to implementation of the professional practice model. Because before and after measures of nurse caring behaviors are not available for comparison, the use of an independent variable does not apply.

METHOD OF DATA COLLECTION
What are the methods of data collection?

> The method used for data collection is not described. The authors do not include how nurses were invited to participate, how the questionnaires were distributed, how the questionnaires were returned or collected, and whether any follow-up measures were used to increase participation. The CBI-24 is an appropriate choice to address the phenomenon of interest, nurse caring behavior. Data collected from the study include demographics (age, gender, location of work-campus and unit, years of practice, initial type of nursing education, and the highest nursing degree held) as well as scores for each of the 24 items on the CBI-24.

Are validity and reliability clearly addressed for prior research and current study, if applicable?

> Reliability data (test–retest reliability and Cronbach alpha) and validity data (convergent validity) for the CBI-24 are presented based on previous studies. However, reliability data for the CBI-24 for the current study is not reported.

Do the measures/instruments address the underlying theoretical concepts or phenomenon of interest?

> Yes the instrument clearly addresses the theoretical concept of nurse caring. The CBI-24 is based on a conceptual definition of nurse caring as an interactive process that occurs between nurses and patients.

Were human rights protected?

> The authors do not identify whether the study was approved by any institutional review board. Confidentiality of the data is also not described. The authors do state that informed consent was implied if a completed questionnaire was returned.

Are other ethical issues identified?

No other ethical issues are apparent or identified in the article.

Is the data-collection method appropriate for research design?

Data collection via the CBI-24 is appropriate for the descriptive research design.

Is there bias in data collection?

The authors do not describe confidentiality for the data collected, nor do they describe who collected the data. Both of these research steps could result in bias if confidentiality of the data or anonymity are not protected.

What is the fidelity of intervention addressed, if applicable?

There is no intervention; therefore, this is not applicable. If the researchers had chosen the pretest–posttest design, which would have been stronger, then the intervention could have been evaluated.

DATA ANALYSIS

Are data analysis techniques described (e.g., statistical tests, methodology for qualitative analysis)?

The authors use SPSS, a well-recognized and used statistical package, for data analysis. Data analysis includes descriptive statistics for demographic variables along with the means and standard deviations for the CBI-24 total and subscale scores.

Does the analysis answer the research question?

The use of the mean for the overall total as well as subscale scores on the CBI-24 is appropriate for the data and does answer the research question of nurse caring behaviors following implementation of a relationship-centered care professional practice model.

Is it appropriate?

The analysis was appropriate.

Is the analysis comprehensive? Are themes identified?

The analysis was comprehensive using descriptive statistics, means, and standard deviations. The authors report a lack of variability in the scores on the CBI-24 precluding statistical correlations between the CBI-24 scores and demographic variables. Analysis of the overview total score and subscores on the CBI-24 does contribute to the theme on nurse caring behaviors, identifying which behaviors are more or less important to nurses.

Is there bias in the analysis (trustworthiness? credibility?)?

The authors do not report how they handled returned questionnaires with incomplete data, which could potentially introduce bias into the analysis.

RESULTS

Are sample characteristics described and fully reported?

Demographics of the sample population, including gender and age, are clearly reported both in narrative and table form. Both the text and table include the percentage of participants who are women (86.1%) as well as the mean age

(39.5 years). The table additionally lists the years of practice/work beginning with less than 1 year up to over 20 years. The collection of data related to the participant's location of work (campus and unit), initial type of nursing education, and highest nursing degree held, are described in the Methods section. However, results for these data are not presented in the text or tables.

The findings of the total and subscale scores on the CBI-24 are clearly presented both in narrative and table form. Standard deviations for the Caring Behavior Subscale scores are also included with the table. The findings of the total and subscale scores on the CBI-24 address the variable on nurse caring behaviors and are clearly related to the research aim of identifying nurse caring behaviors.

Are findings presented related to research aim/objective?

The authors surveyed 1,500 nurses. Five hundred thirty-eight nurses completed the questionnaire for a response rate of 35.9%. The resulting sample of the population is robust. Therefore, the large sample size increases the validity despite the response rate, whicht was less than 50%. It is important to note that this response rate is higher than what would be expected from a survey. It is also important that the sample is representative of the population of nurses working on the clinical units, which is stated by the authors.

Are all outcome variables addressed, if applicable?

The main variable is the nurse caring behaviors. Not only do the authors report the total scores on nurse caring, but they also report the subscale scores, adding richness to the results.

Are results clearly presented in text and/or tables/figures?

Yes, the results are clearly presented in text and tables.

Is significance of results reported, if applicable?

As a purely descriptive study there was no statistical significance reported. The descriptive statistics reported for both nurse caring and the demographic variables are sufficient and appropriate.

DISCUSSION OF RESULTS
Do the authors link the findings to previous research studies?

The authors link the results of this study with previous research findings. Like previous research, this study found that nurses rate aspects of caring very high, with observable aspects of caring receiving the highest ratings.

Are the conclusions comprehensive, yet within the data?

The authors report and discussion of the results do not go beyond the data.

Do the authors interpret the results in the discussion?

An interpretation of the results is offered by the authors, who suggest that education and administration support enhanced staff awareness and implementation of the professional practice model. This is believed to contribute to the overall high perception of caring by nurses.

Are the findings generalizable or transferable?

Because the findings are based upon the use of a professional practice model designed specifically for the site of the study, the results can be generalized only to institutions that utilize the same practice model.

LIMITATIONS
Identified? Accurate? Inclusive?

The authors accurately identify limitations of the study, including the lack of a preimplementation measure. Hence, a knowledge gap remains as to whether the professional practice model enhanced nurses' perceptions of caring. In addition, the authors are accurate to not pursue correlations between nurses' perceptions of caring and demographic variables because a lack of variability in the reported scores on the CBI24 does not permit these analyses.

IMPLICATIONS
Are there implications for practice, education, research?

Implications for both practice and future research are succinctly presented and discussed. This study finds the lowest scores on the subscale of positive connectedness, which has direct implications for nursing practice. Implications for nursing education are not addressed. However, future research on the development of nursing caring behaviors has potential implications for nursing education.

Are there implications for clinical significance?

The study is directly relevant to professional practice model implementation and warrants replication in other venues to determine the influence of implementation of a specific model to increases in nurse caring behaviors. Yet, given the high reports of caring behaviors among nurses in this study and other studies, it is not clear that a change could be determined.

RECOMMENDATIONS
Recommendations for future study/study replication?

Specific and comprehensive recommendations are provided regarding future study of the dimensions of nurse caring. A replication study that includes both a pre- and postimplementation measure would be appropriate. A follow-up study would also be relevant to ascertain whether the professional practice model continues to improve and sustain nurses' high perceptions of caring over time. The authors enumerate multiple venues for future study, including pursuing research to compare nurse and patient perceptions of caring as well as research to explore relationships between nurse caring behaviors and patient outcomes.

CONCLUSION
Is it succinct and does it tie everything together?

No conclusion is presented. A final conclusion would be beneficial to provide an overall synthesis of the research study.

IMPACT OF HEALTH CARE INFORMATION TECHNOLOGY ON NURSING PRACTICE

7

Ronald J. Piscotty, Jr., PhD, RN-BC
Theta Psi, Assistant Professor, Wayne State University College of Nursing,
Detroit, Michigan

Beatrice Kalisch, PhD, RN, FAAN
Rho, Titus Professor, University of Michigan School of Nursing, Ann Arbor, Michigan

Angel Gracey-Thomas
Theta Psi, Research Assistant, Wayne State University College of Nursing, Detroit, Michigan

ABSTRACT

Purpose: To report additional mediation findings from a descriptive cross-sectional study to examine if nurses' perceptions of the impact of health care information technology on their practice mediates the relationship between electronic nursing care reminder use and missed nursing care.

Design: The study used a descriptive design. The sample ($N = 165$) was composed of registered nurses (RNs) working on acute care hospital units. The sample was obtained from a large teaching hospital in southeast Michigan in the fall of 2012. All eligible nursing units ($n = 19$) were included.

Methods: The Missed Nursing Care Survey (MISSCARE), nursing care reminders (NCRs) Usage Survey, and the Impact of Health Care Information Technology Scale were used to collect data to test for mediation. Mediation was tested using the method described by Baron and Kenny. Multiple regression equations were used to analyze the data to determine if mediation occurred between the variables.

Findings: Missed nursing care, the outcome variable, was regressed on the predictor variable, reminder usage, and the mediator variable impact of technology on nursing practice. The impact of health care information technology (IHIT) on nursing practice negatively affected missed nursing care ($t = -4.12$, $p < .001$), explaining 9.8% of variance in missed nursing care. With HIT present, the predictor (reminder usage) was no longer significant ($t = -.70$, $p = .48$). Thus, the reduced direct association between reminder usage and missed nursing care when HIT was in the model supported the hypothesis that HIT was at least one of the mediators in the relationship between reminder usage and missed nursing care.

Conclusions: The perceptions of the IHIT mediates the relationship between nursing care reminder use and missed nursing care. The findings are beneficial to the advancement of health care technology in that designers of HIT systems need to keep in mind that perceptions regarding impacts of the technology will influence usage.

Piscotty, R. J., Jr., Kalisch, B., & Gracey-Thomas, A. (2015). Impact of healthcare information technology on nursing practice. *Journal of Nursing Scholarship,* 47(4), 287–293. doi:10.1111/jnu.12138. Reprinted with permission from Wiley-Blackwell.

Clinical Relevance: Many times, information technology systems are not designed to match the workflow of nurses. Systems built with redundant or impertinent reminders may be ignored. System designers must study which reminders nurses find most useful and which reminders result in the best quality outcomes.

A major challenge facing nurses today is the demand of providing safe and quality care, while still being efficient and cost-effective. Implementation of technology in various aspects of our lives continues. The trend in health care is the introduction of technology to improve both quality of care and decreased costs. Thus, finding methods that can help nurses offer safe and effective care using technology is an absolute necessity. In order to achieve these ambitious goals, the reduction of health care errors is requisite. This includes reducing the occurrence of missed nursing care (required nursing care not delivered or significantly delayed). Missing required nursing care or delaying care contributes to poor patient outcomes (Kalisch & Xie, 2014). Common themes of missed nursing care include basic nursing care such as ambulation, patient turning, feeding, and bathing (Piscotty & Kalisch, 2014a). Technology is being implemented as a tool to prevent health care errors. The technology of interest in this study is the use of clinical decision support systems (CDSS). CDSS have long been used by physicians and are now being used by nurses to guide clinical practice (Choi, Choi, Bae, & Lee, 2011) and to improve patient outcomes (Choi et al., 2011; Piscotty & Kalisch, 2014b; Staggers, Weir, & Phansalkar, 2008). Electronic nursing care reminder usage, a type of CDSS, is related to decreased reports of missed care (Piscotty & Kalisch, 2014c; Piscotty, Kalisch, Gracey-Thomas, & Yarandi, 2015). Technology is meant to augment nurses' clinical reasoning, not replace it. Combining technology and excellent clinical reasoning will more likely lead to a decrease in errors and an improvement in both quality and safety.

The purpose of this study is to report additional mediation findings from a descriptive cross-sectional study that examined the relationship between missed nursing care and electronic NCRs (Piscotty & Kalisch, 2014c). The research question examined in this report is: Do nurses' perceptions of the IHIT on their practice mediate the relationship between electronic nursing care reminder use and missed nursing care? It is hypothesized that nurses who have more favorable perceptions of health care technology will use the technology more readily (e.g., reminders) and therefore sustain decreased amounts of missed nursing care.

KEY WORDS: clinical decision support, missed care, nursing, reminders

LITERATURE REVIEW
Electronic Nursing Care Reminders

Meaningful use of HIT is now a requirement to receive complete reimbursement from both Medicare and Medicaid (HealthIT.gov, n.d.). The objectives of meaningful use include ensuring quality and safety while providing and improving care communication and management (Madison & Staggers, 2011). Even with the meaningful use requirements, embracing the electronic health record (EHR) as a tool in the delivery of care has been challenging (Bove & Jesse, 2010). When nurses view documentation as a difficult and cumbersome task, it often slows the technology's acceptance. Alternatively, if the workflow is designed with the nurse in mind, adoption will be increased (Bove & Jesse, 2010). Several components of the EHR offer advantages in the delivery of complete nursing care. CDSS with NCRs is a specific tool nurses have to provide quality care and is a necessary requirement to attest to meaningful use of HIT.

A review of the current literature did not locate articles that specifically address electronic NCRs. This is a gap in our current understanding of the types of CDSS nurses use, find helpful, or prefer for delivery (Staggers et al., 2008). Choi and colleagues (2011) reported that ICU nurses are more likely to adopt CDSS if integration exists with physiologic monitors. Additionally, they reported that necessary documentation of care must be available in the EHR to improve adoption (Choi et al., 2011). The integration of documentation that eliminates the duplication of work is essential for adoption of the EHR (Bove & Jesse, 2010; Choi et al., 2011). Future research and continuous evaluation of electronic NCRs is necessary in order to ensure accuracy and quality improvement.

Missed Nursing Care

Basic nursing duties, including (but not limited to) feeding, bathing, ambulation, turning, and hygiene, are common nursing care activities that are often missed (Kalisch, 2006). Although the importance of basic nursing care is taught to nurses in their first year of education, these care items are some of the first to not be completed. Pressure ulcer development and pneumonia are just two complications that can be prevented when basic nursing care is delivered in a timely fashion. These complications may result in decreased quality of life for patients and increased health care costs. Reasons nurses do not complete these activities have been found to be related to a lack of staffing and material resources and a decrease in communication with fellow staff and patients (Kalisch, Landstrom, & Williams, 2009).

Three studies have examined solutions in order to reduce the omission of nursing care and improve quality of care (Kalisch, Xie, & Ronis, 2013; Piscotty & Kalisch, 2014c; Piscotty et al., 2015). Kalisch and colleagues (2013) reported that successful teamwork on a unit is significantly related to decreased reports of missed nursing care. NCRs embedded in the EHR have been found to be related to a decrease in the occurrence of missed nursing care (Piscotty & Kalisch, 2014c; Piscotty et al., 2015). In the studies conducted by Piscotty, it was identified that nurses who utilize the electronic NCRs more frequently report less missed care (Piscotty & Kalisch, 2014c; Piscotty et al., 2015).

CONCEPTUAL FRAMEWORK

The conceptual framework chosen for this study is the Structure, Process, and Outcomes Model of Health-Care Quality (Donabedian, 2005). This framework can be used to understand the relationships that NCRs (structure) and their use (process) have on missed nursing care (immediate outcome) and patient and organizational outcomes (distal outcomes; Figure 1). The examination of distal outcomes is beyond the scope of this study and will not be explored. Additionally, a process-mediating variable of nurses' perceptions of the IHIT on practice is included in the model. Conceptual definitions and empirical indicators for each variable are listed in Table 1.

METHODS

The sample, design, measures, and procedures are described in detail in our previous publication (Piscotty & Kalisch, 2014c). A brief summary of methods will be presented here.

Design, Sample, and Setting

The main study utilized a descriptive cross-sectional design with a convenience sample (Piscotty & Kalisch, 2014c). The sample ($N = 165$) consisted of RNs working

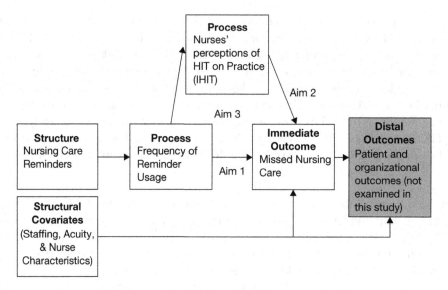

FIGURE 1. Modified structure process outcome model.

IHIT, impact of health care information technology.

TABLE 1. Conceptual Definitions and Empirical Indicators: Dependent, Independent, and Mediating Variables

Dependent variable	Conceptual definition	Empirical indicators
Missed nursing care	Kalisch, Landstrom, & Hinshaw (2009) define missed nursing care in a concept analysis. Missed nursing care is defined as any aspect of Required patient care that is omitted (either in part or whole) or delayed.	Missed nursing care is define Operationally as: The total score On the MISSCARE survey (Kalisch &Williams, 2009).
Independent variable	Conceptual definition	Empirical indicators
Level of use of EHR NCRs	The registered nurses' self-rated level of use of nursing care reminders in their facilities' EHR.	Level of use of nursing care reminders is operationally define as the nurse's total score on the nursing care reminders survey.
Mediating variables	Conceptual definition	Empirical indicators
Impact of health care information technology on nursing practice	Nurses' perceptions of the influence that HIT has on interdisciplinary communication workflow patterns, and satisfaction with HIT applications available in hospitals.	Total score on the IHIT Scale (Dykeset al.,2007).

EHR, electronic health record; HIT, health care information technology; IHIT, impact of health care information technology; MISSCARE, Missed Nursing Care Survey; NCRs, nursing care reminders.

on acute care hospital units in a large teaching hospital in Southeast Michigan in 2012. All eligible nursing units ($n = 19$) were included in the study. Inclusion criteria included that participants had to be RNs that took a daily patient assignment, the EHR had to be implemented for at least 6 months, and the EHR had to include the types of reminders that were examined in the study. Exclusion criteria included non-RN employees (nursing assistants, clerks, patient care associates, nursing students, etc.) and RNs that did not take a daily patient assignment (managers, educators, nursing instructors, case managers, etc.).

Measures

Nursing Care Reminder Usage Survey (NCRS). The NCRS was used to measure frequency of reminder use in this study. The investigators of this study developed the NCRS measurement tool. The survey contains 12 questions regarding usage of NCRs (see Table 2). The following definition regarding NCRs was included in the survey directions: A nursing reminder is an electronic list, prompt, or cue of tasks or procedures that need to be completed by either the nurse or nursing attendant during the shift. Therefore, all questions are asked in the context of electronic reminders. Additional information including instrument validity and reliability has been published elsewhere (Piscotty & Kalisch, 2014c).

Impact of Health Care Information Technology (IHIT) Scale. The IHIT Scale was used to measure nurse perceptions about the impact of HIT on practice (Dykes, Hurley, Cashen, Bakken, & Duffy (2007). The IHIT Scale is composed of 29 items contained in four subscales (Dykes et al., 2007). Additional information, including instrument validity and reliability, has been published elsewhere (Dykes et al., 2007; Piscotty & Kalisch, 2014c).

Missed Nursing Care. The MISSCARE Survey is a two-part survey and a demographics section that measures the extent to which elements of nursing care are missed as well as the reasons for missing care (Kalisch & Williams, 2009). Part A of

---

TABLE 2. Nursing Care Reminders Survey

How frequently do you utilize the following types of NCRs to assist you in completing nursing care activities?
1. A paper list of reminders based on what is in the EHR
2. Printout of list of care activities that serve as a reminder
3. Electronic nursing care orders that serve as a reminder
4. List of nursing care activities in plan of care that serve as a reminder
5. Electronic list of reminders (i.e., task list, documentation checklist, documentation form, work queue, work list)
6. Electronic list of reminders not in the EHR
7. CPOE list that serves as a reminder
8. Electronic documentation in the EHR that serves as a reminder
9. Electronic checklist for documenting care that serves as a reminder
10. Alert of reminder message pop-ups in the EHR
11. How frequently do you utilize NCRs to assist you in completing nursing care activities?
12. How helpful do you find the electronic NCRs?

CPOE, computerized provider order entry; EHR, electronic health record; NCRs, nursing care reminders.

the survey and a demographics section were used in the study to measure elements of missed nursing care (Piscotty & Kalisch, 2014c; Piscotty et al., 2015). Instrument validity and reliability has been published elsewhere (Kalisch & Williams, 2009).

PROCEDURES

Institutional review board approval was obtained prior to the study. Online surveys were used, with links to the surveys sent to each participant via email. Detailed instructions, consent information, and links to the study instruments were included. The surveys were administered using the Qualtrics (Provo, UT, USA) survey software. The surveys were anonymous and no identifying information was collected. Respondent burden was considered to be minimal as the instruments were short and each took less than 10 minute to complete. Nurses were reminded via flyers placed in high-visibility areas on the units. In addition, reminder email messages were sent to all nurses twice a week. Surveys were collected within 1 month from the start of the study.

DATA ANALYSES

Data were analyzed using SPSS 21 (IBM Corp., Armonk, NY, USA). Data were initially examined through descriptive analysis, and total scores were calculated for each of the three main variables in the study. Assumptions for multiple linear regressions were assessed. Missing data were excluded casewise for analysis. The alpha level for all analyses was set at .05 or less.

In order to test for mediation, the method described by Baron and Kenny (1986) was used, in which a variable is considered a mediator (Figure 2) when three criteria are met: (a) variation in the independent variable (reminder usage) accounts for significant variation in the mediator variable (IHIT Scale; path a), (b) variation in the mediator variable (IHIT Scale) accounts for significant variation in the dependent variable (missed care; path b), and (c) when paths a and b are controlled, there is significant reduction in the variance between the independent variable (reminder usage) and dependent variable (missed care; path c). When these three criteria are met, the relationship between the independent variable (reminder usage) and the dependent variable (missed care) must be less in the third equation than in the second (Baron & Kenny, 1986).

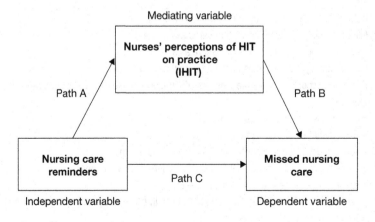

FIGURE 2. General mediation model.

IHIT, impact of health care information technology.

RESULTS
Sample

The sample (N = 165) consisted of staff nurses employed at a large teaching hospital in southeast Michigan. Respondents (69.1%, n = 114) primarily held a baccalaureate degree as their highest level of education, with 66.7% (n = 110) of those participants having a BSN (Piscotty & Kalisch, 2014c). The majority of respondents were female (87.9%, n = 145) and between the ages of 25 and 34 years (37.0%, n = 61; Piscotty & Kalisch, 2014c). The majority of the respondents worked full time (93.3%, n = 154), and over half of the participants in the study (63.0%, n = 104) worked on a medical surgical unit (Piscotty & Kalisch, 2014c).

Surveys

Missed nursing care, reminder usage, IHIT Scale (descriptives). Total missed nursing care scores ranged from a low of 24 to a maximum of 84 (M = 56.09; SD = 11.79) out of a total possible score of 120. NCRs total scores ranged from a low of 11 to a maximum of 50 (M = 29.98; SD = 8.11) out of a total possible score of 60. Total IHIT Scale scores ranged from 28 to 171 (M = 129.32; SD = 22.94) out of a total possible score of 174.

IHIT scale mediation of the effect of reminder usage on missed nursing care. The IHIT was hypothesized in this study as a mediating variable in the relationship between NCRS and missed nursing care. To satisfy the requirements for mediation, three regression equations were computed. To establish mediation, the following conditions had to be satisfied: (a) NCRS must affect IHIT; (b) NCRS must affect missed nursing care in the second equation; and (c) IHIT must affect missed nursing care in the third equation. A strong demonstration of mediation occurs when the relationship between the NCRS and IHIT is not significant (Krause et al., 2010).

In Equation 1, the IHIT Scale, the mediator variable, was regressed on the predictor variable, the NCRS. As noted in Figure 3, results indicated that the NCRS was significantly associated with IHIT (F_{156} = 19.84, p <.001). The NCRS explained 11.3% of the variance in the IHIT scores.

In Equation 2, missed nursing care, the outcome variable, was regressed on the predictor variable, the NCRs. The NCRs was significantly associated with missed nursing care ($F163$ = 5.67, p = .018). The NCRs explained 3.4% of the variance in missed nursing care.

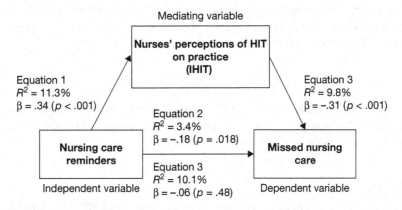

FIGURE 3. Test of the mediation model with regression analyses.

IHIT, impact of health care information technology.

In Equation 3, missed nursing care, the outcome variable, was regressed on the predictor variable, the NCRs, and the mediator variable (IHIT). IHIT negatively affected missed nursing care ($t = -4.12, p < .001$), explaining 9.8% of variance in missed nursing care. With IHIT present, the predictor (NCRs) was no longer significant ($t = -.70, p = .48$). Thus, the reduced direct association between the NCRs and missed nursing care when IHIT was in the model supported the hypothesis that IHIT was at least one of the mediators in the relationship between the NCRs and missed nursing care.

DISCUSSION

Analysis of the mediation results supports the research question that perceptions of the influence of HIT mediates the relationship between reminder use and missed nursing care. Nurses who use the electronic reminders more frequently and have higher perceptions about the impact of HIT on their practice have less missed nursing care than nurses who use the reminders but have neutral or negative perceptions of the impact of HIT.

This is a significant finding because nurses who have more positive perceptions of the impact of HIT on their practice have less missed nursing care than nurses who use the reminders without positive perceptions of their value. This is an important consideration since health care organizations can utilize the IHIT Scale to assess whether or not their nurses have positive perceptions about the technology systems they are required to use. Organizations can then target specific system design or workflow changes to improve nurses' perceptions of the impact of HIT on their practice.

Although the mediating relationship between missed nursing care, perceptions of the impact of HIT, and NCRs had not been previously studied, Dykes et al. (2007) hypothesized that nurses who have positive perceptions of the impact of HIT on their practice would be more likely to use the technology. This hypothesis is supported by the findings from this study. Our findings are similar to previous studies that found that CDSS must be aligned with the nurses' workflow if they are to use the information systems effectively (Choi et al., 2011; Courtney, Alexander, & Demiris, 2008; Piscotty & Kalisch, 2014b; Piscotty & Tzeng, 2011). Saleem et al. (2005) reported that one facilitator to using CDSS by nurses was to integrate the reminders into the nurses' daily clinical workflow.

An alternate explanation for this finding is that nurses who use NCRs already have more positive perceptions of the impacts of HIT on their practice. Nurses who utilize the system may be more accountable and therefore have decreased amounts of missed nursing care to begin with. Organizational or cultural factors may also influence nurses' perceptions of the impact of HIT on their practice.

LIMITATIONS

Limitations included threats to internal and external validity. These threats were addressed through a priori power analysis, using established instruments, and collecting data on multiple nursing units.

CONCLUSIONS

Our study supports that perceptions of the impact of HIT mediates the relationship between nursing care reminder use and missed nursing care. The findings are beneficial to the advancement of health care technology in that designers of HIT systems need to keep in mind that perceptions regarding the impact of the technology will influence usage. Many times, information technology systems are not designed to match the workflow of nurses. Systems built with redundant or impertinent reminders may be ignored. System designers must study which reminders nurses find most useful and which reminders result in the best quality outcomes.

CLINICAL RESOURCES

- The Agency for Healthcare Research and Quality (AHRQ) Patient Safety Network (PSNet) is a national web-based resource featuring the latest news and essential resources on patient safety: http://psnet.ahrq.gov

- The Institute for Healthcare Improvement (IHI) is an independent not-for-profit organization and is a leading innovator, convener, partner, and driver of results in health and health care improvement worldwide: http://www.ihi.org

REFERENCES

Baron, R., & Kenny, D. (1986). The moderator-mediator variable distinction in social psychological research: Conceptual, strategic, and statistical considerations. *Journal of Personality and Social Psychology, 51*(6), 1173–1182.

Bove, L., & Jesse, H. (2010). Worklists: Helping to transform nursing care. *ANIA-CARING Newsletter, 25*(1), 1–7.

Choi, M., Choi, R., Bae, Y., & Lee, S. (2011). Clinical decision support systems for patient safety: A focus group needs assessment with Korean ICU nurses. *Computers, Informatics, Nursing, 29*(11), 671–678.

Courtney, K., Alexander, G., & Demiris, G. (2008). Information technology from novice to expert: Implementation implications. *Journal of Nursing Management, 16*(6), 692–699.

Donabedian, A. (2005). Evaluating the quality of medical care. *Milbank Memorial Fund Quarterly, 83*(4), 691–729, (reprinted from *Milbank Memorial Fund Quarterly, 44*(3), 166–203).

Dykes, P. C., Hurley, A., Cashen, M., Bakken, S., & Duffy, M. E. (2007). Development and psychometric evaluation of the Impact of Health Information Technology (I-HIT) Scale. *Journal of the American Medical Informatics Association, 14*(4), 507–514.

HealtHIT.gov. (n.d.). *EHR incentives & certification: Meaningful use definition and objectives.* Retrieved from http://www.healtHIT.gov/providers-professionals/meaningful-use-definition-objectives.

Kalisch, B. (2006). Missed nursing care: A qualitative study. *Journal of Nursing Care Quality, 21*(4), 306–313.

Kalisch, B., & Xie, B. (2014). Errors of omission: Missed nursing care. *Western Journal of Nursing Research, 36*(7), 875–890.

Kalisch, B., Xie, B., & Ronis, D. L. (2013). Train-the-trainer intervention to increase nursing teamwork and decrease missed nursing care in acute care patient units. *Nursing Research, 62*(6), 405–413.

Kalisch, B. J., Landstrom, G. L., & Hinshaw, A. S. (2009). Missed nursing care: A concept analysis. *Journal of Advanced Nursing, 65*(7), 1509–1517.

Kalisch, B. J., Landstrom, G., & Williams, R. A. (2009). Missed nursing care: Errors of omission. *Nursing Outlook, 57*(1), 3–9.

Kalisch, B. J., & Williams, R. A. (2009). Development and psychometric testing of a tool to measure missed nursing care. *Journal of Nursing Administration, 39*(5), 211–219.

Krause, M., Serlin, R., Ward, S., Rony, R., Ezenwa, M., & Naab, F. (2010). Testing mediation in nursing research: Beyond Baron and Kenny. *Nursing Research, 59*(4), 288–294.

Madison, M., & Staggers, N. (2011). Electronic health records and the implications for nursing practice. *Journal of Nursing Regulation, 1*(4), 54–60.

Piscotty, R., & Kalisch, B. (2014a). Lost opportunities . . . the challenges of "missed nursing care." *Nursing Management, 45*(10), 40–44.

Piscotty, R., & Kalisch, B. (2014b). Nurses' use of clinical decision support: A literature review. *Computers, Informatics, Nursing, 32*(12), 562–568.

Piscotty, R., & Kalisch, B. (2014c). The relationship between electronic nursing care reminders and missed nursing care. *Computers, Informatics, Nursing, 32*(10), 475–481.

Piscotty, R., Kalisch, B., Gracey-Thomas, A., & Yarandi, H. (2015). Electronic nursing care reminders: Implications for nurse leaders. *Journal of Nursing Administration.*

Piscotty, R., & Tzeng, H. (2011). Exploring the clinical information system implementation readiness activities to support nursing in hospital settings. *Computers, Informatics, Nursing, 29*(11), 648–656.

Saleem, J., Patterson, E., Militello, L., Render, M., Orshansky, G., & Asch, S. (2005). Exploring barriers and facilitators to the use of computerized clinical reminders. *Journal of the American Medical Informatics Association, 12*(4), 438–447.

Staggers, N., Weir, C., & Phansalkar, S. (2008). Patient safety and health information technology: Role of the electronic health record. In R. G. Hughes (Ed.), *Patient safety and quality: An evidenced-based handbook for nurses* (pp. 1234–1276). AHRQ Publication No. 08–0043. Rockville, MD: Agency for Healthcare Research and Quality.

IMPACT OF HEALTH CARE INFORMATION TECHNOLOGY ON NURSING PRACTICE

Critique by *Elizabeth A. Madigan*

OVERALL SUMMARY

Health care information technology (HIT) is increasingly used in organizations to improve patient care. This quantitative study utilizes Donabedian's (2005) structure, process, and outcome model to examine how nurses' perceptions of the impact of HIT on their practice influences not only how fully the technology is adopted and used but the frequency of missed nursing care. Utilizing a variety of research instruments for data collection, study findings are particularly relevant for nurses who continue to be challenged by technology systems that increase, rather than improve, their workflow, which reduces the likelihood of disregarding electronic nursing care reminders.

TITLE

Does the title include the key concepts/variables/ phenomenon of interest?

A good title is difficult as the title needs to convey the key concepts in very few words. The title for this manuscript is very broad and could have been improved by including the words "missed nursing care." The authors may have had good reasons to not include this wording. For example, they may not have wanted to limit readers who were looking for the broader approach.

Is it concise (12 words or less) and professionally stated?

The title is concise, nine words, and is professionally stated.

RESEARCHER(S) CREDIBILITY

Educational credentials?

Both the first and second authors are PhD-prepared nurses and nursing faculty at academic institutions.

Prior methodological research experience of the authors (i.e., methodological expertise)?

A review of the reference list indicates that the authors have published on this topic; however, a full determination of methodological expertise would require reading or at least reviewing these cited articles.

Subject matter content experience (prior research on the subject matter)?

A review of the reference list indicates that the authors have published other articles on this topic, indicating that they have content expertise.

ABSTRACT

Does it include the key components (objective/aim, background/rationale, methods, results, and conclusion)?

The key components are present and the headings are in bold, making it easy for the reader to follow the abstract. The abstract for research studies is sometimes the most important part of the manuscript as abstracts are the first-level decision for inclusion in other work (e.g., manuscripts, grant applications). Yet many novice authors do not pay as much attention or focus on the quality of the abstract as compared to the body of the paper.

Does or does not include references?

The abstract does not include references.

Is it concise (150–250 words or less)?

This abstract is 354 words long. Although this is longer than general guidelines, journal requirements are what the authors needed to follow. In addition, when viewed on PubMed, the entire 354 words are present.

Does it entice you to read the rest of the article (interesting)?

The abstract is interesting in that it identifies "missed nursing care" as a key concept, which is a safety issue. The authors do well at identifying what they were testing: whether health information technology reminder usage and missed nursing care was mediated by the impact of technology on nursing practice. Mediation, as a conceptual and statistical concept, can be difficult to explain. The authors did well with explaining this in relatively plain language in the abstract.

INTRODUCTION/PROBLEM

Is the research problem or phenomenon of interest clearly stated?

The authors begin their article by identifying the current state of practice where nurses need to balance safe and high-quality care with efficiency and cost-effectiveness. Later on, the authors make a compelling case for safe nursing care that includes the elements that compromise "missed nursing care." They specify what these elements are under the heading missed nursing care and tie these missed nursing care tasks to patient safety. Thus, they tie their research phenomenon with patient safety.

Is it succinct?

The introduction and purpose statement appear in the third paragraph. This early placement is important so that the reader can follow the rest of the introductory parts of the article.

Does it answer the "so what" question?

The introduction identifies safe and high-quality patient care in a number of places in the introduction but does so without being repetitive. The argument is logically developed.

RESEARCH AIMS/OBJECTIVES

Is the research aim/objective clearly stated?

The authors do well on the study purpose as this is a further analysis of work that has already been published. This is not "salami slicing" or duplicate publication.

Instead they are testing the concept of the mediator and they provide a hypothesis on what they expect to find. Because mediation is not intuitive for those unfamiliar with the concept and approach, it is important that the hypothesis is presented.

Is it concisely written?

The study purpose is concise. The purpose and the explanation of the mediation are captured in one paragraph.

Does it follow logically from the research problem/phenomenon of interest?

There is a very logical flow. One way to determine this is to read the background material and then try to anticipate what the study purpose is. The authors do well at carrying their theme from the abstract through all the introductory material.

SIGNIFICANCE
Is the significance to nursing and health care clearly written?

The key is patient safety and high-quality care, recognizing the challenges that hospital nurses face and how technology needs to be part of the workflow and not an add-on. The significance to nursing and health care is evident.

Does the significance follow from the research aim/objective?

The significance is not a specific section in this article but the significance argument is easy to find.

BACKGROUND
Is there an explicit description of a theoretical perspective or conceptual framework? If not, is it implied?

There is a conceptual framework present and it has a heading, making it easy to find. The authors selected and used the Structure, Process and Outcomes Model of Healthcare Quality (Donabedian, 2005), which is a seminal theory. The authors make explicit how their study concepts are derived from the model. They present Figure 1, which includes the mediation concept that they are testing and identify the relationships being tested by each aim. This is well done and easy to follow. For a study testing mediation, they present Figure 2, which, in conjunction with the text, helps the reader to understand what the potential mediating variable is.

Are there clear theoretical/conceptual definitions of the concepts?

This is particularly well done in this article as Table 1 presents the variables (noting which are independent and which is dependent), the conceptual definitions and the empirical indicators. This level of detail is helpful for the reader who is less experienced at research but benefits all readers who do not need to try to infer understanding of what is being tested.

LITERATURE REVIEW
Primary sources only?

Only primary sources were used.

Current (within the past how many years)?

> The oldest reference was nine years old but was a seminal work on missed nursing care. The inclusion of this reference was appropriate. The other references are most recent, most within the five years prior to the publication date.

Is the search strategy included?

> The search strategy was not identified nor was the source of the search (e.g., which databases were used).

Is literature relevant to the research aims/objectives?

> The literature cited was relevant to the aims and the concepts under study. Although it was brief (four paragraphs), the reader was given sufficient detail to understand the science that drove the present study.

Is it chronologically presented (old to current)?

> The extant research was presented conceptually by the major concepts rather than chronologically. The presentation order was appropriate here as the explanation of the existing research had a logical flow and went from the broad (e.g., meaningful use, the electronic health record [EHR] as an example of meaningful use, adoption of the EHR) to specific discussion of clinical decision support systems (CDSS). Using a chronological explanation of the science here would have resulted in a choppy flow.

Is it comprehensive? If not, is sufficient background literature provided?

> The literature was sufficiently comprehensive to allow the reader to understand what is known in this area and what is unknown.

RATIONALE FOR THE STUDY

Is there a gap in the literature that this study will fill (will it extend prior knowledge)? Is the rationale clearly stated?

> The last sentence of the section discussing the first concept (electronic nursing care reminders) identifies that the research is needed to ensure accuracy and quality improvement. The gap in knowledge is not explicitly stated but can be easily inferred.

Is this a follow-up or replication study?

> This is a study that uses existing data to test a new hypothesis (e.g., the mediation).

RESEARCH QUESTION(S) AND/OR HYPOTHESES

Are these explicitly and clearly stated?

> The research question is clearly stated in the last paragraph prior to the literature review, where the study purpose is stated. The authors also include a directional hypothesis and explain the rationale behind the hypothesis.

Do they include the variables/phenomenon of interest?

> The variables of interest are included in the research question and match clearly with the conceptual framework figure.

Do they follow from the research aim/objective?

> There is clear and logical flow from the study introduction through the literature review and the conceptual model. The conceptual model drives the research questions.

METHODS
Research Design/Paradigm
Is the research design clearly stated?

> The use of a descriptive cross-sectional design is explicitly stated in the first paragraph under the heading "Design, Sample, and Setting." Are all sections referred to within quotes in each chapter?

Is there consistency between the research design and paradigm?

> The quantitative research design is consistent with the positivist paradigm that reality can be known and relationships among variables can be empirically verified.

Is this the best choice of design to address the research problem/phenomenon of interest?

> Considering the state of existing knowledge on this topic, using a descriptive cross-sectional design is appropriate. It would be premature to use a randomized clinical trial or randomized cluster trial (e.g., randomizing the units instead of the nurses) as there is not sufficient descriptive information on whether nurses' perceptions of the influence of HIT has an impact. A longitudinal design would be appropriate for future studies if the investigators wanted to examine whether the introduction of EHRs or CDSS had an influence on missed nursing care, but that is outside the scope of the present study.

Is there rigor in the design?

> Because the research design choice is correct there is rigor in the selection.

SETTING
Is the setting clearly described?

> The setting is clearly described, including the location of the hospital geographically. This information is important because of the potential of regional variation in exposure to EHRs or CDSS.

What biases are introduced as a result of selecting this particular setting?

> The biases are the inability to generalize outside this hospital and this type of hospital. This is one of the trade-offs made when performing research—the use of one hospital limits generalizability to community hospitals (in this case), but the benefit is that there is one EHR in use (versus comparing different systems) and the CDSS is going to be the same within the organization (versus different customized CDSS).

SAMPLING PLAN AND SAMPLE
Is the sampling plan clearly identified?

> The use of a convenience sampling plan is clearly stated. Inclusion and exclusion criteria are reasonable and rationale was provided for exclusions.

Does it represent the population of interest?

> The population of interest is staff nurses with direct patient care and the inclusion criteria specify these nurses.

Is the sampling plan consistent with the research aim/objective?

> There is consistency between the convenience sample and research aim focused on understanding whether the nurses' perception of the impact of HIT on their

practice mediates the relationship between nursing care reminder use and missed nursing care.

Is the sample size sufficient (e.g., power analysis or data saturation)?

There was no power analysis presented so the reader was unable to determine the intended sample size (determined a priori) or whether the actual sample size met the requirement for the number of subjects. This information would have been helpful for future research into this area, particularly effect size where the need for more precise information is helpful. There is a statement at the end that a priori power analysis was done to limit the threats to internal and external validity so the reader had to infer that the power information is contained in prior articles from this study.

VARIABLES

Are variables clearly identified?
Are variables operationally defined and consistent with theoretical concepts?
Are independent and dependent variables identified, if applicable?

Table 1 provides a useful overview of the variables, including which are independent and which is dependent, their conceptual definition and their empirical indicators. This was particularly well done and is not always presented this clearly in other research reports.

METHOD OF DATA COLLECTION

What are the methods of data collection?

Data were collected via an online survey that the nurses responded to. The description of how this was sent to the nurses was provided and was easy to follow.

Are validity and reliability clearly addressed for prior research and current study, if applicable?

There is no explicit detail on the reliability and validity of each instrument but there are references for each instrument. This information is helpful but it would have been beneficial to include at least some information regarding the reliability and validity. The authors may have faced journal requirements limiting the amount of text that they could present and may have chosen to focus on other areas instead.

Do the measures/instruments address the underlying theoretical concepts or phenomenon of interest?

There is congruency between the measures and the concepts.

Were human rights protected?

There is an explicit statement regarding human subjects' approval.

Are other ethical issues identified?

There is a statement that the surveys were anonymous and no identifying information was included. This is important for research with employees who may feel coerced to respond or who may respond more honestly if the information is anonymous.

Is the data-collection method appropriate for research design?

The data collection is appropriate for the descriptive, cross-sectional design. Although readers often want more detailed information (i.e., interviews or focus groups to obtain more details), the study design was appropriate to lay the groundwork on whether nurse perceptions mediate the relationship between nursing care reminders and missed nursing care.

Is there bias in data collection?

There is bias in all data collection. The researcher's job is to recognize and minimize the bias. In this study, there was a 1-month data-collection period although the time of year was not stated. This information may be relevant, as during certain times of a year there may be lower response rates (e.g., December holidays).

What is the fidelity of intervention addressed, if applicable?

Not applicable.

DATA ANALYSIS

Are data analysis techniques described (e.g., statistical tests, methodology for qualitative analysis)?

The authors do very well at describing the analysis for both the descriptive as well as the tests of mediation. Mediation can be a difficult process to explain and the authors provide Figure 3 and the text is explicit. A reader unfamiliar with mediation using regression analysis would be able to follow this explanation.

Does the analysis answer the research question?

The analysis tests the mediation effect and finds that there is indeed mediation from the nurses' perceptions on the relationship between nursing care reminders and missed nursing care.

Is it appropriate?

The analysis was appropriate and the authors cite the source of their approach to mediation.

Is the analysis comprehensive? Are themes identified?

The analysis was comprehensive with the themes identified in the results and discussion sections. Nurses' positive perceptions about the technology they use significantly affect missed nursing care.

Is there bias in the analysis (trustworthiness? credibility?)?

There is no reason to suspect bias in the analysis. Results are reported on each measure and the mediation analysis is detailed. Figure 3 illustrates each step of the mediation analysis, again providing the reader with the information necessary to understand the results. The authors report that they examined the assumptions for multiple regression; this level of detail is common in research reports where most articles do not get into specific details unless they had to make some kind of adjustment based on not meeting the assumptions for the statistical analysis.

RESULTS

Are sample characteristics described and fully reported?

The sample characteristics are sufficiently clear to give the reader an understanding of the nurses responding to the surveys. The response rate is reported (69.1%), which provides information for the reader to use to understand how the response rate may influence the confidence in the findings. There is no "magic" response rate and while researchers may want 100% response, a 69% response rate to a web-based survey is reasonable.

Are findings presented related to research aim/objective?

The findings on the mediation analysis are presented in a clear way, are detailed and explain the results.

Are all outcome variables addressed, if applicable?

There was only one outcome variable, missed nursing care, and it was addressed.

Are results clearly presented in text and/or tables/figures?

The authors provide both Figure 3 and text on the mediation analysis. This was helpful information for the reader to follow along with the three regression equations needed to evaluate mediation analysis.

Is significance of results reported, if applicable?

Statistical significance of each step in the regression analysis was reported as were the R^2 and the standardized regression coefficients.

DISCUSSION OF RESULTS

Do the authors link the findings to previous research studies?

The authors link their findings to previous studies in the third paragraph under Discussion. Their study findings are consistent with past research, which indicates that nurses' positive perceptions of the impact of HIT on their practice and CDSS aligned with their workflow make it more likely that information systems will be used effectively.

Are the conclusions comprehensive, yet within the data?

The discussion is sufficiently comprehensive and does not go beyond the data. The authors also provide an alternative explanation for the findings in the fourth paragraph under Discussion, which provides important context for the findings.

Do the authors interpret the results in the discussion?

The interpretation of the results is presented in the first and second paragraphs of the discussion. The interpretation is clear and follows from the Results section.

Are the findings generalizable or transferable?

There is nothing explicit in the discussion about the generalizability of findings.

LIMITATIONS

Identified? Accurate? Inclusive?

Very limited and generic information is presented on the limitations. More details would have been helpful for the reader who looks to the limitations section of existing studies to help avoid challenges and problems faced by prior investigators and investigations.

IMPLICATIONS
Are there implications for practice, education, research?
Are there implications for clinical significance?

> The journal requires a section called Clinical Resources, which is provided but there is no section specific to the implications for clinical significance, practice, education, and research.

RECOMMENDATIONS
Recommendations for future study/study replication?

> There is no specific section that identifies future studies that need to be done. This may have been helpful to guide future research but the space limitations may have prevented the authors from providing this kind of detail.

CONCLUSION
Is it succinct and does it tie everything together?

> The conclusion is well done—succinct, ties the introductory section, literature review, and study purpose back to the results and makes recommendations on how to improve the electronic nursing reminder systems to improve patient care. This is a strong close.

GERIATRIC NURSING HOME FALLS: A SINGLE INSTITUTION CROSS-SECTIONAL STUDY

8

Isadora Botwinick
Montefiore Medical Center, Albert Einstein College of Medicine and Jacobi
Medical Center, Department of Surgery, 111 East 210th Street, Bronx, NY
10467, United States

Joshua H. Johnson
Albert Einstein College of Medicine, 1300 Morris Park Avenue, Bronx, NY 10461, United States

Saman Safadjou
Albert Einstein College of Medicine and Jacobi Medical Center, Department of Surgery, 1400 Pelham
Parkway South, Bronx, NY 10461, United States

Wayne Cohen-Levy
Albert Einstein College of Medicine, 1300 Morris Park Avenue, Bronx, NY 10461, United States

Srinivas H. Reddy
Albert Einstein College of Medicine and Jacobi Medical Center, Department of Surgery, 1400 Pelham
Parkway South, Bronx, NY 10461, United States

John McNelis
Albert Einstein College of Medicine and Jacobi Medical Center, Department of Surgery, 1400 Pelham
Parkway South, Bronx, NY 10461, United States

Sheldon H. Teperman
Albert Einstein College of Medicine and Jacobi Medical Center, Department of Surgery, 1400 Pelham
Parkway South, Bronx, NY 10461, United States

Melvin E. Stone, Jr.
Albert Einstein College of Medicine and Jacobi Medical Center, Department of Surgery, 1400 Pelham
Parkway South, Bronx, NY 10461, United States

ABSTRACT

Background: Falls are the leading cause of fatal injury in geriatric patients. Nursing
home falls occur at twice the rate of community falls, yet few studies have compared
these groups. We hypothesized that nursing home residents admitted for fall would be
sicker than their community counterparts on presentation and have worse outcomes.

Botwinick, I., Johnson, J. H., Safadjou, S., Cohen-Levy, W., Reddy, S. H., McNelis, J., . . . Stone, M. E., Jr.
(2016). Geriatric nursing home falls: A single institution cross-sectional study. *Archives of Gerontology and
Geriatrics, 63,* 43–48. doi:10.1016/j.archger.2015.12.002. Reprinted with permission from Elsevier.

Methods: Records of 1,708 patients, age 65 years and older with a documented nursing home status, admitted to our center between 2008 and 2012 were reviewed. Clinical data including injury severity score (ISS), admission Glasgow Coma Scale (GCS), in-hospital complications, length of stay (LOS), and in-hospital mortality were collected. Continuous data were analyzed using Mann–Whitney tests and categorical data using Fisher exact tests. Variables in the univariate tests were analyzed in a multivariate logistic regression.

Results: Nursing home patients were older than community patients, presented with lower GCS, lower hemoglobin, higher international normalized ratio (INR) and a higher percentage of patients with body mass index (BMI) <18.5. LOS for nursing home patients was longer, and they suffered higher rates of in-hospital complications. ISS, rates of traumatic brain injury (TBI), operative intervention and mortality were not significantly different. In a multivariate logistic regression, ISS, GCS, and age, but not nursing home status, were significant predictors of in-hospital mortality.

Conclusions: In comparison to their community counterparts, nursing home patients presenting after fall are more debilitated and have increased morbidity as evidenced by more in-house complications and increased LOS. However, nursing home residency was not a significant predictor of mortality.

KEYWORDS: fall; nursing home; in-hospital mortality

BACKGROUND

One in every three adults older than 65 years of age will fall each year, making falls a significant problem in the geriatric population (Tromp et al., 2001). In addition to being the leading cause of traumatic brain injury (TBI) and bony fracture, falls are the leading cause of fatal injuries in the elderly (Rubenstein, Josephson, & Robbins, 1994). Consequently, geriatric falls result in significant cost to the United States health care system. In the year 2000, $12 billion was spent on hospitalizations for adults over 65 years of age who fell (Stevens, Corso, Finkelstein, & Miller, 2006). As the elderly population grows in the United States, this financial burden continues to increase with geriatric falls exacting $30 billion in 2010 in direct medical costs (Stevens et al., 2006). Nursing home falls occur at twice the rate of community falls, causing further disability in an already dependent population (Rubenstein et al., 1994). However, it remains unclear if the more dependent nursing home population has different outcomes when compared to their community counterparts. While there are multiple studies focusing on fall risk and prevention in both community and nursing home patients, surprisingly, there is scant literature that directly compares the post-fall outcomes of these two disparate populations. The aim of our study was to directly compare the outcomes between elderly patients who fall in the nursing home and their community counterparts after presentation to a Level 1 trauma center. We hypothesized that nursing home residents admitted for a fall would have more comorbidities and would present with greater physiologic derangements than their community counterparts on presentation and would therefore have worse outcomes—specifically, in regards to mortality and complication rate.

METHODS

We obtained institutional review board (IRB) approval for a cross-sectional study. We included all patients age 65 years or older who presented after a fall, for whom information on nursing home status was available. If we could not clearly identify whether a patient was living in the community or in a nursing home, then that patient was excluded from the study. The trauma registry was queried to identify all ground level fall patients age 65 years and older who presented to Jacobi Medical Center, a Level 1 trauma facility, from 2008 to 2012. Patient clinical characteristics at admission were then collected after review of the medical chart. Clinical data collected included: age, sex, body mass index (BMI), injury severity score (ISS), admission Glasgow Coma Score (GCS), along with admission systolic blood pressure (SBP) and hemoglobin. We chose to analyze BMI, GCS, and international normalized ratio (INR) in a dichotomous fashion to emphasize the most relevant parameters: those which would be considered "abnormal" by a practicing clinician. For BMI, we chose 18.5 because this is defined as underweight by the National Institutes of Health (NIH). We chose GCS <15 because we felt that any alteration in mental status was a clinically relevant finding. We chose an INR >1.2 because this is considered abnormal by our laboratory standards and might merit clinical investigation and possible treatment if an invasive procedure were planned. Additionally, platelet count and coagulation parameters at admission were also collected. Outcome data of interest included: in-hospital complications, including transfusion requirements, length of stay (LOS), operative intervention, and in-hospital mortality. Patient comorbidities and in-hospital complications were based on those defined by the National Trauma Data Bank (NTDB). Comorbidities included: alcoholism, bleeding disorder, chronic renal failure, congestive heart failure, current smoker, cancer and/or chemotherapy, cerebrovascular incident, dementia, diabetes, drug abuse, history of myocardial infarction, hypertension, obesity, respiratory disease, and steroid use. In-hospital complications included: acute kidney injury (AKI), *Clostridium difficile* colitis, sepsis, decubiti, deep vein thrombosis, respiratory failure (defined as tracheotomy and/or need for mechanical ventilation), and urinary tract infections. TBI on presentation was also included as a post-fall outcome variable. TBI was strictly defined as any patient with CT findings of intracranial hemorrhage upon admission. The total cohort was then divided into two groups for comparison: nursing home and community patients. A nursing home patient was defined as a patient residing in nursing home at the time of the fall; community patients were defined as all patients not residing in a nursing home at the time of the fall. Continuous nonparametric data and categorical data were analyzed using Mann–Whitney test and Fisher's exact test, respectively. In order to identify variables independently associated with mortality, a multivariate logistic regression analysis was performed using variables in the univariate analysis with p <.02; in addition, nursing home residency (yes/ no) and ISS were included. Statistical significance for all analyses was set at p <.05. Inclusion criteria are shown in Figure 1. In total, 1,765 fall patients were identified, of which 1,708 patients had nursing home status data available. These 1,708 patients were included in the univariate analysis. For the multivariate analysis, only patients with complete data for each of the variables were included, for a total of 1,296 patients.

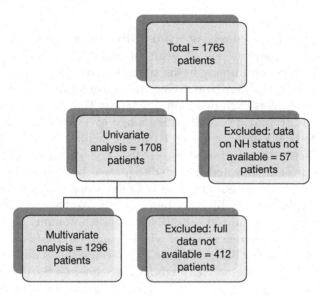

FIGURE 1. Inclusion by analysis.

NH, nursing home.

RESULTS

In the 5-year study period, 1,765 patients 65 and older (age range 65–102 years) were admitted to our institution for ground level fall. Of the total cohort included in the analysis, 9.5% (163/1,708) were nursing home residents. Clinical data and patient characteristics are shown in Tables 1 through 4. Nursing home patients were older than community patients, and presented with lower SBP, lower hemoglobin, and higher INR (Table 1). The percentage of patients with an abnormal GCS on presentation was significantly higher in the nursing home group, as was the percentage of patients who had a BMI less than 18.5. ISS was not significantly different between both groups, nor was the rate of TBI. Additionally, there was no difference in the need for an operative intervention between the two groups; frequency of specific fall-associated injuries such as operative hip fractures were not significantly different either.

Individual comorbidities are shown in Table 2. Nursing home patients had significantly higher rates of cerebrovascular disease and dementia, while community patients had a slightly higher rate of diabetes when compared to the nursing home cohort. Our Trauma Registry is not currently designed to collect all data required for a Charlson comorbidity score, but based on our results as shown in Tables 1 and 2, we calculated an average Charlson comorbidity score for the nursing home patients at 5.2 compared to an average score of 4.8 for the community patients. Outcome data are shown in Tables 3 and 4. Median LOS was one day longer in nursing home patients compared to community patients. As mentioned, admission GCS was lower for the nursing home group; however, the incidence of TBI on presentation was similar between both groups. Nursing home patients also had a significantly higher overall rate of complications.

Individual complication rates are shown in Table 4. Patients from nursing homes had significantly higher rates of pneumonia, sepsis, unplanned intubation, and urinary tract infections, when compared to patients admitted from home. However, LOS in intensive care was similar between groups.

Notably, in-hospital mortality was not significantly different between the two groups. In the logistic regression model of the total cohort (Table 5) ISS, admission GCS, SBP, and age were significant independent predictors of in-hospital mortality after fall. Odds ratio for in-hospital mortality was lower with increasing SBP and higher admission GCS, while odds ratio for mortality was higher with increased age and ISS. BMI, hemoglobin, and nursing residency status were not significant independent predictors of mortality. Only patients for whom complete data were available were included in the multivariate analysis; Table 6 demonstrates that the subsets of nursing home and community patients included in the multivariate analysis were not significantly different from the cohorts included in the univariate analysis.

TABLE 1. Clinical Data and Baseline Characteristics

	Nursing Home *n* = 163 Patients	Community *n* = 1,545 Patients	Total Cohort *n*	*P* value
Age	84 (76–90)	80 (73–87)	80 (73–87)	.0002
Male gender	48 (29%)	471 (30%)	519 (30%)	NS
ISS	9 (4–9)	8 (4–9)	9 (4–9)	NS
GCS <15	45 (36%)	196 (15%)	241 (17%)	<.0001
BMI <18.5	16 (13%)	80 (6%)	96 (7%)	.01
Temperature	97.2 (96.4–98)	97.2 (96.6–98)	97.2 (96.6–98)	NS
Heart rate	86 (73–96)	82 (71–95)	82 (71–95)	NS
SBP	147 (127–165)	153 (138–172)	153 (136–171)	.002
Hemoglobin	11.7 (10.7–13)	12.4 (11.4–13.5)	12.3 (11.3–13.5)	<.0001
INR >1.2	21 (17%)	133 (11%)	154 (11%)	.03
PTT	24.3 (22.7–22.7)	24.4 (22.5–26.5)	240 (191–289)	NS
Platelet count	250 (196–305)	239 (189–287)	240 (191–289)	NS
Drugs/alcohol use	2 (1.2%)	24 (1.6%)	26 (1.5%)	NS

BMI, body mass index; GCS, Glasgow coma score; INR, international normalized ratio; ISS, injury severity score; NS, nonsignificant; PTT, partial thromboplastin time; SBP, systolic blood pressure. Data reported as median or number of patients with interquartile range or percentage of total patients shown in parentheses.

TABLE 2. Patient Comorbidities

	Nursing Home *n* = 163	Community *n* = 1,545	Total Cohort *n* = 1,708	*P* value
Alcoholism	9 (5.5%)	99 (6.4%)	108 (6.3%)	NS
Bleeding disorder	4 (2.3%)	71 (4.6%)	75 (4.4%)	NS

(continued)

TABLE 2. Patient Comorbidities (*continued*)

	Nursing Home *n* = 163	Community *n* = 1,545	Total Cohort *n* = 1,708	*P* value
Chronic renal failure	5 (3.1%)	31 (2%)	36 (2.1%)	NS
Congestive heart failure	23 (14.1%)	165 (10.7%)	188 (11%)	NS
Current smoker	4 (2.5%)	94 (6.1%)	98 (5.7%)	NS
Cerebrovascular incident	30 (18.4%)	189 (12.2%)	219 (12.8%)	.035
Dementia	77 (47.2%)	242 (15.7%)	319 (18.7%)	<.0001
Diabetes	36 (22.1%)	467 (30%)	503 (29.4%)	.03
Cancer/ chemotherapy	4 (2.5%)	26 (1.7%)	30 (1.8%)	NS
Drug abuse	2 (12%)	15 (0.97%)	17 (1.0%)	NS
History of myocardial infarction	14 (8.6%)	101 (6.5%)	115 (6.7%)	NS
Hypertension	107 (65.6%)	1046 (67.7%)	1153 (67.5%)	NS
Obesity	3 (1.8%)	48 (3.1%)	51 (3.0%)	NS
Respiratory disease	14 (8.6%)	189 (12.2%)	203 (11.9%)	NS
Steroid use	2 (1.2%)	27 (1.7%)	29 (1.7%)	NS

Data reported as median or number of patients with interquartile range or percentage of total patients shown in parentheses. NS, nonsignificant.

TABLE 3. Post-Fall Outcomes

	Nursing Home	Community	Total Cohort	*P* value
LOS	6 (3–10)	5 (3–9)	5 (3–9)	.03
Complications	53 (32.5%)	313 (20.3%)	366 (21.4%)	.0006
TBI	16 (9.8%)	155 (10.0%)	171 (10.0%)	NS
Operative intervention	49 (30.0%)	539 (34.9%)	588 (34.4%)	NS
In-hospital mortality	9 (5.5%)	55 (3.6%)	64 (3.7%)	NS
New nursing home placement	–	569 (36.8%)		–

Data reported as median or number of patients with interquartile range or percentage of total patients shown in parentheses.

LOS, length of stay; NS, nonsignificant; TBI, traumatic brain injury.

DISCUSSION

These data show that nursing home patients who fall are significantly more debilitated than their community counterparts on admission. Not surprisingly, nursing home falls are associated with worse outcomes, including increased complication rates and prolonged LOS, when compared to geriatric falls in the community. However, this study did not show a difference in mortality between nursing home falls and community falls among patients age 65 and older. Several findings in our study support the notion that nursing home patients are significantly more debilitated on presentation after a fall than their community counterparts, and therefore, have worse outcomes. First and foremost, the nursing home patients were simply older than the community patients, and the literature is replete with evidence that increased age is associated with poorer outcomes following injury (Bergeron et al., 2006). With this increased age one might expect more underlying dementia and cognitive deficits. Indeed, we found a higher incidence of dementia associated with the nursing home group. Additionally, prior studies suggest that underlying dementia can impact the admission GCS score; for example, a patient may be unable to follow commands at baseline secondary to chronic cognitive impairment, resulting in a lower GCS score (Panisset, Saxton, & Boller, 1995; Sporer et al., 2013). Arguably, a lower GCS would be suggestive of TBI; however, the rate of TBI was similar between nursing home and community patients. We hypothesize that decreased GCS likely represents a lower level of premorbid cognitive function. While dementia per se may not be directly associated with poor outcomes, it certainly might affect discharge disposition. For example, cognitively impaired patients are more likely to be discharged to long-term rehabilitation or nursing homes than discharged to home (Luppa et al., 2010).

TABLE 4. Individual In-Hospital Complications

	Nursing Home $n = 163$	Community $n = 1,545$	Total Cohort	P value
AKI	13 (8.0%)	99 (6.4%)	112 (6.6%)	NS
C. *difficile* colitis	4 (2.5%)	13 (0.8%)	17 (1.0%)	NS
Decubitus	5 (3%)	23 (1.5%)	28 (1.6%)	NS
Deep vein thrombosis	2 (1.2%)	28 (1.8%)	30 (1.8%)	NS
Myocardial infarction	1 (0.6%)	30 (1.9%)	31 (1.8%)	NS
Pneumonia	21 (12.9%)	85 (5.5%)	106 (6.2%)	.0009
Respiratory failure	5 (3%)	20 (1.3%)	25 (1.5%)	NS
Sepsis	11 (6.7%)	22 (1.4%)	33 (1.9%)	.0001
Unplanned intubation	13 (8%)	61 (3.9%)	74 (4.3%)	.0243
Urinary tract infection	23 (14%)	114 (7.4%)	137 (8.0%)	.0056
Transfusion	132 (19%)	233 (15%)	365 (21.4%)	NS

Data reported as median or number of patients with interquartile range or percentage of total patients shown in parentheses.

AKI, acute kidney injury. NS, nonsignificant.

TABLE 5. Logistic Regression Analysis of Factors Associated with in-Hospital Mortality

Risk Factor	Odds Ratio	Lower 95%	Upper 95%	P value
Age	1.0018	1.0006	1.0030	.003
ISS	1.0069	1.0052	1.0086	p <.0001
BMI	1	0.9984	1.0020	NS
Hemoglobin	1	0.9902	1.0022	NS
Nursing home vs. community	1	0.9676	1.0389	NS
GCS score	0.9616	0.9553	0.9679	p <.0001
SBP	0.9996	0.9993	1.0000	.04

BMI, body mass index; GCS, Glasgow Coma Score; ISS, injury severity score; NS, nonsignificant; SBP, systolic blood pressure.

Nursing home patients were significantly more likely to have BMIs less than 18.5. Low BMI can be a surrogate marker for being underweight and undernourished. The World Health Organization (WHO) defines a healthy body weight range as a BMI between 18.5 and 24.9 (Winter, MacInnis, Wattanapenpaiboon, & Nowson, 2014). A recent meta-analysis showed that low BMI is associated with poor outcomes—in particular, all-cause mortality—for adults older than 65 years of age with a BMI <23 (Woodman, Ferrucci, & Guralnik, 2005). Moreover, anemia and undernourishment and/or low BMI are sometimes related (Woodman et al., 2005); not unexpectedly, the nursing home group was more anemic than the community group. Anemia is common in the elderly population, affecting over 10% of patients older than 65 years old (Beghe, Wilson, & Ershler, 2004; Woodman et al., 2005). Several studies suggest that anemia both predisposes patients to falls, and predicts post-fall mortality (Al Tehewy, Amin, & Nassar, 2015; Beghe et al., 2004; Hannan, Mendeloff, Farrell, Cayten, & Murphy, 1995). In sum, anemia and low BMI could indicate underlying conditions that predispose the nursing home patient to more in-hospital complications and prolonged LOS.

SBP and INR were slightly lower and higher, respectively, in the nursing home patients than in the community group; however, it is unclear whether these factors contributed significantly to poorer outcomes in nursing home patients. There was no significant difference in transfusion requirements between groups, so it is unlikely that the lower blood pressure is the result of traumatic blood loss and subsequent hypovolemia. It may be the case that this difference only represents improved adherence to blood pressure medication regimens in the nursing home patients (Hughes & Goldie, 2009). The slight difference in INR could be attributed to several factors, which include more nursing home patients on anticoagulation, more nursing home patient compliance with anticoagulation regimens, a higher rate of hepatic synthetic function abnormalities among older and debilitated nursing home patients, or diet changes in the nursing home. Again, given that the transfusion requirement was similar between both groups, this slight difference in INR does not seem to be clinically significant or to have played a large role in outcome differences between both groups.

The nursing home group had a longer LOS overall, but did not have a significantly longer ICU stay, which might suggest that the extra days spent in the hospital were

TABLE 6. Comparison of Univariate and Multivariate Data Set

	Univariate NH	Multivariate NH	*P* value	Univariate Community	Multivariate Community	*P* value
Age	84 (76–90)	85 (76–91)	NS	80 (73–87)	80 (73–87)	NS
ISS	9 (4–9)	9 (4–10)	NS	8 (4–9)	9 (4–9)	NS
BMI	16 (13.0%)	14 (13.9%)	NS	80 (6.4%)	73 (6.6%)	NS
Hemoglobin	11.7 (10.7–13)	11.8 (10.8–13)	NS	12.4 (11.4–13.5)	12.4 (11.4–13.5)	NS
GCS	45 (36%)	39 (33.9%)	NS	196 (15.9%)	185 (15.7%)	NS
SBP	147 (127–165)	147 (129–165)	NS	153 (138–172)	153 (137–172)	NS

Data reported as median or number of patients with interquartile range or percentage of total patients shown in parentheses. NS, nonsignificant.

not necessarily related to higher injury acuity on presentation. However, nursing home patients did have a higher rate of in-hospital complications, which may also account for the prolonged LOS relative to community patients. Additionally, in our institution's experience, discharge back to a nursing home facility is usually easier and less time consuming for the nursing home patient who already has an established bed/space—as opposed to the "fresh" community patient who now needs to fulfill new financial and logistical requirements for disposition to a nursing home which can prolong the hospital stay. This reality lends more support to the assumption that more in-hospital complications may have played a significant role in prolonged LOS in the nursing home group. That said, relative to other published data, our LOS for fall patients was relatively short; a recent study demonstrated an average LOS of 14 days for patients older than 70 years of age who presented after a fall (Close et al., 2012). Regardless, of cause or amount, most will agree any increase in LOS remains an undesirable outcome. Billions of dollars are spent on hospitalization for adults older than 65 years of age who fall; and hospital admission is a significantly more costly expenditure than outpatient and emergency room care for fall-related incidents (Stevens, Corso, Finkelstein, & Miller, 2006).

Pneumonia, sepsis, urinary tract infection, and unplanned intubation were the specific in-hospital complications which were more frequent in the nursing home group. These particular complications can have a significant negative impact on patient prognosis. A large retrospective study of over 5,000 trauma patients recently demonstrated that development of a urinary tract infection, one of the most common complications noted in this study, is associated with increased mortality, particularly in older patients (Monaghan et al., 2011). Hospital-acquired pneumonia, another common complication for the nursing home group, is also known to increase mortality among elderly patients who have been admitted after a fall (Siracuse et al., 2012).

Interestingly, despite being more debilitated with more in-hospital complications—in particular, complications that are associated with higher mortality—the nursing home group was found to have the same in-hospital mortality as the community group.

At first glance, this finding appears counter-intuitive and difficult to reconcile— how does the more debilitated nursing home group have the same mortality rate as the community group? The answer to this question may be explained by the low ISS scores found in both cohorts. Our multivariate analysis did demonstrate that ISS was an independent risk factor for mortality and ISS has been shown to have a positive correlation with mortality—in short, higher ISS scores are associated with higher mortality (Baker, O'Neill, Haddon, & Long, 1974). However, both patient groups, nursing home and community, had very low and similar ISS scores (medians of 9 and 8, respectively). Therefore, not surprisingly, both groups had similar—and relatively low—mortality rates of 6% and 4%, respectively. Additionally, it is important to note that while ISS was an independent predictor for mortality, nursing home residency did not predict mortality in the regression model.

While nursing home residency did not predict mortality, we did identify several variables in the regression analysis which were independently associated with the risk of in-house mortality: SBP, GCS, and age. However, despite differences in these variables between the two study groups, as noted previously, overall mortality remained the same for both nursing home and community patients. While the nursing home patients did present with lower SBP, the median SBPs for both groups was essentially in the normotensive range, and so most likely the effect size of a low SBP on mortality was fairly limited. The lower GCS found in the nursing home may be more indicative of underlying dementia, rather than TBI. Thus, similar to SBP, the lower GCS found in the nursing home group may have little to no effect on mortality in this group. Of these three variables, age alone and its difference between the two groups likely had a significant impact on mortality. As mentioned previously, increased age is associated with poorer outcomes (Bergeron et al., 2006).

The findings of this study must be interpreted in the context of the study's limitations. This is a retrospective study, making it difficult to control for confounding variables. Additionally, there was a large discrepancy in the size of the study groups, and it remains unclear if a larger nursing home group would have resulted in different findings. On the other hand, despite the group size discrepancy, both group characteristics were consistent with national trends. For instance, in both nursing home and community populations, the majority of patients were female (Jones, Dwyer, Bercovitz, & Strahan, 2004). Further, our study's community mortality rate of 4% is consistent with a recent analysis by Spaniolas et al. of 32,320 elderly ground level fall patients from the NTDB, which demonstrated a 4.4% mortality rate (Spaniolas et al., 2010). While our data set is significantly smaller, our similar mortality rate suggests our results may be applicable to a larger population. An additional limitation, arguably, is that this study represents a single-center experience. However, the single-center study design did allow for uniformity of postpresentation management between both groups, particularly as the majority of elderly fall patients at our institution are admitted to one service. Elderly fall patients with isolated orthopedic injuries, such as hip fractures, are admitted not to orthopedics but to the trauma service, because our institution has previously demonstrated that this policy improves mortality in our patient population (Stone, Barbaro, Bhamidipati, Cucuzzo, & Simon, 2007). Moreover, the single-center experience may also decrease the possibility of differences in postpresentation management which might influence patient outcomes.

CONCLUSION

These data demonstrate that nursing home patients presenting after fall have more comorbid conditions and more debilitated on presentation than their community counterparts. Consequently, nursing home patients had poorer outcomes, as evidenced by longer LOS and increased in-hospital complications, when compared to community patients. However, mortality was similar between both groups and nursing home residency was not a significant predictor of mortality. Further investigation would benefit from the inclusion of frailty measures. We were unable to collect data to calculate scales such as the frailty index or the phenotype of frailty (Bouillon et al., 2013) given the retrospective nature of our study. The frailty index and other scoring systems like it allow a way to objectively quantify an elderly patient's frailty and debility. Further prospective studies might include the frailty index to further elucidate the relationship between geriatric patients who fall in the community and their nursing home counterparts. One of the most pertinent questions for future investigation will be how to prevent the morbidity and mortality of falls in elderly patients. Most likely a two-pronged approach will be required. On one hand is the need for preventative measures. As our data show, nursing home patients bear the brunt of post-fall morbidity. It might be wise to focus antifall measures on the nursing home community, possibly in the form of increased supervision, or balance training. For community patients, home visits to assess the safety of the patient's living environment might help reduce risk. On the other hand is the issue of harm reduction once a fall has already occurred—how can we prevent in-hospital morbidity and mortality, and how can we prevent recidivism once a patient has fallen and been discharged from the hospital? More prospective, multicenter studies are warranted, including some form of community outreach to better investigate the success of interventions in the populations we are trying to serve.

Conflicts of interest

None of the authors have any conflicts of interest to declare. No outside funding received.

Financial support

None.

Authors' contributions

Isadora Botwinick: literature search, study design, data analysis, data interpretation, writing, critical revision; Joshua Johnson: study design, data collection, critical revision; Wayne Cohen-Levy: data collection, writing, critical revision Srinivas H. Reddy: data interpretation, critical revision John McNelis: data interpretation, critical revision Sheldon H. Teperman: data interpretation, critical revision Melvin E. Stone Jr.: literature search, study design, data analysis, data interpretation, writing, critical revision.

Meetings

This research was presented September 10th, 2014, at the Scientific Poster Session at the Annual Meeting of the American Association for the Surgery of Trauma in Philadelphia, Pennsylvania.

Institutional review

The Albert Einstein College of Medicine IRB approved this study. Requirement of informed consent was waived.

ACKNOWLEDGMENTS

Special thanks to Chuck Mikell for his assistance with manuscript preparation and Janet Cucuzzo, Joseph Roche and Francine Ciarletta for providing registry data.

All listed authors were provided with access to the de-identified data. Joshua Johnson and Wayne Cohen-Levy accessed the medical records to collect the data.

Isadora Botwinick had full access to all the data in the study and takes responsibility for the integrity of the data and the accuracy of the data analysis.

REFERENCES

Al Tehewy, M. M., Amin, G. E., & Nassar, N. W. (2015). A study of rate and predictors of fall among elderly patients in a University Hospital. *Journal of Patient Safety, 11* (December (4)), 210–214.

Baker, S. P., O'Neill, B., Haddon, W. Jr., & Long, W. B. (1974). The injury severity score: a method for describing patients with multiple injuries and evaluating emergency care. *Journal of Trauma, 14*(3), 187–196.

Beghe, C., Wilson, A., & Ershler, W. B. (2004). Prevalence and outcomes of anemia in geriatrics: a systematic review of the literature. *The American Journal of Medicine, 116*(Suppl. 7A), 3S–10S.

Bergeron, E., Clement, J., Lavoie, A., Ratte, S., Bamvita, J. M., Aumont, F., et al. (2006). A simple fall in the elderly: not so simple. *Journal of Trauma, 60*(2), 268–273.

Bouillon, K., Kivimaki, M., Hamer, M., et al. (2013). Measures of frailty in population-based studies: an overview. *BMC Geriatrics, 13,* 64.

Close, J. C., Lord, S. R., Antonova, E. J., Martin, M., Lensberg, B., Taylor, M., et al. (2012). Older people presenting to the emergency department after a fall: a population with substantial recurrent healthcare use. *Emergency Medicine Journal, 29*(9), 742–747.

Hannan, E. L., Mendeloff, J., Farrell, L. S., Cayten, C. G., & Murphy, J. G. (1995). Multivariate models for predicting survival of patients with trauma from low falls: the impact of gender and pre-existing conditions. *Journal of Trauma, 38*(5), 697–704.

Hughes, C. M., & Goldie, R. (2009). I just take what I am given: adherence and resident involvement in decision making on medicines in nursing homes for older people: a qualitative survey. *Drugs & Aging, 26*(6), 505–517.

Jones, A. L., Dwyer, L. L., Bercovitz, A. R., & Strahan, G. W. (2004). The National nursing home survey: overview. National Center for Health Statistics. *Vital and Health Statistics, 13*(167), 2009.

Luppa, M., Luck, T., Weyerer, S., Konig, H. H., Brahler, E., & Riedel-Heller, S. G. (2010). Prediction of institutionalization in the elderly. A systematic review. *Age and Ageing, 39*(1), 31–38.

Monaghan, S. F., Heffernan, D. S., Thakkar, R. K., Reinert, S. E., Machan, J. T., Connolly, M. D., et al. (2011). The development of a urinary tract infection is associated with increased mortality in trauma patients. *Journal of Trauma, 71*(6), 1569–1574.

Panisset, M., Saxton, J., & Boller, F. (1995). End-stage Alzheimer's disease: Glasgow Coma Scale and the neurologic examination. *Archives of Neurology, 52*(2), 127–128.

Rubenstein, L. Z., Josephson, K. R., & Robbins, A. S. (1994). Falls in the nursing home. *Annals of Internal Medicine, 121*(6), 442–451.

Siracuse, J. J., Odell, D. D., Gondek, S. P., Odom, S. R., Kasper, E. M., Hauser, C. J., et al. (2012). Health care and socioeconomic impact of falls in the elderly. *The American Journal of Surgery, 203*(3), 335–338 discussion 338.

Spaniolas, K., Cheng, J. D., Gestring, M. L., Sangosanya, A., Stassen, N. A., & Bankey, P. E. (2010). Ground level falls are associated with significant mortality in elderly patients. *Journal of Trauma, 69*(4), 821–825.

Sporer, K. A., Solares, M., Durant, E. J., Wang, W., Wu, A. H., & Rodriguez, R. M. (2013). Accuracy of the initial diagnosis among patients with an acutely altered mental status. *Emergency Medicine Journal*, *30*(3), 243–246.

Stevens, J. A., Corso, P. S., Finkelstein, E. A., & Miller, T. R. (2006). The costs of fatal and non-fatal falls among older adults. *Injury Prevention*, *12*(5), 290–295.

Stone, M. E. Jr., Barbaro, C., Bhamidipati, C. M., Cucuzzo, J., & Simon, R. (2007). Elderly hip fracture patients admitted to the trauma service: does it impact patient outcome? *Journal of Trauma*, *63*(6), 1348–1352.

Tromp, A. M., Pluijm, S. M., Smit, J. H., Deeg, D. J., Bouter, L. M., & Lips, P. (2001). Fall- risk screening test: a prospective study on predictors for falls in community-dwelling elderly. *Journal of Clinical Epidemiology*, *54*(8), 837–844.

Winter, J. E., MacInnis, R. J., Wattanapenpaiboon, N., & Nowson, C. A. (2014). BMI and all-cause mortality in older adults: a meta-analysis. *The American Journal of Clinical Nutrition*, *99*(4), 875–890.

Woodman, R., Ferrucci, L., & Guralnik, J. (2005). Anemia in older adults. *Current Opinion in Hematology*, *12*(2), 123–128.

GERIATRIC NURSING HOME FALLS: A SINGLE INSTITUTION CROSS-SECTIONAL STUDY

Critique by *Margaret McCarthy*

OVERALL SUMMARY

Patient falls are of concern across all health care institutions, especially among older adults and also especially in long-term care facilities such as nursing homes. Falls are of particular concern because of the resultant outcomes; it is often difficult for older adults to recover from the fall and again be independent in activities of daily living. The researchers conducted a retrospective review of more than 1,700 older adults' records comparing those in nursing homes to a community cohort. As expected, they found that nursing home residents had more negative outcomes than community-dwelling older adults. Various outcome factors were analyzed, made possible by the substantial sample size. The study results lead to better understandings of the complexity associated with both aging itself and falls among the elderly. The researchers identify future research needed for both preventative measures related to falls and for interventions to reduce morbidity among nursing home residents in particular. Overall there is clarity in the research, particularly in the background and study rationale. The complexity of the outcome variables in the study, often evident in clinical research, requires the novice researcher to carefully consider the study implications for future research and practice. The researchers clearly identify the challenges inherent in clinical research of this nature, particularly when studying a phenomenon, such as falls, that can be linked to several factors in addition to primary place of residence.

TITLE

Does the title include the key concepts/variables/ phenomenon of interest?

The title does include several key variables: geriatric, nursing home, falls, type of study (cross-sectional). It does not state a comparison to community falls or anything about the outcomes of interest.

Is it concise (12 words or less) and professionally stated?

The title is concise (nine words).

RESEARCHER(S) CREDIBILITY

Educational credentials?

No educational credentials are provided for authors, other than their place of employment/professional affiliation.

Prior methodological research experience of the authors (i.e., methodological expertise)?

Methodological expertise is not stated and is not clear. However, the paper does provide author contributions, which is desirable, and consistent with current standards of publication. The authors and their contributions are as follows: Isadora Botwinick: literature search, study design, data analysis, data interpretation, writing, critical revision; Joshua Johnson: study design, data collection, critical revision; Wayne Cohen-Levy: data collection, writing, critical revision; Srinivas H. Reddy: data interpretation, critical revision; John McNelis: data interpretation, critical revision; Sheldon H. Teperman: data interpretation, critical revision; Melvin E. Stone, Jr.: literature search, study design, data analysis, data interpretation, writing, critical revision.

Subject matter content experience (prior research on the subject matter)?

A search of MEDLINE reveals the following about each author: Isadora Botwinick: none in subject area; Joshua H. Johnson: none in subject area; Saman Safadjou: none in subject area; Wayne Cohen-Levy: none in subject area; Srinivas H. Reddy: none in subject area. John McNelis: has a previous related publication in which the morbidity and mortality of geriatric falls were evaluated. Sheldon H. Teperman has previous publications, including an analysis of trauma registry. Melvin E. Stone, Jr. was an author on a retrospective cohort study in similar falls content area in which registry data were analyzed.

ABSTRACT

Does it include the key components (objective/aim, background/rationale, methods, results, and conclusions)?

The structured abstract includes background, methods, results, and conclusion. It does not include the study objective or aim but does provide hypothesis. The structured components of the abstract are those prescribed by the journal (*Archives of Gerontology and Geriatrics*).

Does or does not include references?

The abstract does not include references.

Is it concise (150–250 words or less)?

The abstract is concise at 250 words.

Does it entice you to read the rest of the article (interesting)?

It was interesting due to fact that hypothesis was not supported, so it draws the reader in for an explanation.

INTRODUCTION/PROBLEM

Is the research problem or phenomenon of interest clearly stated?

The authors state the problem of falls, the prevalence, cost, and that rates of falls in the nursing home are twice the rate of falls in the community. Thus, the problem is stated unambiguously and is easy to identify.

Does the problem have significance for nursing?

Falls among geriatric patients are of significance to nursing no matter the residence of the individual who falls. To determine the differences in fall rates between nursing home residents and community dwelling elders would help to understand some aspects of geriatric falls. The researchers hypothesized that nursing home residents' falls would be a significant predictor of mortality, but this hypothesis was not supported. Nursing home residence was a significant predictor of morbidity. This alone is significant for nursing and health care.

Is it succinct?

Yes the problem statement is succinct at one paragraph.

Does it answer the "so what" question?

Because nursing home patients fall twice as often as community dwellers, it is important to determine whether, after a fall, they have worse outcomes. However, it does not address pre-fall prevention in this section, or any discussion of characteristics of patients before a fall, except for their place of residence.

RESEARCH AIMS/OBJECTIVES

Is the research aim/objective clearly stated?

The aim of study is clearly stated, although the sentence describing the research aim could have been written more clearly. The authors state the aim is to directly compare "outcomes between elderly patients who fall in the nursing home and their community counterparts." It could have been made clearer that the comparison was between those who lived and fell in nursing home, with those who lived and fell in the community.

Is it concisely written?

Yes, the aim is concisely written in one sentence.

Does it follow logically from the research problem/phenomenon of interest?

Yes, the aim of comparing post-fall outcomes follows the background and significance of falls, especially falls that occur in nursing homes.

SIGNIFICANCE

Is the significance to nursing and health care clearly written?

This section notes significance of the prevalence of falls and cost of falls to the health care system. The significance is also noted about a growing elderly population and the greater cost of treating falls. It does not state the significance specifically to nursing.

Does the significance follow from the research aim/objective?

Yes the significance follows directly from the research aim. If nursing home residents have more complications, their length of stay (LOS) will be longer and will cost more. The questions the authors pose is that it is unclear whether nursing home patients will have worse outcomes. It is not stated what the significance to the health care system or nursing will be if we find out nursing home residents have worse outcomes. Will the hospital care differ if a nursing home patient is admitted for a fall, as opposed to a community dwelling patient? We already know they fall twice as often as community dwellers, which speaks more to preventive efforts.

BACKGROUND

Is there an explicit description of a theoretical perspective or conceptual framework? If not, is it implied?

There is no specific mention of a theoretical basis or conceptual model for the study. One can assume that the researchers used a biomedical model for guiding the research in that the outcome variables that were identified were morbidity and mortality.

Are there clear theoretical/conceptual definitions of the concepts?

There are no definitions of concepts.

LITERATURE REVIEW
Primary sources only?

In reviewing each reference, there are 15 primary studies, two overviews, two systematic reviews, one meta-analysis, and one commentary. Therefore, the majority of the sources contain primary data.

Current (within the past how many years)?

The references range from 1974 to 2015. Some of the data are from papers more than 20 years old and up to 40 years old.

Is the search strategy included?

There was no search strategy included.

Is literature relevant to the research aims/objectives?

Data were provided that were relevant to the research aims. However, some of these data were old and more recent data would be more relevant to the research problem.

Is it chronologically presented (old to current)?

The data were not presented in any chronological order.

Is it comprehensive? If not, is sufficient background literature provided?

The background section was very brief (one paragraph), even for this journal, in which backgrounds of three to five paragraphs are common.

RATIONALE FOR THE STUDY
Is there a gap in the literature that this study will fill (will it extend prior knowledge)? Is the rationale clearly stated?

Authors do state that there is little literature on directly comparing post-fall outcomes of these two populations. Exactly why this is important to compare is not clearly stated. What appears left out is the focus on nursing home falls, since they occur more frequently.

Is this a follow-up or replication study?

The authors did not state that this was a follow-up or replication study. In fact, the authors state there is scant literature that directly compares the post-fall outcomes of these two populations, but no other studies are referenced, so it is not clear what the "scant" literature includes, or if there is none.

RESEARCH QUESTION(S) AND/OR HYPOTHESES
Are these explicitly and clearly stated?

The research aims were clearly stated. However, the authors state, "The aim of our study was to directly compare the outcomes between elderly patients who fall in the nursing home and their community counterparts after presentation to a Level 1 trauma center," without stating what outcomes they are comparing. But the hypothesis does expand on what outcomes they are comparing: mortality and complication rate.

Do they include the variables/phenomenon of interest?

The variables of interest are not stated in the aims.

Do they follow from the research aim/objective?

The hypothesis directly follows the study aims. The authors believe nursing home residents will have more comorbidities as they enter the hospital for a fall, and therefore do worse while hospitalized.

METHODS
Research Design/Paradigm
Is the research design clearly stated?

This was a cross-sectional study with data gathered over a 4-year period (2008–2012). This is clearly stated in the first sentence of the Methods section. The authors state they obtained institutional review board (IRB) approval for a cross-sectional study.

Is there consistency between the research design and paradigm?

As stated previously, as there is no explicit conceptual model or paradigm, it is not possible to assess whether the design matched the conceptual model.

Is this the best choice of design to address the research problem/phenomenon of interest?

The research question was to assess whether nursing home patients who experienced a fall were more likely to have poorer outcomes as compared to their community counterparts. The data were taken from the medical record for the hospital stay after the fall. Although the LOS was significantly longer for nursing home residents than community counterparts (mean = 6; range, 3–10 vs. mean = 5; range, 3–9), the LOS was short to assess outcomes. This may explain why, despite nursing home residents having more complications, there were no significant differences in in-hospital mortality between the two groups.

Is there rigor in the design?

This was a secondary analysis of previously collected medical record data. As in all secondary analyses, this limits the research question to include only the data available. They did use all patients who were admitted with a fall, excluding only those with missing data, which resulted in a large sample. But there is no mention of sample size calculations or power analysis to determine an adequate sample size to answer the research question.

The authors based comorbidities and in-hospital complications on the National Trauma Data Bank (NTDB), which is the largest collection of trauma data in the United States. The NTDB uses an extensive data dictionary to establish a national standard of trauma registry data.

They chose to dichotomize three independent variables (body mass index, Glasgow Coma Scale, and international normalized ration [INR]) based on what would be considered "abnormal" by a practicing physician. This was based on clinical judgement, but lacks a theoretical basis. However, dichotomizing continuous data creates problems in interpretation of the data. For example, a body mass index of 18.4 is considered abnormal, but 18.6 would be normal. An INR of 1.3 is abnormal, and so is an INR of 3.0. We know there is a clinical difference in these two INR values, but not much difference in the body mass values. There is valuable information lost when you dichotomize continuous data.

The design was cross-sectional, taken at one point in time, which limits our ability to establish causation, such as that the independent variables (clinical and demographic data) caused the dependent variable (in-hospital complications and mortality) to occur. A stronger design would have followed the two cohorts of participants prospectively, into the future.

SETTING
Is the setting clearly described?

The setting was Jacobi Medical Center, a major Level 1 trauma center. There were no other details given about the hospital, geographic area, or typical patient population.

What biases are introduced as a result of selecting this particular setting?

When only one setting is chosen, we do not know whether similar results would be found in another setting, even another trauma center. There may be important differences in the setting, patient population, staff, workload, and geographic area that may affect results.

SAMPLING PLAN AND SAMPLE
Is the sampling plan clearly identified?

The sampling plan included all patients who were admitted for a fall to this facility from 2008 to 2012. The sampling plan thus was inclusive of the entire population of interest.

Does it represent the population of interest?

The sample represented the entire population for the specified time period. The population of interest was adults older than 65 years who experienced a ground-level fall, either as nursing home or community resident. This was the sample of the study, for which data were extracted from the medical record.

Is the sampling plan consistent with the research aim/objective?

Yes, the sampling plan is consistent with the aim of assessing differences in fall outcomes between the two populations. The plan was to include every patient who presented to the trauma center over a period of 4 years.

Is the sample size sufficient (e.g., power analysis or data saturation)?

It is unknown whether the sample size is sufficient since there were no sample size calculations mentioned. Therefore, we do not know whether there were no differences between the groups in the outcome "in-hospital mortality" because of the study design (length of follow-up), or whether the sample was not large enough to detect a difference, or whether there really was no difference. The authors could have conducted sample size calculations prior to setting their sampling plan, which might have led them to choose a longer time period to study. Furthermore, the difference in the sample sizes between groups should be noted. The nursing home group was much smaller ($n = 163$) than the community dwelling group ($n = 1,545$). A larger sample of nursing home patients may have changed the results.

VARIABLES
Are variables clearly identified?

The authors state, "Outcome data of interest included: in-hospital complications, including transfusion requirements, LOS, operative intervention, and in-hospital mortality." They proceed to define what are included as complications using definitions from the NTDB. Similarly, they list what are considered comorbidities (as an independent or predictor variable).

Are variables operationally defined and consistent with theoretical concepts?

Variables are operationally defined, although consistency with theoretical concepts cannot be assessed since there were no theoretical concepts identified.

Are independent and dependent variables identified, if applicable?

Yes, both independent and dependent variables have been identified. The authors also define what constitutes a nursing home and community patient. The authors do not state what variables they controlled for, the variables that might confound, or confuse, the relationship between nursing home status and outcomes. However, they do include in the multivariate analysis, in addition to nursing home status, the injury severity score (ISS). This score may confound the relationship between nursing home status and the outcome. If the community dwellers had more severe injuries that may partly explain their outcomes. So, although they do not use the term, they did address a potential confounder.

METHOD OF DATA COLLECTION
What are the methods of data collection?

All data were extracted from the patients' medical records.

Are validity and reliability clearly addressed for prior research and current study, if applicable?

For this study, two authors (Johnson and Cohen-Levy) were noted to have conducted the data collection. There are no details on the process of data collection, nor on any measures to assure accuracy and consistency between the two researchers.

Do the measures/instruments address the underlying theoretical concepts or phenomenon of interest?

All data are medical record data. No other instruments or measures are used. The measures address the phenomena of interest.

Were human rights protected?

At the end of the paper, IRB approval is noted. No consent was required.

Are other ethical issues identified?

There is no mention of de-identifying the data obtained from the medical record.

Is the data-collection method appropriate for research design?

Yes, the data collected were sufficient to address the aims of the study and were appropriate for the design.

Is there bias in data collection?

Two authors completed data collection, but there is no discussion on the process of data collection or how reliability was established between the two researchers.

What is the fidelity of intervention addressed, if applicable?

There was no intervention in this study.

DATA ANALYSIS

Are data analysis techniques described (e.g., statistical tests, methodology for qualitative analysis)?

At the end of the Methods section, there are several sentences about the data analysis that was conducted. This includes the specific tests used to compare the two groups (Mann–Whitney test and Fisher's exact test). The Mann-Whitney test is the nonparametric equivalent of the independent t-test, and the Fisher's exact test is an alternative to chi-square when sample sizes are small. Because no sample size calculations or power analyses were conducted, it is unknown why the authors chose these tests. Although the outcome of the multivariate analysis is not stated in the text here, we can see from Table 5 the outcome is in-hospital mortality. In-hospital complications were compared between the two groups of patients.

Does the analysis answer the research question?

Yes, the analysis does address the aims: comparing the outcomes (in-hospital complications and mortality) between the two groups of elderly patients who present with a fall. However, the logistic regression answers the question: what are the independent factors related to the outcome (in-hospital mortality), after controlling for other variables. Logistic regression provides the odds ratios for each independent variable as it relates to the dependent variable. This was not stated specifically as an aim. The authors did not conduct logistic regression analyses for the other outcome variable, in-hospital complications, which was significantly different between the two groups.

Is the analysis comprehensive?

As for the aims stated, the completed analyses were sufficient to compare the two groups.

Are themes identified?

Not applicable.

Is there bias in the analysis (trustworthiness? credibility?)?

For these quantitative analyses, there appears to be no bias.

RESULTS

Are sample characteristics described and fully reported?

Table 1 describes and compares the clinical data and the baseline characteristics of the whole sample, as well as each group (nursing home and community dweller). Table 2 describes the prevalence of the comorbidities in the whole sample, as well as each group. The p-value on Tables 1 and 2 tells us whether there are significant differences ($p < .05$ as statement in methods) between the two groups in each variable.

Are findings presented related to research aim/objective?

The findings were presented as per the aim of the study. Authors provided data on comorbidities, in-hospital complications, and in-hospital mortality.

Are all outcome variables addressed if applicable?

As per the aims, the analyses include the comparison of the prevalence of in-hospital complications and mortality.

Are results clearly presented in text and/or tables/figures?

The data are presented in table format.

Is significance of results reported, if applicable?

Tables 2 and 3 list the differences between the two groups' comorbidities and post-fall outcomes. Table 4 lists the difference in individual complications. The p-values in each table tell us whether there are any significant differences between the groups in each variable.

DISCUSSION OF RESULTS

Do the authors link the findings to previous research studies?

The discussion begins with a summary of the findings. The authors then compare their results with previous evidence, for example, the findings on older age, increased incidence of dementia, lower body mass index, LOS, and complications.

Are the conclusions comprehensive, yet within the data? Do the authors interpret the results in the discussion?

Yes, for example, the authors discuss the finding that nursing home patients did not have higher mortality than the community dwellers, despite being more debilitated and having a higher rate of complications. The authors went beyond the findings to hypothesize the reason for this inconsistency might have been the low ISS for each group. They note that higher ISS scores have been associated with high mortality in the past (though note that the reference is from 1974). The authors do proceed to explain the remaining factors associated with in-hospital mortality (e.g., systolic blood pressure, Glasgow Coma Scale).

Are the findings generalizable or transferable?

The authors note that both groups' characteristics are consistent with national trends, which may make the data generalizable to a larger population.

LIMITATIONS

Identified? Accurate? Inclusive?

Limitations are identified, accurate, and inclusive. They note sample size discrepancy between the two groups, retrospective design limiting their ability to adjust for confounders, and the single center for data collection. However, they note this last limitation also had the benefit of limiting differences in post-fall management as most elderly fall patients are admitted to the same service.

IMPLICATIONS

Are there implications for practice, education, research? For clinical significance?

The authors address several research implications related to clinical care. These include adding a frailty index to a future prospective study to quantify an elderly patient's frailty. Second, future investigations should focus on preventing morbidity and mortality. The authors noted this would have a two-pronged approach: preventing falls and reducing harm after a fall has occurred.

RECOMMENDATIONS
Recommendations for future study/study replication?

The authors suggest multicenter studies are warranted, including visits to the community to assess how well interventions are working.

CONCLUSION
Is it succinct and does it tie everything together?

The conclusion is succinct and summarizes the study's key findings while pointing toward potential research questions for the future.

RESILIENCE AND PROFESSIONAL QUALITY OF LIFE AMONG MILITARY HEALTH CARE PROVIDERS

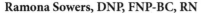

9

Colleen Leners, DNP, FNP-BC, RN
VA Medical Center, Combat, Complex, and Casualty Clinic, San Diego, California, USA

Ramona Sowers, DNP, FNP-BC, RN
VA Medical Center, Durham, North Carolina, USA

Mary T. Quinn Griffin, PhD, RN, FAAN
Case Western Reserve University, Frances Payne Bolton School of Nursing, Cleveland, Ohio, USA

Joyce J. Fitzpatrick, PhD, RN, FAAN
Case Western Reserve University, Frances Payne Bolton School of Nursing, Cleveland, Ohio, USA

ABSTRACT

The retention of qualified military health care providers is a top priority for Department of Defense (DoD) leaders. The purpose of this study is to examine the relationship between resilience and professional quality of life (ProQoL) and to explore differences among providers who had been deployed and those who had never been deployed. Results indicated high resilience scores among all providers, and significant relationships between dimensions of ProQoL and resilience. There were significant differences in ProQoL based on deployment. Recommendations for future research are included, particularly as retention is an important issue for the DoD.

Retention of qualified military health care providers is a top priority for the U.S. Department of Defense (DoD). Military medical professionals are in demand due to the operational requirements of two wars, the increasing number of retirees accessing the military health system, and the inability to meet recruiting and retention requirements. The DoD is experiencing shortfalls in the recruitment of physicians, nurses, and other medical officers (U.S. Government Accountability Office, 2010). Various factors present challenges to retention including, for example, work-related stressors, workplace adversity, deployment to a war zone, multiple deployments, increasing acuity of the patient population, and multiple relocations necessary for career advancement. Military operations place health care providers in combat arenas where they experience stressful situations involving danger to themselves while

Leners, C., Sowers, R., Quinn Griffin, M. T., & Fitzpatrick, J. J. (2014). Resilience and professional quality of life among military healthcare providers. *Issues in Mental Health Nursing*, 35(7), 497–502. doi:10.3109/01612840.2014.887164. Reprinted with permission from Taylor & Francis Ltd.

needing to care for patients with life-threatening situations (Gibbons, Barnett, & Hickling, 2012; Hickling, Gibbons, Barnett, & Watts, 2011). Shea et al. (2010) reported that combat veterans have experienced psychological problems as a result of such experiences. In a 2006 survey of military providers, 15% of all providers reported that burnout, or compassion fatigue, affected their overall performance. In this same survey, 45% of primary care providers and 33% of mental health providers reported experiencing burnout (Mental Health Advisory Team-III, 2006). Preventing burnout and increasing resilience of military health care providers is of particular importance in high stress times such as those associated with war and repeated deployments.

Address correspondence to Joyce J. Fitzpatrick, Case Western Reserve University, Frances Payne Bolton School of Nursing, 10900 Euclid Avenue, Cleveland, OH 44106 USA. E-mail: jjfitzpatrick@hotmail.com.

BACKGROUND

Based on recommendations from a 2004 study of 52,000 participants, in which 18% of health care professionals and 27% of medical doctors reported burnout, the U.S. Army Medical Command (MEDCOM) implemented resiliency training for all health professionals. Participants indicated that the program was valuable (Adams, Camarillo, Lewis, & McNish, 2010), but there were no studies of the effects of the program on retention, burnout, or mental health variables.

Hagerty et al. (2011) reported that a significant percentage (20%–30%) of deployed military personnel reported psychological effects, including compassion fatigue. While this study was not focused on military health providers, it is important in its emphasis on deployed personnel. In an earlier qualitative study of nurses who served in either Iraq or Afghanistan, researchers found that these nurses showed signs of compassion fatigue (Scannell-Desch & Doherty, 2010).

Although there are few studies of resilience among active military personnel, there have been three studies of veterans. Vogt and Tanner (2007) evaluated postwar risk factors of posttraumatic stress syndrome (PTSS) and resilience among 308 veterans who served in Gulf War 1. Resilience accounted for 64% of the variance in PTSS. Researchers from the Netherlands studied 1,561 veterans and found that resilience associated with the cognitive processing of war experiences was associated with more personal growth following military deployment (Schok, Kleber, Gerty, & Lensvelt-Mulders, 2010). The third study (Pietrzak et al., 2010) included 285 veterans surveyed within 2 years of deployment ($N = 285$). The researchers found that protective factors, including resilience, social support, and the military unit's postdeployment support, served as psychosocial buffers for PTSS and depressive symptoms (Pietrzak et al., 2010).

In addition to research on resilience among military personnel, there have been studies focused on behavioral health issues related to deployment. Adler and colleagues (2005) found that the length of deployment was positively related to higher levels of stress and depression. Further, compassion fatigue has been directly and positively related to job stress (Kenny & Hull, 2008), and burnout has been related to past trauma (Whealin, Batzer, Morgan, Detwiler, Schurr, & Friedman, 2007). Hoge and colleagues (2004) found that those deployed to Iraq had greater posttraumatic stress disorder (PTSD) symptoms after duty than those deployed to Afghanistan (Hoge, Castro, Messer, McGurk, Cotting, & Koffman, 2004). In a recent study of combat health care providers' coping, Gibbons and colleagues (2013) found that providers believed that a sense of control and a sense of purpose contributed to their ability to cope (Gibbons, Shafer, Aramanda, Hickling, & Benedek, 2013). Given the repeated trauma witnessed by military health care providers, these findings from prior studies are particularly important. Also, given the high deployment of military providers within the past decade, differences in the key variables based on whether individuals had ever been deployed were of particular interest to the investigators.

In summary, although there are a number of studies of behavioral health issues, including resilience, among military health care providers, there are no prior studies linking resilience and professional quality of life (ProQoL) (compassion satisfaction, burnout, and compassion fatigue/secondary trauma) among military health care providers. In prior research, differences were found based on deployment status of the providers. The purpose of the present study is to examine these relationships and to explore differences between providers who had been deployed and those who had never been deployed.

METHODS

The study used a descriptive, correlational, quantitative design. Data were collected at a convention of the American Military Surgeons of the United States (AMSUS) in San Antonio, Texas. The convention is attended by active duty and reservist medical personnel from the four armed forces services: Navy, Air Force, Army, and Marines.

Sample

There were approximately 3,248 attendees at the 2011 AMSUS meeting. Approximately 50% of the attendees were enlisted or international delegates and were not eligible to participate in the study. Inclusion criteria for the study were having a minimum education of a bachelor's degree in nursing (for the nurse participants) or an MD (for physicians), and being on active duty or having reserve officer status in the armed forces. There were 548 nurses (including APNs) and 339 physicians in attendance who were eligible to participate in the study.

Instruments
Resilience Scale

The Resilience Scale (RS), a 25-item questionnaire developed by Wagnild (2009), was used to measure resilience. The RS is scored on a positively worded 7-point scale (1 = disagree, 7 = agree); scores range from 25 to 175, with higher scores indicating higher levels of resilience. The RS has been widely used, and has been shown to be valid and reliable; reliabilities range from .75 to .95 (Ahern, Kiehl, Sole, & Byers, 2006). In the present study the Cronbach alpha reliability was .95. Resilience was measured by the total score on the RS.

Professional Quality of Life Instrument

The ProQoL instrument is a 30-item questionnaire that evaluates three components of ProQoL. The three subscales are (a) compassion satisfaction, the pleasure you derive from being able to do your work (higher scores on this subscale represent greater satisfaction with being a caregiver, or greater pleasure derived from doing a good job at work); (b) burnout, which measures feelings of hopelessness, difficulty dealing with work, or difficulty being effective at one's job (higher scores on this scale indicate a higher risk of burnout); and (c) compassion fatigue/secondary trauma, which relates to extreme work-related trauma exposure, either directly imposed, as in military or police service, or indirectly, such as an emergency room employee or social worker (higher scores may indicate that something in the workplace environment is traumatic). The alpha reliability scores in prior research were as follows: Compassion satisfaction, $r = .87$; burnout, $r = .72$; compassion fatigue, $r = .80$ (Stamm, 2010). In the present study the reliabilities were: compassion satisfaction, $r = .90$; burnout, $r = .77$; and compassion fatigue, $r = .85$. The total scores on each of the three subscales of the ProQoL instrument were used to measure key variables in this study.

The following background data were collected: gender, age, race/ethnicity, branch of service, service rank, and number and location of deployments.

Procedure

Approval to conduct the study at AMSUS was granted by the convention education coordinator. Institutional review board (IRB) approval was obtained; anonymity and confidentiality were assured. Individuals were approached at the conference, and if they met inclusion criteria for the study, they were asked to complete the questionnaires.

Statistical Analysis

All data were directly entered and coded into the Statistical Package for the Social Sciences (SPSS) through the Survey Monkey integration and Excel spreadsheet. Preliminary frequencies were computed to determine out-of-range responses. Descriptive, univariate analysis was performed on the data set for the results related to the sample characteristics. Cronbach alpha coefficients were computed for the RS and ProQoL sub-scales. These scores were examined for mean, median, measures of central tendency, and variance. Bivariate, correlational tests were used to determine the relationships among resilience and the ProQoL subscale scores. Further analyses using analysis of variance (ANOVA) were undertaken to determine differences between groups based on deployment status.

RESULTS

Sample Characteristics

There were 168 surveys completed, 71 by nurses, 42 by advanced practice nurses, and 47 by physicians. The total response rate was 19%, with the response rate among nurses being 20.6% and among physicians, 13.9%.

Gender distribution was 46.4% ($n = 78$) male and 53.6% ($n = 90$) female. The age range was from 23 to 66+ years old. The following ranks of military officer were represented: commander, lieutenant colonel, 33.3%, $n = 60$; lieutenant commander, major, 26.2%, $n = 44$; lieutenant, captain, 21.4%, $n = 36$; colonel, captain, 11.9%, $n = 20$; lieutenant junior grade, 2nd lieutenant, 4.8%, $n = 8$; and ensign, 1st lieutenant, 2.4%, $n = 4$. All branches of the service were represented. Detailed background characteristics are included in Table 1.

The participants were from a range of specialties within nursing and medicine. These results are included in Table 2.

TABLE 1. Sample Characteristics (N = 168)

	Frequency	Percentage
Gender		
Male	78	46.4
Female	90	53.6
Age Range		
23–39	49	29.1
40–55	96	57.1
55–66+	23	13.6
Race/Ethnicity		
White	123	73.2
Asian	20	11.9
Hispanic	10	6.0
Black	5	3.0
Pacific Islander	3	1.8
Native American	3	1.8
Multiple	4	2.4
Missing	1	
Marital Status		
Married	125	74.4
Divorced	20	11.9
Never married	19	11.3
Missing	4	
Rank		
05 Commander/Lt Colonel	60	33.3
04 Lt Commander, Major	44	26.2
03 Lieutenant, Captain	36	21.4
02 Lieutenant Jr. Grade, 2nd Lieutenant	20	11.9
01 Ensign, 1st Lieutenant	4	2.4
Missing	4	2.4

Regarding deployment, 67.9% (n = 114) had been deployed; 32.1% (n = 54) had deployed to Iraq; and 20.8% (n = 60) been deployed, but to countries other than Iraq. Almost one third (32.1%, n = 54) had never been deployed.

Relationship Between Resilience and Professional Quality of Life

The mean score on the RS was 147.93 (SD = 18.92; range: 41–175). The scores on the ProQoL subscales were: Compassion Satisfaction: Mean = 41.80 (SD = 5.40; range: 23–50); Burnout: Mean = 20.45 (SD = 4.90; range: 10–34); and Compassion Fatigue/Secondary Trauma: Mean = 19.28 (SD = 5.66; range: 10–42). These results are shown in Table 3.

TABLE 2. Providers by Type (N = 168)

Provider Type	Specialty	Frequency	Percentage
Nurses	Medical/Surgical	32	41
	Critical Care	17	22
	Emergency	15	19.2
	Community Health	8	10.1
	Operating	3	3.8
	Psychiatric	2	2.7
	Flight	1	1.3
Advanced	Nurse Anesthetist	18	42.9
Practice	Family	17	40.5
Nurses	Adult	5	11.9
	Acute Care	1	2.4
	Midwife	1	2.4
Physician	Orthopedic Surgeon	13	27.7
	Flight Surgeon	7	14.9
	Family Medicine	7	14.9
	General Surgeon	4	8.5
	Specialty Surgeon	4	8.5
	Internal Medicine	4	8.5
	Emergency	3	6.4
	Anesthesiology	2	6.4
	Psychiatry	2	4.7
Missing		2	4.7

Pearson correlations were used to determine the relationships among resilience and the ProQoL subscale scores. There were statistically significant relationships between resilience and compassion satisfaction (r = .45, p <.001.); resilience and burnout (r = −.37, p <.001); and resilience and compassion fatigue/secondary trauma (r = −.29, p <.001).

TABLE 3. Descriptive Statistics for Resilience and Professional Quality of Life Variables

Variable	Mean	SD	Range
Resilience	147.93	18.92	41–175
Compassion Satisfaction	41.80	5.40	23–50
Burnout	20.44	4.90	10–34
Compassion Fatigue/Secondary Trauma	19.18	5.66	10–42

Further analyses were undertaken to determine differences based on deployment status. The first analysis was between those who had never deployed (n = 54) and those who had been deployed (n = 114) independent of country of deployment. There were significant differences between deployed providers versus those who had never deployed on all of the variables: Resilience: $F = 2.73, p = .05$; Compassion Satisfaction: $F = 4.95, p < .01$; Burnout: $F = 9.25, p < .01$; and Compassion Fatigue/Secondary Trauma: $F = 9.19, p < .001$. Those who had never deployed had higher resilience scores, higher compassion satisfaction, lower burnout, and lower compassion fatigue/secondary trauma than those who had deployed.

The results were examined further by comparing those deployed to Iraq (n = 54), those deployed to all other sites (n = 60), and those never deployed (n = 54). There were no significant differences in resilience among these groups. Significant differences were found between groups on Compassion Satisfaction, $F = 4.02, p < .05$; Burnout, $F = 4.54, p < .01$; and Compassion Fatigue/Secondary Trauma, $F = 5.59, p < .01$. On these ProQoL variables, those deployed to Iraq were significantly different from those never deployed but were not significantly different from those deployed elsewhere. Those deployed to Iraq had lower compassion satisfaction, higher burnout, and higher compassion fatigue/secondary trauma than the two other groups. Those deployed to somewhere other than Iraq were not significantly different from those who had never deployed on any of the variables.

DISCUSSION

There are no prior studies of resilience and ProQoL among military health care providers; however, the results of the present study are consistent with research on other groups of health care providers who have experienced trauma. Hooper et al. (2010) studied components of ProQoL among emergency nurses compared to nurses in other highly stressful inpatient units. These researchers found that 20% of all staff scored low for compassion satisfaction, 26.6% were at risk for burnout, and 28.4% were at risk for compassion fatigue. Kenny and Hull (2008) noted that 82% of critical care nursing staff expressed a need for emotional support due to the increased stress and workload caring for those evacuated from the front line. They also indicated that in-service education for compassion fatigue and PTSD was needed. Adams et al. (2010), using the ProQoL scale, noted that in a survey sent out during the MHAT-II study (2005) of approximately 52,000 military medical personnel, 18% reported burnout. Both physicians (27%) and enlisted (23%) reported burnout. Participants in the present study had moderately high resilience scores. This result would be expected based on their years of military and professional experience (21+ years), yet there is no prior research specifically among military health care personnel.

Interestingly, resilience scores were higher in those who had not deployed. This warrants further investigation in a larger study with a focus on deployment experience by rank and experience. This finding of higher resilience in nondeployed personnel has not been considered in previous research. Differences in ProQoL variables (lower compassion satisfaction, higher burnout, and higher compassion fatigue/secondary trauma) among those deployed to Iraq compared to those deployed elsewhere are consistent with the work of Hoge and colleagues (2004) who compared those deployed to Iraq and those deployed to Afghanistan. The finding that the deployed group reported lower resilience scores strongly supports the need for resilience training for military health care providers, particularly as a means of addressing personnel retention. Resiliency is an important factor in buffering or preventing PTSD. Maguen and colleagues (2008), in a study of 328 U.S. Air Force health care providers, reported that 87% of respondents had at least one potentially traumatic event prior to deployment. Predeployment PTSD symptoms were strongly associated with predeployment stressors and lifetime trauma over and above resiliency. Maguen et al. (2008) postulate that these predeployment risk factors outweigh the benefits of resiliency. Perhaps this may account for the lower resiliency scores among the deployed group found in the current study. This is an area that warrants further investigation.

Ahmed (2007) suggests that involvement in creative activities along with strategies to identify needs of health care personnel and interventions to meet these identified needs with support can promote resilience. Gibbons and colleagues (2013) found that calming activities that enhanced self-reflection were useful for combat health care providers. Applewhite and Arincorayan (2009) recommended that DoD leaders act to prevent compassion fatigue by increasing the number of mental health providers in each brigade, clarifying the health care providers' role, and giving the providers more authority. They also recommended building resilience by implementing mental health education programs, combat operational stress control training, Army provider resiliency programs, and social support networks.

There is a major role for health care providers to develop and provide these supports and programs to military health care providers. Often the health care providers are so involved in doing this work for other military providers they may neglect to provide these same supports and programs for their own health care provider group. There is a need for these supports and programs to be formalized and made available to all military health care personnel, particularly those with low resiliency scores. Social support networks of friends and work colleagues, along with a strong work team spirit, are important in helping to increase resilience (La Salle, 2000). Ongoing evaluation of resiliency can be implemented and interventions can be targeted to enhance resiliency of health care providers as well as all military personnel.

Limitations of the Study

The limitations of the study are related to the sample and the method of data collection, lack of random sampling, and some sample characteristics that make the study results not generalizable to the broader military health care provider population. The sample included a larger percentage of individuals of higher rank than the population of military health care providers. Senior officers comprise 37% of the active duty force. This is in contrast with the sample, where 71.4% were senior officers. This very elite group would be expected to be different that enlisted health care providers and certainly warrants future research.

Recommendations for Future Research

There are several potential areas for future research. The study should be repeated among junior officers to see if there are differences based on years of military and professional experience. Also, the study should be conducted with a larger, randomized sample, particularly one including enlisted personnel. Replication among providers in the Veterans Administration health care system also would be an important addition to the literature, and it would be useful to compare civilians to military health care providers.

This study highlighted the need for the DoD to evaluate ProQoL for military health care providers, as compassion fatigue, burnout, and compassion satisfaction may directly impact the ability of the DoD to retain highly trained health care providers.

Declaration of Interest: The authors report no conflicts of interest. The authors alone are responsible for the content and writing of the paper.

REFERENCES

Adams, S., Camarillo, C., Lewis, S., & McNish, N. (2010). Resiliency training for medical professionals. *The Army Medical Department Journal, April–June*, 48–55.

Adler, A. B., Huffman, A. H., Bliese, P. D., & Castro, C. A. (2005). The impact of deployment length and experience on the well-being of male and female soldiers. *Journal of Occupational Health Psychology, 10*(2), 121–137.

Ahern, N., Kiehl, E., Sole, M., & Byers, J. (2006). Review of instruments measuring resilience. *Comprehensive Pediatric Nursing, 29*(2), 103–125.

Ahmed, A. S. (2007). Post-traumatic stress disorder, resilience, and vulnerability. *Advances in Psychiatric Treatment, 13*, 369–375. doi:10.1192/apt.bp.106.003236

Applewhite, L. L., & Arincorayan, D. L. (2009). Provider resilience: The challenge for behavioral health providers assigned to brigade combat teams. *The Army Medical Department Journal, April–June*, 24–30.

Gibbons, S. W., Barnett, S. D., & Hickling, E. J. (2012). Family stress and posttraumatic stress: The impact of military operations on military healthcare providers. *Archives of Psychiatric Nursing, 26*(4), e31–e39. doi: 10.1016/j.apnu.2012.04.001

Gibbons, S. W., Shafer, M., Aramanda, L., Hickling, E. J., & Benedek, D. M. (2013). Combat healthcare providers and resiliency: Adaptive coping mechanisms during and after deployment. *Psychological Services*. [epub ahead of print]

Hagerty, B. M., Williams, R. A., Bingham, M., & Richard, M. (2011). Military nurses and combat-wounded patients: A qualitative analysis of psychosocial care. *Perspectives in Psychiatric Care, 47*(2), 84–92.

Hickling, E. J., Gibbons, S., Barnett, S. D., & Watts, D. (2011). The psychological impact of deployment on OEF/OIF healthcare providers. *Journal of Traumatic Stress, 24*(6), 726–734. doi: 10.1002/jts.20703

Hoge, C. W., Castro, C. A., Messer, S. C., McGurk, D., Cotting, D. I., & Koffman, R. L. (2004). Combat duty in Iraq and Afghanistan, mental health problems, and barriers to care. *The New England Journal of Medicine, 351*(1), 13–22.

Hooper, C., Craig, J. J., Wetsel, M. A., & Reimels, E. (2010). Compassion satisfaction, burnout, and compassion fatigue among emergency nurses compared with nurses in other selected inpatient specialties. *Journal of Emergency Nursing, 36*(5), 420–427.

Kenny, D. J., & Hull, M. (2008). Critical care nurses' experiences caring for the casualties of war evacuated from the front line: Lessons learned and needs identified. *Critical Care Nursing Clinics of North America, 20*, 41–49.

La Salle, M. A. (2000). Vietnam nursing: The experience lives on. *Military Medicine, 165*(9), 641–646.

Maguen, S., Turcotte, D. M., Peterson, A. A., Dremsa, T. L., Garb, H. N., McNally, R. J. & Litz, B. T. (2008). Description of risk and resilience factors among military medical personnel before deployment to Iraq. *Military Medicine 173*(1), 1–9.

Mental Health Advisory Team-II. (2005). Operation Iraqi Freedom. Report Chartered by U. S. Army Surgeon General, Washington, DC.

Mental Health Advisory Team-III. (2006). Operation Iraqi Freedom 04-06. Report Chartered by U.S. Army Surgeon General, Washington, DC.

Pietrzak, R. H., Johnson, D. C., Goldstein, M. B., Malley, J. C., Rivers, A. J., Morgan, C. A., & Southwick, S. M. (2010). Psychosocial buffers of traumatic stress, depressive symptoms, and psychosocial difficulties in veterans of Operations Enduring Freedom and Iraqi Freedom: The role of resilience, unit support, and postdeployment social support. *Journal of Affective Disorders, 120*, 188–192.

Scannell-Desch, E., & Doherty, M. E. (2010). Experiences of U.S. military nurses in Iraq and Afghanistan wars, 2003–2009. *Journal of Nursing Scholarship, 42*(1), 3–12. doi: 10.1111/j.1547-5069.2009.01329.x

Schok, M., Kleber, R., Gerty, J. L., & Lenvelt-Mulders, L. (2010). A model of resilience and meaning after military deployment: Personal resources in making sense of war and peacekeeping experiences. *Aging & Mental Health, 14*(3), 328–338. doi: 10.1080/13607860903228812

Shea, M., Vujanovic, A., Mansfiels, A., Sevin, E., & Lui, F. (2010). Posttraumatic stress disorder symptoms and functional impairment among OEF and OIF National Guard and Reserve veterans. *Journal of Traumatic Stress, 23*(1), 100–107.

Stamm, B. (2010). The Concise ProQoL Manual (2nd ed.). Pocatello, ID: ProQoL.org.

United States Government Accountability Office. (2010). Enhanced collaboration and process improvements needed for determining military treatment facility medical personnel requirements. Washington, DC: Author.

Vogt, D. S., & Tanner, L. R. (2007). Risk and resilience factors for posttraumatic stress symptomology in Gulf War I veterans. *Journal of Traumatic Stress, 20,* 27–38.

Wagnild, G. M. (2009). The Resilience Scale user's guide for the US English version. Worden, MT: The Resilience Center.

Whealin, J., Batzer, W. B., Morgan, C. A., Detwiler, H. F., Schnurr, P. P., & Friedman, M. J. (2007). Cohesion, burnout and past trauma in tri-service medical and support personnel. *Military Medicine, 172*(3), 266–272.

RESILIENCE AND PROFESSIONAL QUALITY OF LIFE AMONG MILITARY HEALTH CARE PROVIDERS

Critique by *Andrew P. Reimer*

OVERALL SUMMARY

The topic of resilience and professional quality of life among military health care professionals is of great interest, particularly as preassessment data that might lead to intervention designs. Although this study is purely descriptive with limited generalizability due to the convenience sample, it adds to the knowledge base among this targeted vulnerable group, particularly as related to deployment status. The research is logically and clearly presented. The analyses are appropriate and results are presented in detail in text and tables. Importantly, the researchers describe the results in relation to prior research and make strong recommendations about future research and educational implications. Overall, the study is straightforward, clearly presented, and adds to our understanding of the variables under study.

TITLE

Does the title include the key concepts/variables/ phenomenon of interest?

The title clearly indicates the key concepts (resilience, quality of life) and study population (military health care providers).

Is it concise (12 words or less) and professionally stated?

The title is 10 words and is concise and professionally stated.

RESEARCHER(S) CREDIBILITY

Educational credentials?

All authors hold doctoral degrees in nursing and have the educational credentials for the research. The team represents a pairing of those with professional doctorates (DNP) and those with research doctorates (PhD).

Prior methodological research experience of the authors (i.e., methodological expertise)?

The first and second authors have appropriate educational backgrounds, but have a limited research and publishing track record. They have the content expertise for research among military personnel. The third and fourth authors have the methodological expertise.

Subject matter content experience (prior research on the subject matter)?

In this case, it appears that the first and second authors are content and practice experts, who are supplemented by senior and highly experienced coauthors (authors three and four).

ABSTRACT

Does it include the key components (objective/aim, background/rationale, methods, results, and conclusions)?

The article includes a concise unstructured abstract. Each major component of an abstract is included in self-contained sentences from the background (first sentence) and the purpose (second sentence). However the abstract does not mention details of the research methods, including sample or measurement. The significant finding of the study is stated, and the conclusion that is presented is the recommendation for future research.

Does or does not include references?

There are no references included in the abstract.

Is it concise (150–250 words or less)?

This is a concise abstract at 99 words.

Does it entice you to read the rest of the article (interesting)?

The abstract contains just enough information to garner the reader's attention. The last sentence especially entices further reading.

INTRODUCTION/PROBLEM

Is the research problem or phenomenon of interest clearly stated?

The primary problem is clearly stated in the first paragraph of the introduction.

Is it succinct?

The authors present an introductory paragraph that is slightly long and presents some background literature. The introductory paragraph could be more concise. The authors link the need for baseline data on resilience and professional quality of life to retention. This is consistent with prior literature.

Does it answer the "so what" question?

The introduction answers the "so what" question by addressing the issue of retention among military providers, and linking this issue to the phenomena of interest, resilience.

RESEARCH AIMS/OBJECTIVES

Is the research aim/objective clearly stated?

The research aim (purpose) is described in the last sentence of the background section. Although appropriately introduced, the sentence is not clear referring to "these relationships" without identifying the relationships of interest. It can be assumed that the authors are referring to the relationships between resilience and professional quality of life, the two main variables in the study.

Is it concisely written?

Yes, the research aim is concisely written but as stated, the relationships that are of interest are not clear. The differences that the researchers will examine between providers who have been deployed and those who have not been deployed are clearly and concisely stated.

Does it follow logically from the research problem/phenomenon of interest?

The research aim flows logically from the problem statement, the need to understand resilience and professional quality of life among military providers.

SIGNIFICANCE

Is the significance to nursing and health care clearly written?

The significance is clearly established in the first sentence of the manuscript, and then supported throughout the introductory paragraph and the background literature review. The important component of the study is to learn about the key variables that may be related to retention. Although the study does not examine retention, the relationship between the key variables and retention points to the significance of the study.

Does the significance follow from the research aim/objective?

The significance is related to the research aims and follows directly from the intention of knowing some factors that might influence retention of military providers.

BACKGROUND

Is there an explicit description of a theoretical perspective or conceptual framework? If not, is it implied?

There is no mention of a theoretical or conceptual framework guiding the study. After reading the introduction and the background one can deduce the implied relationships between resilience and deployment affecting professional quality of life. The assumption is that the professional quality of life component is related to the broader concept of retention in that it includes the components of compassion satisfaction, burnout, and compassion fatigue.

Are there clear theoretical/conceptual definitions of the concepts?

There are no conceptual definitions provided in the article.

LITERATURE REVIEW

Primary sources only?

Only primary sources are used to delineate the background literature.

Current (within the past how many years)?

The earliest article cited was from 2000, with a majority of the articles ranging between 2005 and 2010. This article was published in 2014 so there is a gap of four years from the time the literature was reviewed and the publication of this work occurred. It would have been useful to conduct another literature review related to this topic as more than 4 years have passed from the last article in the literature review (2010) and the publication date (2014).

Is the search strategy included?

Although no details are provided on the search strategy or resources used to conduct the literature, this is not an uncommon omission from articles that are publishing study results and not focused on extensive review of the literature.

Is literature relevant to the research aims/objectives?

> The background (Literature Review) section is clearly laid out for the reader to develop an overall understanding of the related literature in short order. The literature reviewed is directly relevant to the research aims of the study.

Is it chronologically presented (old to current)?

> The background literature is presented chronologically within the categories of interest to the research aims.

RATIONALE FOR THE STUDY
Is there a gap in the literature that this study will fill (will it extend prior knowledge)?

> The authors identify the gap that this study is addressing in the first sentence of the concluding paragraph of the background section.

Is the rationale clearly stated?

> The rationale for the study is clearly stated in this identification of the gap.

RESEARCH QUESTIONS AND/OR HYPOTHESES
Are these explicitly and clearly stated?

> The research questions are not explicitly stated, making the reader infer exactly what the authors are testing. To identify what is being tested you have to revisit the purpose statement and then work through what the questionnaires that are employed are measuring.

Do they include the variables/phenomena of interest?

> Because there are no explicit research questions there are no explicit variables identified; these can be inferred from the purpose statement.

Do they follow from the research aim/objective?

> The research purpose statement provides direction for the design and analysis.

METHODS
Research Design/Paradigm
Is the research design clearly stated?

> The research design is clearly stated as a descriptive, correlational, quantitative design. This was included in the first sentence of the Methods section.

Is there consistency between the research design and paradigm?

> The quantitative research design is consist with positivism, a prevailing paradigm that guides quantitative research.

Is this the best choice of design to address the research problem/phenomenon of interest?

> Although there is no theoretical or conceptual framework presented, the evidence from prior work in the literature review and intended purpose of this study align with a quantitative approach. Enough is known on the topic of interest that an exploratory qualitative investigation would not be warranted. Because this study

is employing validated instruments that collect discrete self-reported data from individuals, a questionnaire-based study is the most appropriate data-collection methodology.

Is there rigor in the design?

The design has rigor for a descriptive quantitative research study.

SETTING

Is the setting clearly described?

The setting for survey administration is described in the Methods paragraph as a military convention that is attended by active and reservist medical providers from four branches of the military.

What biases are introduced as a result of selecting this particular setting?

This approach to data collection represents a convenience sample, introducing two potential biases. The first is that you are only capturing members who are attending a professional conference, which means that these are people who are engaged and active in their profession—potentially providing a bias if you would compare data collected from those that are not active and do not attend conferences or other professional events. Second, the other potential bias is that those who might score low on resilience and have poorer professional quality of life may not attend conferences due to their current situation. Thus data collection at the conference may not capture those who might score poorly, limiting the generalizability of the findings to the broader population of interest. Both of these biases are evident in the results of this study with the sample characteristics having an over-representation of higher ranking senior officers, who are expected to have higher scores than lower ranking individuals.

SAMPLING PLAN AND SAMPLE

Is the sampling plan clearly identified?

The authors chose a convenience sample approach and clearly identified this as their approach.

Does it represent the population of interest?

Although this approach improves feasibility of accomplishing data collection in a time efficient manner, the limitations and potential of introducing bias as described previously a increase.

Is the sampling plan consistent with the research aim/objective?

Again, the biases introduced in the sampling plan (collection of data at a conference, thereby limiting the type of participants) influence the results and therefore the consistency with the overall research aims.

Is the sample size sufficient (e.g., power analysis or data saturation)?

The available pool of potential study participants (N = approximately 3248) is sufficient to obtain the sample. The final sample consisted of 168 participants, a 19% response rate of the actual number surveyed. No power analysis is presented.

VARIABLES
Are variables clearly identified?

> The variables were not clearly identified, but the reader can identify the key variables through the Instruments section of the paper.

Are variables operationally defined and consistent with theoretical concepts?

> The variables are operationally defined in the Instruments section of the paper. Because there were no theoretical concepts explicitly stated it is not possible to determine consistency between theoretical and operational definitions.

Are independent and dependent variables identified, if applicable?

> This is a descriptive study and no independent and dependent variables are identified; this identification is not relevant to the study.

METHOD OF DATA COLLECTION
What are the methods of data collection?

> The researchers administered a survey to conference participants who were individually approached by the primary researcher. The conference was an annual national conference attended by military health care personnel, the target population.

Are validity and reliability clearly addressed for prior research and current study, if applicable?

> The authors discuss the psychometric qualities (validity and reliability) of each of the two instruments as assessed in prior studies. Appropriate reliability statistics (Cronbach's alpha) are provided for each instrument from previous studies, and assessed in the current study as well. The reliability estimates in the current study are even higher than reported in the literature, supporting the reliable use of these questionnaires in the present study.

Do the measures/instruments address the underlying theoretical concepts or phenomenon of interest?

> In the Instruments section the authors provide a description of each of the questionnaires used. Because there is no explicit identification of the study variables with associated conceptual definitions, it is difficult to assess whether there is consistency between the concepts and the operational measures. At face value, it appears as if these instruments measure the phenomena of interest, resilience, and professional quality of life (which includes the three subscales of compassion satisfaction, burnout, and compassion fatigue).

Were human rights protected?

> The authors state that institutional review board approval was obtained and that the conference organizers provided approval for the researchers to collect data at the conference.

Are other ethical issues identified.

> No other ethical issues were identified.

Is the data-collection method appropriate for research design?

> Data collection via survey is appropriate for a quantitative research design such as used in this study.

Is there bias in data collection?

The bias in data collection is as referred to previously, the fact that those attending the conference may present as a biased sample, as they are likely to be both of higher military rank and also more engaged, and thus score higher on the two variables of interest.

What is the fidelity of intervention addressed, if applicable?

There is no intervention; therefore, this is not applicable.

DATA ANALYSIS

Are data analysis techniques described (e.g., statistical tests, methodology for qualitative analysis)?

The handling and analysis of data are adequately described in the statistical analysis paragraph of the article. The authors used a standard software package for data analysis.

Does the analysis answer the research question?

Although no research questions are explicitly stated, the employed questionnaires and associated statistical tests provide the information necessary to address the primary purpose of this study.

Is it appropriate?

The statistical analyses, descriptive statistics for the background and demographic variables, Pearson correlations for the relationships between resilience and professional quality of life, and analysis of variance for the differences between deployed and not-deployed groups are appropriate to answer the research purpose.

Is the analysis comprehensive? Are themes identified?

The analysis as described previously was comprehensive.

Is there bias in the analysis (trustworthiness? credibility?)?

No bias was detected in the analysis.

RESULTS

Are sample characteristics described and fully reported?

The sample characteristics section provides adequate sample description to understand who composed the study sample. The article contains what is considered a "standard" Table 1, which presents the sample demographics that most all studies report. The second paragraph could have been shortened by not describing the military ranks that are also present in Table 1. This extra text is redundant and does not add additional information to presentation of the results, and thus should be avoided.

Are findings presented related to research aim/objective?

There are two primary results sections labeled Relationship Between Resilience and Professional Quality of Life, and Differences Based on Deployment Status, each section providing the results for the primary aims of the study as stated in the purpose statement in the abstract.

Are all outcome variables addressed, if applicable?

> All of the outcome variables, resilience, and professional quality of life, are addressed in the two main results sections of the paper.

Are results clearly presented in text and/or tables/figures?

> The study results are clearly presented in both the text and tables. There is considerable detail provided on the background characteristics of the providers, both presented in Tables 1 and 2. Table 3 includes the descriptive statistics on each of the main variables. The significance values and the results of the inferential statistics are not presented in table form, but are included in the text.

Is significance of results reported, if applicable?

> The significant results and associated F scores and p-values are provided with summary result statistics presented in Table 3. Overall the results section is well written, but could have benefited from providing an additional table listing the values for the other statistical tests that are discussed in the text with no reported F or p-values.

DISCUSSION OF RESULTS

Do the authors link the findings to previous research studies?

> The authors clearly situate their findings within the broader literature and maintain fidelity to only discussing their findings. The second paragraph presents an in-depth discussion on an unanticipated finding. Although the authors point out that this was an unexpected finding, no details or discussion was provided by the authors to clearly explicate why this was an unexpected finding, but simply state that it was.

Are the conclusions comprehensive yet does done go beyond the data?

> The authors discussion of the results does not go beyond the data.

Do the authors interpret the results in the discussion?

> Yes, the authors interpret the results and discuss both the high resilience scores and and the differences in resilience scores between the deployed and nondeployed military health care personnel. They interpret the unexpected finding that resilience scores were higher in the nondeployed personnel. The authors interpret their results in relation to previous studies of health care personnel who have experienced trauma.

Are the findings generalizable or transferable?

> The convenience sample limits generalizability and the authors acknowledge this as a limitation. Yet, because this is the first study of the two main variables among military health care providers, it provides important baseline data from which to build future research and educational programs.

LIMITATIONS

Identified? Accurate? Inclusive?

> This first sentence of the Limitations section offers a general indication that there are limitations related to the sample, the method of data collection, and the lack of random sampling. The only additional information provided is related to details about the

sample characteristics. Additional explanation of the method of data collection and lack of random sampling are warranted due to the potential for introducing bias.

IMPLICATIONS
Are there implications for practice, education, research?

The implications for practice are adequately discussed as the authors indicate that there is a need to identify strategies for enhancing resilience among military health care personnel. They recommend that formal supports and programs be initiated to enhance resiliency among these providers. There is no explicit attention to implications for education, but it is implied that educational programs would be part of the support provided to enhance resilience. The implications for research are discussed in a specific section of the paper. These recommendations for research address several potential future research areas, including study replication to expand generalizability, and attention to designing future research that would address the limitations of this study.

Are there implications for clinical significance?

There is clinical significance in the findings, particularly as they can be interpreted in relation to health care providers who experience other types of trauma. The main study variables, resilience and professional quality of life, are important variables to consider for all health care professionals who are repeatedly exposed to trauma, particularly as related to retention.

RECOMMENDATIONS
Recommendations for future study/study replication?

The authors state recommendations for future research both in the Discussion section and in the Limitations section. In the Limitations section the authors indicate that future research should address the limitation of an over representation of senior officers in the sample. In addition, the last section of the paper is Recommendations for Future Research, and contains additional recommendations for future research to further assess the findings from this study and continue to broaden the reach of the study to include additional populations to increase generalizability.

CONCLUSION
Is it succinct and does it tie everything together?

Although this article does not contain a distinct conclusion section, the last sentence of the Recommendations for Future Research section serves as a concluding sentence that is succinct and summative of the main study finding and future work to be done.

EVALUATION OF A MEDITATION INTERVENTION TO REDUCE THE EFFECTS OF STRESSORS ASSOCIATED WITH COMPASSION FATIGUE AMONG NURSES

10

Julie A. Hevezi, RN, MSN, CNL, CHTP,
is a staff nurse at Thornton Hospital Progressive Care Unit, University of
California San Diego Health System.

ABSTRACT

Purpose of Study: This pilot study evaluated whether short (<10 minutes) structured meditations decrease compassion fatigue and improve compassion satisfaction (CS) in oncology nurses.

Design of Study: A nonrandomized, pre–post intervention study.

Methods Used: Participants used specific meditations designed to establish a sense of calm, relaxation, and self-compassion 5 days a week for 4 weeks. Meditations were provided on an audio CD after brief individual instruction. The Professional Quality of Life Survey (ProQOL), Version 5, was administered pre- and postintervention along with supplementary questions.

Findings: Fifteen nurses participated in the study over a 6-month period in 2014. Paired t test revealed that the intervention demonstrated a statistically significant increase in CS scores (mean difference = −2.66, 95% confidence interval [CI] = [−4.98, −0.36], $t[14] = −2.48$, $p = .027$, $d = 0.63$) and decreases in burnout (mean difference = 4.13, 95% CI = [1.66, 6.60], $t[14] = 3.581$, $p = .003$, $d = 0.92$) and secondary trauma (mean difference = 3.00, 95% CI = [0.40, 5.96], $t[14] = 2.174$, $p = .047$, $d = 0.56$) scores. All participants reported increased feelings of relaxation and well-being on supplemental questions.

Conclusions: Even in this small sample, the practice of short breathing and meditation exercises was effective in improving nurse outcomes. A larger study is warranted including tracking sustained effects relative to maintaining a meditation practice.

KEY WORDS: compassion fatigue; nurses; stress and coping

The stressors involved in caring for patients with complex life-limiting or terminal diagnoses can lead to compassion fatigue (CF) and burnout in nurses. The physical, mental, and psychological effects of CF and burnout adversely affect nurse satisfaction and quality of care (Boyle, 2011; Lombardo & Eyre, 2011; Yoder, 2008). Research has demonstrated the effectiveness of mind–body techniques in reducing stress and

Hevezi, J. A. (2016). Evaluation of a meditation intervention to reduce the effects of stressors associated with compassion fatigue among nurses. *Journal of Holistic Nursing*, 34(4), 343–350. doi:10.1177/ 0898010115615981. Reprinted by Permission of SAGE Publications, Ltd.

enhancing a subjective sense of well-being (Bazarko, 2013; Hofmann, Sawyer, & Oh, 2010). A small pilot study was conducted in the setting of an intermediate care oncology unit. The purpose of this study was to evaluate the potential impact of brief (<10 minutes) structured meditations on CF and compassion satisfaction (CS) in oncology nurses.

LITERATURE REVIEW

Searches using the key words CF, burnout, meditation, mindfulness, compassion, and loving kindness were conducted in the PubMed, CINHAL, Cochrane Library, and Google Scholar databases. The literature is replete with articles on stress, burnout, CF, and coping strategies among nurses. Joinson first described the phenomenon of CF in 1992 while studying the emotional effects of burnout in emergency room nurses. The term was adopted and more formally defined by Figley in 1995 (Coatzee & Klopper, 2010; Neville & Cole, 2013). The terms CF, secondary traumatic stress (STS), and burnout describe the negative effects of one's quality of professional life, and definitions can vary in the literature according to contextual and conceptual frameworks (Coetzee & Klopper, 2010; Neville & Cole, 2013; Stamm, 2010). For the purpose of this pilot study, CF describes the state of physical, emotional, and spiritual depletion experienced by caregivers of seriously ill or traumatized patients. CF is often used synonymously with STS, in which caregivers indirectly experience the trauma of their patients (Lombardo & Eyre, 2011; Melvin, 2015; Neville & Cole, 2013).

CF VERSUS BURNOUT

CF is related to burnout and shares many of the physical and emotional signs and symptoms experienced by caregivers, which can include feelings of apathy, detachment, and ineffectiveness at one's job. Both CF and burnout result from ineffective or depleted coping resources and both negatively affect quality of patient care, nurse satisfaction and retention (Lombardo & Eyre, 2011; Romano, Trotta, & Rich, 2013; Stamm, 2010; Yoder, 2008). The major difference between CF and burnout is the cause. CF is a consequence of repeated exposure to suffering when emotional depletion surpasses a person's ability to recuperate. Burnout is the result of long-term exposure to workplace stressors including patients' suffering, excessive workload, short-staffing, and unchecked workplace conflict (Boyle, 2015; Mathieu, 2014). CF also appears to be more relational in nature, as it is linked to the empathy and compassion inherent in those in the healing professions. It is a consequence of caring for others in distress. CF usually has an acute onset and shorter recovery, whereas burnout typically has a gradual onset in reaction to persistent work environment stressors and can occur in any type of work (Hunsaker, Chen, Maughan, & Heaston, 2015; Lombardo & Eyre, 2011). According to Stamm (2010), the quality of one's professional life contains both negative (CF) and positive (CS) aspects in which CF comprises the components burnout and STS. The ProQOL, Version 5, used in this study measures the separate constructs of CS, STS, and burnout.

CS describes the positive emotions derived from helping others. Nurses can experience this when they feel they are contributing to the well-being of their patients (Stamm, 2010). Compassion is foundational to nursing practice and satisfaction can be derived by the positive feelings generated by benevolence, kindness, and a sense of contributing to the benefit of others, even in a stressful environment. There are few published studies describing the relationship between CF/STS, burnout, and CS. Literature suggests that nurses with higher levels of CS may experience less CF and burnout (Hunsaker et al., 2015; Ray, Wong, & Heaslip, 2013).

Strategies for combating CF and burnout include recognizing what is occurring and intervening early. Workplace resources such as employee assistance programs are often available. However, creating and adhering to a self-care plan is essential for nurses, particularly those working in areas at risk for developing CF and burnout. Self-care plans can include regular exercise, proper nutrition, maintaining social support networks, artistic pursuits, spirituality, and mind–body techniques that teach mindfulness such as yoga and meditation (Boyle, 2011; Kravits, McAllister-Black, Grant, & Kirk, 2010; Malloy, Thrane, Winston, Virani, & Kelly, 2013). Sanso et al. (2015) conducted a study that demonstrated a positive correlation between self-care and CS and a negative correlation between self-care and CF.

Mindfulness is described as a state of active, focused attention to what one is experiencing in the mind and body at the present moment. It is the observation of thoughts and feelings without judgment in order to detach, label, and gain insight from them. Using mindfulness techniques in stressful situations can create a gap between the experience and reaction to it—allowing a choice to be made on how to respond (Kabat-Zinn, 1990).

There is a growing body of research demonstrating the effectiveness of mindfulness-based meditation practices on reducing the physical, emotional, and mental effects of stress among health care workers (Goodman & Schorling, 2012; Hofmann et al., 2010). Derived from Buddhist practices, meditations that focus on breathing can quiet the mind and balance the sympathetic and parasympathetic nervous systems, thus decreasing the physical and mental symptoms of stress (Davies, 2008; Hanson, 2009; Orly, Berger, Eckshtein, & Segal-Engelchin, 2012; Kabat-Zinn, 1990). The well-known mindfulness-based stress reduction (MBSR) program pioneered by Jon Kabat-Zinn usually consists of eight weekly learning sessions of several hours and daily practice of mindful meditation or movement (yoga). This time commitment may dissuade nurses from pursuing MBSR courses (Mackenzie, Poulin, & Seidman-Carlson, 2006). Indeed, informal discussions during the planning stages with project unit nurses consistently revealed concern with the time commitment involved with learning and practicing meditation. There are a few published studies demonstrating the effectiveness of alternative forms of stress management training at least for the short term including brief MBSR and Institute of HeartMath biofeedback training (Foureur, Besley, Burton, Yu, & Crisp, 2013; LaRose, Danhauer, Feldman, Evans, & Kemper, 2010; Mackenzie et al., 2006; Ruotsalainen, Verbeek, Marine, & Serra, 2014).

The loving kindness meditation (LKM), also derived from ancient Buddhist practices, is designed to cultivate an emotional state of unconditional kindness to all beings. The meditation, which can be relatively short, generally consists of directing aspirations and good feelings to others of various degrees of interpersonal relationships to one's self. Studies have demonstrated that the practice of LKM enhances positive emotions, decreases negative affect, and may reduce stress and immune response (Hofmann, Grossman, & Hinton, 2011; Pace et al., 2011). Cultivating self-compassion is an essential part of self-care as nurses often ignore their own needs at the expense of their physical, mental, emotional, and spiritual well-being (Bazarko, 2013; Malloy et al., 2013). In addition, self-compassionate individuals appear to experience less depression and anxiety and exhibit better psychological health and strengths (Neff & Gerner, 2013).

METHOD
Procedure

Approval was obtained from the University of California San Diego institutional review board. Registered nurses (RNs) on the designated pilot unit were eligible to participate, and recruitment was performed through email, staff meeting announcements, and word of mouth.

Design

A nonrandomized, pre–post intervention study to evaluate the effectiveness of breathing and meditation techniques on reducing CF and improving CS among oncology nurses in an academic medical center. All participants received the intervention; there was no control group.

Sample

This was a convenience sample of self-identified nurses from the pilot unit. A total of 17 RNs employed at the designated pilot unit were recruited. One left her position and was lost to follow-up. One participant withdrew before actually starting the meditation practice. Enrollment was ongoing over a 6-month period. All participants were female. While demographic variables were not considered in this study, the age and years of nursing experience were reflective of the overall makeup of the pilot unit staff.

Measures

Participants completed the ProQOL, Version 5 survey prior to beginning and at the end of 4 weeks of practicing the intervention exercises. The ProQOL, Version 5, survey is a 30-question Likert-type scale of 1 to 5, where 1 is *never* and 5 is *very often*. The instrument measures three separate constructs related to positive and negative aspects of working in fields that support people who are experiencing traumatic events: CS, burnout, and STS (considered by the instrument's authors as the component parts of CF). Use of this tool and its validity and reliability have been well established in the literature (Stamm, 2010). Four subjective, supplemental questions and an opportunity for free text response were also completed with the postintervention ProQOL.

Intervention

During a one-on-one educational session, informed consent was obtained, and each participant was given a folder that contained a printed version of an educational PowerPoint describing CF, CS, burnout, self-care, and mindfulness. The folder also contained an author-made audio CD containing a (4-minute) mindful breathing technique for immediate stress reduction introduced at the end of a realistic work-based scenario, an (8-minute) breathing meditation for relaxation, and a (4-minute) LKM (designed to cultivate self-compassion). The folder also contained information on the study itself and the CD exercises. The meditations were purposely short as prestudy casual conversations with the progressive care unit nurses revealed conceptions that meditation "took too long," "I don't think I do it right," and so on. These meditation exercises were designed to demonstrate that stress reduction and cultivating self-compassion did not necessarily take much time.

Participants committed to practicing the meditations 5 days per week for a 4-week period. The ProQOL was completed just prior to starting the meditations. Participants were casually questioned on how the meditations were going and if there were any issues that arose during the first weeks of their study period. At the end of the fourth week, participants were reminded to complete the post-ProQOL and supplemental questions contained in their folders.

Results

Fifteen nurses participated in the study. Paired t test of the ProQOL constructs revealed that the intervention demonstrated a statistically significant increase in CS scores (mean difference = −2.66, 95% confidence interval [CI] = [−4.98, −0.36], $t[14]$ = −2.48, p = .027, d = 0.63) and decreases in burnout (mean difference = 4.13, 95% CI = [1.66, 6.60], $t[14]$ = 3.581, p = .003, d = 0.92) and secondary trauma (mean difference = 3.00, 95% CI = [0.40, 5.96], $t[14]$ = 2.174, p = .047, d = 0.56) scores. The effect size, which measures the magnitude of the treatment effect, was large (d >0.5), despite the small sample. Data are summarized in Table 1.

On the supplementary questions, all participants reported increased feelings of relaxation; developing sense of self-compassion; positive changes in physical, emotional, and mental reactions to stress; and a high likelihood of incorporating meditation into their self-care plans (Figures 1–4).

Nine participants responded to the free text on the supplementary questions. Four described the benefits of the breathing exercises with two nurses reporting incorporating them into bedside care. Two participants described feeling less stress at work. Two described emotional difficulty when starting the LKM, in realizing the extent to which they thought of others but not themselves.

Discussion

Positive results in this small pilot project demonstrate the effectiveness of meditation practices on the well-being of the nurse participants by reducing stress and cultivating self-compassion. This study originated from a personal desire to help coworkers learn tools for coping with the myriad of occupational stressors encountered on a daily basis in the care of complex, often critical or terminal patients. Recurrent generation of the energy that enables nurses to provide compassionate care is essential. The physical, emotional, and mental demands in caring for this population exact a toll, which negatively affects nurse satisfaction and quality of patient care. During informal discussions prior to the start of this study, nurses on the project unit reported occupational related signs and symptoms of stress. The nurses who engaged in these prestudy discussions conveyed interest in learning basic mindfulness stress reduction techniques. However, the majority of them expressed concern with not having "enough time" to learn or practice meditation between their demanding work and home lives. The study was designed with these concerns in mind.

TABLE 1. Summary of ProQOL Pre- and Postintervention Scores

Subscale	Mean Before	Mean After	Confidence Interval (%)	*p*-Value
Compassion satisfaction	36.6	39.3	95	.027
Burnout	26.4	22.2	95	.003
Secondary trauma score	25.3	22.2	95	.047

ProQOL, Professional Quality of Life Survey.

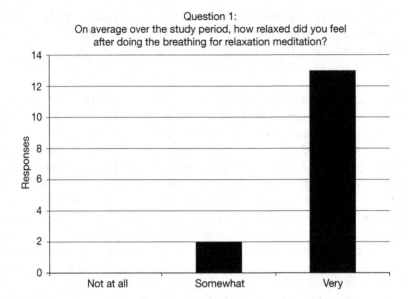

FIGURE 1. Responses to supplemental question 1.

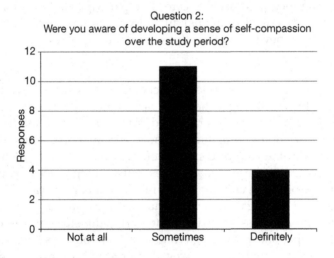

FIGURE 2. Responses to supplemental question 2.

Unlike the traditional MBSR courses that meet weekly for 8 weeks and require a daily commitment to practice, the exercises in this study were purposely short and consisted of home-based learning. Even so, several nurses interested in participation expressed concern over the 5 days/week, 1-month time commitment and did not enroll. Several nurses had to delay their start time after enrolling until their schedules permitted their time commitment.

The one time individualized instruction took place at the work site. A location outside of work would have been ideal; however, work schedules and driving distances precluded this option. Any future instruction should be conducted in a more private area with time to foster an environment of quiet, acceptance, and healing as a basis from which the participants could practice on their own.

The meditation-based intervention appears to have been successful as demonstrated by statistically significant improved ProQOL scores, a large effect size despite

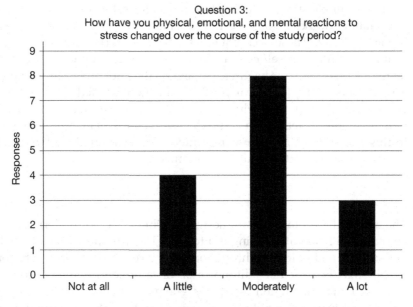

FIGURE 3. Responses to supplemental question 3.

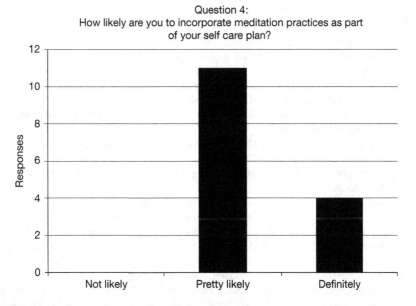

FIGURE 4. Responses to supplemental question 4.

the small sample size, and self-reported enhanced feelings of well-being. However, the small sample size and lack of a control group make it difficult to generalize these results to a larger population. In addition, while many of the participants indicated a likelihood of continuing using meditation as part of a self-care regimen, subsequent timed postintervention questionnaires were not part of the study design. Therefore, the long-term effects of the interventions are not known.

Results of the study as well as the project CD have been shared with colleagues across the nursing spectrum at the pilot unit medical center at both formal and informal venues demonstrating a clear interest in learning and incorporating these relatively simple stress-reducing techniques for self-care. In addition, once learned and embraced, these skills are translatable to the bedside, as several participants reported doing. These techniques can be introduced during new graduate RN training modules on self-care as well as in the development of caregiver support teams. Discussions have begun to expand on the pilot project into other nursing units under a more complex research design, including timed follow-up questionnaires and a control group. In conclusion, short meditation exercises conducted for 30 days with brief preinstruction and audio CD were successful in improving nurse outcomes in this pilot project. More research studies are warranted for the well-being of our fellow nurses, yet initial results are promising.

ACKNOWLEDGMENTS

The author thanks JoAnn Daugherty, RN, PhD, CNL, for undertaking the statistical analysis and help with putting it into plain English; Judith Davidson, RN, DNP, for her support and guidance throughout the project process; Lori Johnson, MSN, RN, OCN, AHN-BC, for her editorial assistance, guidance, and encouragement; and Andrew Laub, meditation instructor, energy and sound healer, for his invaluable insight into teaching meditation. Please address correspondence to Julie A. Hevezi, RN, MSN, CNL, CHTP, email: jhevezi@ucsd.edu.

REFERENCES

Bazarko, D. (2013). The impact of an innovative mindfulness-based stress reduction program on the health and well-being of nurses employed in a corporate setting. *Journal of Workplace Behavioral Health, 28,* 107–133.

Boyle, D. (2011). Countering compassion fatigue: A requisite nursing agenda. *Online Journal of Issues in Nursing, 16*(1), 2. doi:10.3912/OJIN.Vol16No01Man02

Boyle, D. (2015). Compassion fatigue: The cost of caring. *Nursing, 45*(7), 48–51. doi:10.1097/01. NURSE.0000461857.48809.a1

Coetzee, S. K., & Klopper, H. C. (2010). Compassion fatigue within nursing practice: A concept analysis. *Nursing & Health Sciences, 12*(2), 235–243.

Davies, W. (2008). Mindful meditation healing burnout in critical care nursing. *Holistic Nursing Practice, 22*(1), 32–36.

Foureur, M., Besley, K., Burton, G., Yu, N., & Crisp, J. (2013). Enhancing the resilience of nurses and midwives: Pilot of a mindfulness based program for increased health, sense of coherence and decreased depression, anxiety and stress. *Contemporary Nurse, 45*(1), 114–125.

Goodman, M., & Schorling, J. (2012). A mindfulness course decreases burnout and improves well-being among health-care providers. *International Journal of Psychiatry in Medicine, 43*(2), 119–128.

Hanson, R. (2009). *Buddha's brain.* Oakland, CA: New Harbinger.

Hofmann, A., Sawyer, A., & Oh, D. (2010). The effect of mindfulness-based therapy on anxiety and depression: A meta-analytic review. *Journal of Consulting and Clinical Psychology, 78,* 169–183. doi:10.1037/a0018555

Hofmann, S., Grossman, P., & Hinton, D. (2011). Loving-kindness and compassion meditation: Potential for psychological interventions. *Clinical Psychological Review, 31,* 1126–1132. doi:10.1016/j.cpr.2011.07.003

Hunsaker, S., Chen, H.C., Maughan, D., & Heaston, S. (2015). Factors that influence the development of compassion fatigue, burnout, and compassion satisfaction in emergency department nurses. *Nursing Scholarship, 47,* 186–194.

Kabat-Zinn, J. (1990). *Full catastrophe living: Using the wisdom of your body and mind to face stress, pain, and illness.* New York, NY: Delta Trade Paperbacks/Bantam Bell.

Kravits, K., McAllister-Black, R., Grant, M., & Kirk, C. (2010). Self-care strategies for nurses: A psycho-educational intervention for stress reduction and the prevention of burnout. *Applied Nursing Research, 23,* 130–138.

LaRose, A., Danhauer, S., Feldman, J., Evans, G., & Kemper, K. (2010). Brief stress-reduction training in an academic health center. *Journal of Alternative and Complementary Medicine, 16*, 935–936. doi:10.1089/acm.2010.0338

Lombardo, B., & Eyre, C. (2011). Compassion fatigue: A nurse's primer. *Online Journal of Issues in Nursing, 16*(1), 3. doi:10.3912/OJIN.Vol16No01Man03

Mackenzie, C., Poulin, P., & Seidman-Carlson, R. (2006). A brief mindfulness-based stress reduction intervention for nurses and nurse aides. *Applied Nursing Research, 19*, 105–109. doi:10.1016/j.apnr.2005.08.002

Malloy, P., Thrane, S., Winston, T., Virani, R., & Kelly, K. (2013). Do nurses who care for patients in palliative and end of life settings perform good self care? *Journal of Hospice and Palliative Nursing, 15*, 99–106. doi:10.1097/NJH.0b013e31826bef72

Mathieu, F. (2014). Occupational hazards: Compassion fatigue, vicarious trauma and burnout. *Canadian Nurse, 19*(2), 12–13.

Melvin, C. (2015). Historical review in understanding burnout, professional compassion fatigue, and secondary traumatic stress disorder from a hospice and palliative nursing prospective. *Journal of Hospice and Palliative Nursing, 17*, 66–72.

Neff, K., & Gerner, C. (2013). A pilot study and randomized controlled trial of the mindful self-compassion program. *Journal of Clinical Psychology, 69*(1), 28–44. doi:10.1002/jclp.21923

Neville, K., & Cole, D. A. (2013). The relationships among health promotion behaviors, compassion fatigue, burnout, and compassion satisfaction in nurses practicing in a community medical center. *Journal of Nursing Administration, 43*, 348–354.

Orly, S., Berger, R., Eckshtein, R., & Segal-Engelchin, D. (2012). Are cognitive-behavioral interventions effective in reducing occupational stress among nurses? *Applied Nursing Research, 25*, 152–157. doi:10.1016/j.apnr.2011.01.004

Pace, T., Negi, L., Adame, D., Cole, S., Sivilli, T., Brown, T., … Raison, C. (2009). Effect of compassion meditation on neuroendocrine, innate immune and behavioral responses to psychosocial stress. *Psychoneuroendocrinology, 34*(1), 87–98.

Ray, S., Wong, C., & Heaslip, K. (2013). Compassion satisfaction, compassion fatigue, work life conditions, and burnout among frontline mental health care professionals. *Traumatology, 19*(4) 255–267. doi:10.1177/1534765612471144

Romano, J., Trotta, R., & Rich, V. (2013). Combating compassion fatigue: An exemplar of an approach to nursing renewal. *Nursing Administration Quarterly, 37*, 333–336. doi:10.1097/NAQ.Ob013e3182a2f9ff

Ruotsalainen, J., Verbeek, J., Marine, A., & Serra, C. (2014). *Preventing occupational stress in healthcare workers.* Retrieved from http://www.cochrane.org/CD002892/OCCHEALTH_preventing-occupational-stress-in-healthcare-workers

Sanso, N., Galiana, L., Oliver, A., Pascual, A., Sinclair, S., & Benito, E. (2015). Palliative care professionals' inner life: Exploring the relationships among awareness, self-care, and compassion satisfaction and fatigue, burnout, and coping with death. *Journal of Pain and Symptom Management, 50*, 200–207.

Stamm, B. H. (2010). *The concise ProQOL manual* (2nd ed.). Retrieved from http://www.proqol.org/uploads/ProQOL_Concise_2ndEd_12-2010.pdf

Yoder, E. (2008). Compassion fatigue in nurses. *Applied Nursing Research, 23*, 191–197. doi:10.1016/j.apnr.2008.09.003

EVALUATION OF A MEDITATION INTERVENTION TO REDUCE THE EFFECTS OF STRESSORS ASSOCIATED WITH COMPASSION FATIGUE AMONG NURSES

Critique by *Jacqueline Rhoads and Joyce J. Fitzpatrick*

OVERALL SUMMARY

This meditation intervention study and its effects on nurses' compassion fatigue (CF) is of interest to the discipline for two reasons: (a) the interest in complementary therapies, and (b) strategies to reduce CF among nurses and thus potentially increase retention. The research is logically and clearly presented aside from an indirect attention to stress reduction which is implied. The authors should have described this as a pilot study as the sample and aspects of the design are exploratory. The researchers do explain that the setting is a pilot unit, but other aspects of the design also should be labeled the same. Other details are missing, which may be related to the fact that this paper was published in a clinical journal rather than a research journal. As indicated by the researchers the intervention holds promise for future research.

TITLE

Does the title include the key concepts/variables/ phenomenon of interest?

The title includes key concepts of an intervention (meditation), outcome variables (stress reduction), and the population of interest (nurses with CF). Yet in reading the article, the focus is on reduction of CF and compassion satisfaction (CS). The study is not about stressors associated with these outcome variables, thus the title is misleading.

Is it concise (12 words or less) and professionally stated?

The title is professionally stated but a bit lengthy (17 words). The words that could be eliminated are "Evaluation of ... the effects of stressors associated with" and the title could be changed to read: "Meditation Intervention: Effects on Compassion Fatigue and Satisfaction Among Oncology Nurses" thus reducing to 11 words and clearly reflecting the focus of the study.

RESEARCHER(S) CREDIBILITY

Educational credentials?

The sole author is a master's-prepared nurse; thus, she has no terminal degree in nursing or another discipline.

Prior methodological research experience of the authors (i.e., methodological expertise)?

The author does not have prior research experience. She acknowledges others who assisted with the manuscript, specifically the statistical analyses and editorial guidance. Two of the individuals acknowledged have doctoral degrees and the research background necessary for this work.

Subject matter content experience (prior research on the subject matter)?

The author is certified as both a clinical nurse leader (CNL) and a holistic touch practitioner and thus would have the clinical expertise for this clinical study on a holistic modality. She does not have prior research on the subject.

ABSTRACT

Does it include the key components (objective/aim, background/rationale, methods, results, and conclusions)?

The abstract is structured to include the following components: purpose, design, methods, findings, and conclusions. It is very detailed and addresses the main features of the study. The abstract also includes details of the results (the difference scores, the statistical test results, and the probability values). Generally, this amount of detail is not included in an abstract. The background/rationale for the study is not included.

Does or does not include references?

The abstract does not include references.

Is it concise (150–250 words or less)?

The abstract contains approximately 200 words and thus is concise.

Does it entice you to read the rest of the article (interesting)?

This is a small study with positive outcomes on stress reduction using the meditation intervention. The reader is enticed to read on due to the significant findings.

INTRODUCTION/PROBLEM

Is the research problem or phenomenon of interest clearly stated?

The problem statement was consistent with the study title (with the addition of a new variable, CS) and was stated unambiguously; it is easy to identify as it is clearly stated in the first paragraph. This unambiguous statement is consistent with that stated in the abstract but not in the article title.

Does the problem have significance for nursing?

Yes, both CF and CS are of great interest to nursing and there is much research on this topic. The population of study here is oncology nurses, a population of nurses who might experience high stress.

Is it succinct?

Yes, the problem statement is succinct; it is one paragraph.

Does it answer the "so what" question?

Yes, the author indicates that CF is of concern for oncology nurses and there is a need to enhance CS. The arguments presented by the author are supported by references.

RESEARCH AIMS/OBJECTIVES
Is the research aim/objective clearly stated?

The research aim was clearly stated in the last sentence of the first paragraph of the article.

Is it concisely written?

The purpose statement is concise (one sentence).

Does it follow logically from the research problem/phenomenon of interest?

Yes, the research statement flows logically from the research problem stated in the same paragraph, although there is no mention specifically of meditation in the problem statement. Rather there is reference to mind–body techniques to reduce stress. Again, there seems to be an implied notion that reducing CF and enhancing CS reduces stress. The authors do not provide explicit support for this assertion in the problem statement. More important, the study is not about stress reduction per se.

SIGNIFICANCE
Is the significance to nursing and health care clearly written?

There is no separate significance section in the paper, but the author identifies the significance in the introductory paragraph of the article.

Does the significance follow from the research aims/objectives?

Yes, the significance is directly related to the research objectives of the study.

BACKGROUND
Is there an explicit description of a theoretical perspective or conceptual framework? If not, is it implied?

There is no explicit theoretical framework described in the article. Based on the author's insertion of stress reduction as an element related to CF, a stress/coping theoretical framework is implied.

Are there clear theoretical/conceptual definitions of the concepts?

The theoretical/conceptual definitions of the concepts, CF, and CS are presented in the literature review (first paragraph) supported by appropriate references.

LITERATURE REVIEW
Primary sources only?

Only primary sources are cited in the literature review.

Current (within the past how many years)?

The literature review includes citations from 2006 to 2014, and thus is relatively current, spanning a 9-year period. The article was published in December 2016. Articles published more recently, 2015–2016 were thus not included.

Is the search strategy included?

Some aspects of the search strategy were included, specifically the key words and the search engines used. There was no information provided regarding the years covered by the search process although the author indicated that there were some references to CF as early as 1992.

Although the majority of the literature review is directly relevant to the research aims, there is some tangential information presented. For example, the author provides too much detail about some of the interventions that are related to but not central to the study.

The literature is not chronologically presented, although in some of the content subheadings there is attention to the chronological development of the body of knowledge.

RATIONALE FOR THE STUDY

Is there a gap in the literature that this study will fill (will it extend prior knowledge)?

This is an original study not a replication. The author identifies the gap in the literature as the limited studies on stress management among nurses. Again, this stress management concept that is implied as a conceptual framework appears in the article. The author, however, does not sufficiently weave together the focus on stress and the intervention and the outcome variables.

Is the rationale clearly stated?

There is no clear statement about the gap that the author is trying to address. The assumption is that this intervention (a short meditation intervention) had not previously been studied with oncology nurses to determine the effect on diminishing CF and increasing CS.

RESEARCH QUESTION(S) AND/OR HYPOTHESES

Are these explicitly and clearly stated?

No specific research questions or hypotheses are included, but in the Design section there is a statement of the intent to evaluate the effectiveness of breathing and meditation techniques on reducing CF and improving CS among oncology nurses. This can be presumed to be the research question. One inconsistency introduced here is the specification of "breathing and meditation techniques" as this is the first mention of breathing techniques. It is not clear that this is one and the same or two separate interventions although the assumption is that the intervention will include both.

Do they include the variables/phenomena of interest?

There are no variables identified in research questions or hypotheses, but rather these are embedded in the purpose statement and the previous statement included in the Design section.

Do they follow from the research aim/objective?

If we assume that the statement in the Design section is the research question, then it follows from the research purpose (objective). The research purpose is a bit different and more specific in identifying the intervention: "to evaluate the potential impact of brief (less than 10 minutes) structured meditation on CF and CS in oncology nurses."

METHODS
Research Design/Paradigm
Is the research design clearly stated?

> The research design, a nonrandomized, pre–post intervention study is clearly stated.

Is there consistency between the research design and paradigm?

> There is consistency between the research design and the paradigm underlying quantitative research.

Is this the best choice of design to address the research problem/phenomenon of interest?

> This is an adequate design to address the research problem.

Is there rigor in the design?

> Based on the sample size and selection and the identification of the setting as a "pilot unit" this may best be described as a pilot study. The study would be more rigorous if formalized and described as a pilot study.

SETTING
Is the setting clearly described?

> The setting is described only as a pilot unit; no other details are provided. One assumes that this pilot unit is an oncology unit as the nurses recruited are oncology nurses.

What biases are introduced as a result of selecting this particular setting?

> It is not clear whether the author is employed by the setting and, if so, in what role. The investigator role could introduce bias.

SAMPLING PLAN AND SAMPLE
Is the sampling plan clearly identified?

> The sampling plan is clearly identified. The study involved a convenience sample of self-identified nurses from the pilot unit. A total of 17 RNs employed at the designated pilot unit were recruited (15 completed the study). Although demographic variables were not considered in this study, the age and years of nursing experience were reflective of the overall makeup of the pilot unit staff.

Does it represent the population of interest?

> Yes, the sampling plan represents oncology nurses, the population of interest.

Is the sampling plan consistent with the research aim/objective?

> Since the objective was to test the intervention with oncology nurses, then the sampling plan was consistent with the objective.

Is the sample size sufficient (e.g., power analysis or data saturation)?

> The sample size was small ($N = 15$) and more reflective of a pilot study. There was no power analysis reported.

VARIABLES
Are variables clearly identified?

The CD used in the intervention variable was described in detail, as was the initial one-to-one session in which participants were provided with a folder with an educational PowerPoint describing the outcome measures, and the mindfulness intervention. The variables of CS and CF are described in the Measures section of the article. Yet the author mentions three scores obtained from the Professional Quality of Life instrument and does not make it clear which of the scores are being used. It is unclear whether the burnout subscale is used or just the CS and CF components of the scale.

Are variables operationally defined and consistent with theoretical concepts?

Although the variables are consistent with the concepts being studied, there are no operational definitions presented. The reader can assume that the researcher is using the total score on the CS and the total score on the CF subscales of the Professional Quality of Life instrument.

Are independent and dependent variables identified, if applicable?

There is not explicit identification of independent and dependent variables, but the design assumes the intervention is the independent variable and the CF and CS are the dependent variables. The researcher mentions four additional, subjective questions that were added and these variables are not clearly defined or included in any of the prior discussion. The assumption is that they also are dependent variables.

METHOD OF DATA COLLECTION
What are the methods of data collection?

The methods used to gather the data for this study were explained. The intervention was conducted in one-on-one introductory sessions, then through use of a CD for follow-up interventions. Data were collected over a 6-month period. The researcher described the intervention that was introduced, and participants were expected to practice the meditation (and the breathing although this is not specified) 5 days per week for a 4-week period. There was no clear information regarding how many times a day the participants should use the intervention, and no effort was made to capture these data. The outcome variables were assessed before the implementation and at the end of the fourth week.

Are validity and reliability clearly addressed for prior research and current study, if applicable?

The author made a general statement that the ProQOL questionnaire validity and reliability have been well established in the literature, with one reference citation. There was no mention of the specific psychometric specifics for this instrument. Further there was no assessment of the reliability of the ProQOL in the present study. There also was no discussion of the validity and reliability of the intervention variable. Since the intervention was introduced over a 6-month period, it is possible that some of the participants began using the intervention before their pretest. There also was no control on how many times the intervention should be used per day.

Do the measures/instruments address the underlying theoretical concepts or phenomenon of interest?

The measures address the phenomena of interest, the meditation intervention, and the CF and CS outcome variables.

Were human rights protected?

Institutional review board approval was obtained prior to implementation of the study.

Are other ethical issues identified?

No other ethical issues were identified, although the author does not address any dropout rate other than the initial loss of the two participants. It is assumed that the participants knew they could dropout and that this would not affect their employment.

Is the data-collection method appropriate for research design?

This design is more appropriate for a pilot study, with the small sample size and the new intervention being tested.

Is there bias in data collection?

There may have been bias due to the fact that the researcher was employed in the study site, and this may have influenced the responses to the questionnaires, and the overall outcome responses.

What is the fidelity of intervention addressed, if applicable?

The fidelity of the intervention is not directly addressed. Because the study was conducted over a 6-month period with ongoing enrollment, it is not clear what cross-over effects might have occurred, such as the nurses participating earlier may have influenced the nurses who enrolled later. Also, even though the participants were to practice the meditation 5 days per week there was specific way of evaluating this practice.

DATA ANALYSIS

Are data analysis techniques described (e.g., statistical tests, methodology for qualitative analysis)?

Although there was no specific section detailing the data analysis plan, the results of the data analysis were reported in detail.

Does the analysis answer the research question?

Yes, the analysis answers the research questions. Yet there is another variable added in the Analysis section that was not clearly presented or discussed in the presentation of the variables. The third score on the ProQOL scale is a measure of burnout. Although in the Measures section the researcher indicates that the two scores, burnout and secondary traumatic stress, are considered components of CF by the instrument author, this is not clearly stipulated throughout the manuscript. This confusion would have been clarified if the author presented clear conceptual and operational definitions. In fact, in the conceptual definition the author indicated that CF is often used synonymously with secondary traumatic stress. If this is the case, then why also use the burnout measure? This lack of clarity could have been avoided if the author merely used the three scores separately as was done in the analysis.

Is it appropriate?

The analysis of difference scores from time 1 to time 2 was appropriate to determine the effects of the intervention.

Is the analysis comprehensive? Are themes identified?

> The analysis was comprehensive for the research design and to answer the research purpose statement/question.

Is there bias in the analysis (trustworthiness? credibility?)?

> There is not bias detected in the analysis.

RESULTS

Are sample characteristics described and fully reported?

> There were no demographic data collected. The researcher indicated that all participants were female. The researcher also indicated in a general statement that the age and education of the participants were reflective of the overall pilot unit staff. If would be helpful to know the specifics in these domains, but for the population (i.e., how many nurses worked on the pilot unit and what percentage participated), and the sample in the study.

Are findings presented related to research aim/objective?

> Findings related to the research objectives are presented. Additional findings related to the four qualitative questions also are presented.

Are all outcome variables addressed, if applicable?

> All outcome variables are presented but again the confusion exists as to the measure of CF. Is it reflected in the two separate scores of burnout and secondary traumatic stress or is it somehow the combination of these scores. In the analysis and results, the scores of the two variables are presented independently.

Are results clearly presented in text and/or tables/figures?

> There is one clearly presented table with the quantitative scores pre and post on the ProQOL scale. These results also are presented in detail in the text so there is redundancy. The results of the four qualitative questions are presented clearly in four figures.

Is significance of results reported, if applicable?

> The significance levels for all analyses are presented in the results in the text and table.

DISCUSSION OF RESULTS

Do the authors link the findings to previous research studies?

> The author does not link the findings to previous research in this area. No other studies are cited in the Discussion section. This is a major flaw in the research report as it is expected that the researcher findings will be linked to prior research.

Are the conclusions comprehensive, yet within the data?

> The Discussion section is beyond a discussion of the study findings. Rather it also includes some aspects that were previously presented in earlier sections of the paper, for example, the specifics of the intervention and the data collection plans. The Discussion section also includes other information gleaned from the participants that was not part of the study, for example, reasons why some nurses did not enroll for the study. Overall, this section should have been much tighter.

Do the authors interpret the results in the discussion?

> There is interpretation of the results in the Discussion section, but more detail is provided on related aspects of the overall study.

Are the findings generalizable or transferable?

> The generalizability is limited due to the small sample size. Yet the impressive significant results make the transferability and generalizability of interest.

LIMITATIONS
Identified? Accurate? Inclusive?

> There is no specific section describing the study limitations. Rather the author presents some of the study limitations, for example, small sample size, challenges in recruitment, and therefore perhaps a biased sample, and the single-site pilot unit.

IMPLICATIONS
Are there implications for practice, education, research?

> The author indicates several recommendations for practice, for education of clinicians, and for future research. The value of this condensed version of meditation holds potential for decreasing CF among nurses in many clinical areas.

Are there implications for clinical significance?

> The clinical significance is also related to the potential for reducing CF and enhancing CS among nurses.

RECOMMENDATIONS
Recommendations for future study/study replication?

> There was no specific section on recommendations for future research. Throughout the Results and Discussion sections, the author repeated the need for follow-up research and for a larger sample size to evaluate the same variables.

CONCLUSION
Is it succinct and does it tie everything together?

> A formal concluding statement is not evident but throughout the Results and Discussion sections the author repeated the need for follow-up and larger sample size.

PATIENT SAFETY CULTURE AND NURSE-REPORTED ADVERSE EVENTS IN OUTPATIENT HEMODIALYSIS UNITS

Charlotte Thomas-Hawkins, PhD, RN,
School of Nursing, Rutgers University, Newark, New Jersey

Linda Flynn, PhD, RN, FAAN,
College of Nursing, University of Colorado-Denver

ABSTRACT

Aims: Patient safety culture is an important quality indicator in health care facilities and has been associated with key patient outcomes in hospitals. The purpose of this analysis was to examine relationships between patient safety culture and nurse-reported adverse patient events in outpatient hemodialysis facilities.

Methods: A cross-sectional correlational, mailed survey design was used. The analytic sample consisted of 422 registered nurses who worked in outpatient dialysis facilities in the United States. The Handoff and Transitions and the Overall Patient Safety Grade Scales of the Agency for Healthcare Research and Quality's (AHRQ) Hospital Patient on Safety Survey were modified and used to measure patient safety culture in outpatient dialysis facilities. Nurse-reported adverse patient events were measured as a series of questions designed to capture the frequency with which nurses report that 13 adverse events occur in the outpatient dialysis facility setting.

Results: Handoff and transitions safety during patient shift change in dialysis centers was perceived negatively by a majority of nurses. On the other hand, a majority of nurses rated the overall patient safety culture in their dialysis facility as good to excellent. All relationships between patient safety culture items and adverse patient events were in the expected direction. Negative ratings of handoffs and transitions safety were independently associated with increased odds of frequent occurrences of vascular access thrombosis and patient complaints. Negative ratings of overall patient safety culture in dialysis units were independently associated with increased odds of frequent occurrences of medication errors by nurses, patient hospitalization, vascular access infection, and patient complaints.

Conclusion: Findings from this analysis indicate that a positive patient safety culture is an important antecedent for optimal patient outcomes in ambulatory care settings.

KEY WORDS: patient safety culture; hemodialysis; adverse events; quality of care

Thomas-Hawkins, C., & Flynn, L. (2015). Patient safety culture and nurse-reported adverse events in outpatient hemodialysis units. *Research and Theory for Nursing Practice, 29,* 53–65. doi:10.1891/1541-6577.29.1.53. Republished with permission of Springer Publishing Company.

A vast majority of health care in the United States takes place in outpatient or ambulatory care settings (Agency for Healthcare Research and Quality, 2012). Despite this fact, efforts to improve patient safety have focused largely on inpatient settings, and less is known about safety culture in care settings outside of the hospital. Outpatient hemodialysis centers are a type of ambulatory care setting that is the most common site of long-term hemodialysis therapy for persons with chronic kidney failure. Nearly 90% of persons with this condition in the United States receive hemodialysis treatments three times a week in 6,000 outpatient dialysis centers (United States Renal Data System, 2013). Currently, more than 60 million hemodialysis treatments in outpatient settings are performed annually in the United States. Although hemodialysis in an outpatient setting is a routine mode of treatment, it is a complex and potentially hazardous procedure (Holley, 2010). Moreover, it is well established that there are major gaps in the safety net around this procedure (Himmelfarb, 2010), and there has been little research dedicated to assessing and improving the safety of patients in this critical outpatient setting.

ADVERSE EVENTS IN HEMODIALYSIS PATIENTS

Multiple patient safety risks and adverse events are readily apparent in outpatient hemodialysis units. In the past decade, surveys of dialysis professionals and patients that focused on safety issues in dialysis units revealed these outpatient settings share important patient safety risks including patient falls, medication errors, failure to follow established policies, errors in dialysis machine preparation, lapses in infection control, vascular access-related events, excess blood loss/prolonged bleeding, and lapses in communication (DeVivo, 2001; Renal Physicians Association, 2007). In addition, a review of adverse events in four outpatient hemodialysis units during an 18-month period revealed a total of 88 events over this time span, including infiltration of the vascular access, medication errors, dialysis circuit clotting, and falls in the dialysis unit after the treatment (Holley, 2006). A lack of adherence to the prescribed hemodialysis session length (shortened treatments) and to the session schedule (skipped treatments) are also frequent adverse events among persons receiving long-term hemodialysis treatments and significant contributors to hospitalization and mortality (Saran et al., 2003; Tapolyai et al., 2010). Likewise, findings from an investigation of nurse-reported adverse patient events in outpatient hemodialysis facilities (Thomas-Hawkins, Flynn, & Clarke, 2008) revealed nurse reports of frequent occurrences of adverse patient events in their dialysis units such as skipped and shortened dialysis treatments, hypotensive episodes during the dialysis procedure, and patient complaints. These findings support the assertion that hemodialysis can be potentially hazardous for patients. In addition, there has been little research dedicated to assessing and improving the safety of patients in this critical outpatient setting.

PATIENT SAFETY CULTURE IN HEMODIALYSIS UNITS

To improve patient safety, the Institute of Medicine (IOM, 2004) recommends that all health care facilities across the care continuum develop and maintain a culture of patient safety. According to AHRQ (2014), a culture of safety is a commitment at all levels of the organization to minimize adverse patient events in the face of inherently complex and potentially hazardous procedures. AHRQ has conceptualized patient safety culture as a multidimensional concept, and two dimensions were examined in this study. The first of these is employees' "overall grade" of patient safety, from excellent to failing, in their workplace. Importantly, an emerging body of research indicates that employees' fair to failing ratings of patient safety in their hospitals are associated with adverse patient events such as medication errors (Chang & Mark, 2011; Hofman & Mark, 2006) and iatrogenic pneumothorax and infections following surgical procedures (Mardon, Khanna, Sorra, Dyer, & Famolaro, 2010).

The second patient safety culture dimension examined in this study was "patient handoff and transitions." An effective patient handoff and transition within and across health care settings is a process that includes interactive communication, up-to-date accurate information, limited interruptions, a process for verification, and an opportunity to review any relevant patient data (The Joint Commission, 2010). Ineffective transitions and handoffs, however, are common and have been linked with adverse patient events such as misdiagnosis, incorrect treatments, and failure to communicate follow-up with patients (Gandhi, 2005; Mardon et al., 2010). Unlike patient handoffs and transitions that occur during "nurse change-of-shift" periods in hospital settings, "patient shift change" in outpatient hemodialysis units is a common patient transition period. During these patient changeover periods that occur multiple times per day in a single hemodialysis unit, cohorts of patients concurrently transition in or out of the hemodialysis unit before or after their treatments. A patient shift change goal is to safely terminate hemodialysis treatments for a group of patients while simultaneously safely initiating treatment for the next shift of incoming patients. Notably, patient transition periods in outpatient hemodialysis facilities provide ample opportunity for misinformation, miscommunication, and error. Moreover, increased interruptions and demands on nurses' time during patient transition periods can threaten patient safety and lead to adverse patient events (Clancy, 2011; IOM, 2004).

THEORETICAL FRAMEWORK

Despite the patient safety challenges in outpatient hemodialysis units, little attention has been allocated to assessing the patient safety cultures of these health care settings. Consequently, there is little evidence on which to guide strategies to ensure patient safety during peak patient transition times. The nursing organization and outcomes model (Aiken, Clarke, & Sloane, 2002) provides a particularly efficient explanation of how patient safety culture in dialysis units influences adverse patient events. The model postulates that a high-quality work environment is an organizational feature that influences positive patient outcomes. One characteristic of a high-quality work environment is the presence of a culture that supports and fosters patient safety. The model also posits that high-quality work environments enhance the quality of nursing care processes, such as care provided during patient transitions in dialysis units. In turn, safe care processes result in superior patient outcomes. For this study, a high-quality work environment was represented as nurses' grades for patient safety in their dialysis unit. Quality nursing care processes were represented as nurses' ratings of patient transition safety during patient shift change, and patient outcomes were represented as nurse-reported adverse patient events.

STUDY PURPOSE

Little is known regarding the state of patient safety in outpatient hemodialysis settings, nor is there any evidence regarding the impact of safety cultures on the frequency of adverse event occurrences among patients receiving hemodialysis treatments in outpatient settings. The purpose of this study was to investigate associations among staff nurses' ratings of patient transition safety, nurses' grade for patient safety in their dialysis unit, and the odds of nurse reports of adverse patient events in their dialysis units. This study was designed to address the following research questions:

1. What percentage of nursing staff in dialysis facilities report positive ratings of (a) patient transition safety and (b) patient safety?
2. What are the associations between nurse-rated patient transition safety and the odds of nurse-reported adverse patient events in outpatient hemodialysis units?
3. What are the associations between nurses' patient safety grade and the odds of nurse-reported adverse patient events in outpatient hemodialysis units?

METHODS

A cross-sectional, correlational design was used for this study. The analysis of nurses' patient safety grade for their dialysis units, nurses' rating of patient transition safety, and nurse-reported adverse patient events described here uses secondary data collected between September 2007 and November 2007 in a parent study conducted in the United States that was designed to disentangle the relationships among nurse staffing, omitted care, and outcomes in outpatient hemodialysis settings (Flynn, Thomas-Hawkins, & Clarke, 2009; Thomas-Hawkins et al., 2008). The Rutgers University Institutional Review Board approved the study.

Sample

A modified Dillman survey method was used for data collection in the parent study (Dillman, 2007). Two thousand registered nurses (RNs) who identified themselves as staff nurses in hemodialysis settings were randomly selected from the American Nephrology Nurses' Association's (ANNA) membership list to receive survey packets mailed to their homes. Rather than mailing potential participants an advance notice letter prior to receipt of the full survey, the Dillman method was modified. Participants were initially mailed the full survey with a cover letter that described the study purpose and indicated their completion of the questionnaire served as consent to participate. One week after the initial mailing, nonresponders were sent a reminder postcard. Two weeks later, nonresponders were mailed a full survey with a follow-up reminder postcard 1 week later. A survey response rate of 52% resulted in data from 1,015 nephrology RNs across the United States. Among these, 422 RNs representing 47 of the 50 states indicated they worked as staff RNs at an outpatient hemodialysis unit, and therefore, comprised the analytic sample for this analysis. The demographic characteristics of the study sample are presented in Table 1.

Measures

Nurse-reported adverse events were measured as a series of survey items designed to capture the frequency with which 13 adverse patient events occurred in the dialysis unit in the past year. The adverse patient events reported in the survey are common among hemodialysis patients and have been identified as important patient safety indicators in outpatient hemodialysis units (Holley, 2006; Port et al., 2004; Saran et al.,

TABLE 1. Characteristics of Study Sample

	M	SD
Age (years)	48.6	8.1
Years in current position	7.8	6.8
Years working for current employer	10.4	9.2
Years in nephrology nursing	13.2	8.6
Gender	*n*	%
Female	394	93.4
Male	26	6.2
Not reported	2	0.5
Race	*n*	%
African American/Black	29	6.9
Asian/Pacific Islander	31	7.4
Hispanic	8	1.9
White	346	82.0
Other	5	1.1
Not reported	3	0.7
Nursing education	*n*	%
Diploma	76	18.0
Associate degree	153	36.3
Baccalaureate degree	173	41.0
Baccalaureate degree	11	2.6
Not reported	9	2.1

2003). Event frequency was rated on a 7-point scale ranging from 1 (*never*) to 7 (*every day*), with higher scores indicating higher frequencies of adverse events.

Two scales of the Hospital Survey on Patient Safety Culture (HSOPS; Sorra & Nieva, 2004) were used to measure patient safety culture in the parent study. The four-item Handoff and Transitions Scale of the HSOPS was used to measure nurses' ratings of dialysis patient transitions safety during patient shift change. A slight modification was made to the wording of each scale item. The wording "when transferred to another unit" or "shift change" in scale items was replaced with "during patient shift change" to reflect the time of patient transitions in outpatient hemodialysis units. Nurses were asked to rate their level of agreement or disagreement with each item on a scale of 1 (*strongly agree*) to 5 (*strongly disagree*); higher scores indicate higher ratings of safe patient transitions. Alpha reliability for the scale in this study was 0.91. Prior to data analysis, total composite scores were dichotomized so that scores of 3.50 or greater (*disagree* or *strongly disagree* with item) indicated a safe patient transition rating and composite scores less than 3.50 indicated an unsafe patient transition rating.

The patient safety grade single item rating on the HSOPS (Sorra & Nieva, 2004) was used to measure nurses' grades for patient safety in their dialysis units. Nurses were asked to give their dialysis unit an overall grade on patient safety (A = *excellent*, B = *good*, C = *fair*, D = *poor*, F = *failing*). Prior to data analysis, patient safety grades were dichotomized so that grades of fair/poor/failing indicated an unfavorable patient safety rating and grades of excellent/good indicated a favorable patient safety rating.

Data Analysis

Frequency distributions and descriptive statistics of study variables were computed and examined. A series of 13 unadjusted and adjusted logistic regression models were estimated to determine the individual and independent effects of patient transition safety and patient safety grade on the odds of nurses' reporting frequent adverse patient events. In the unadjusted models, fair to failing patient safety grades and unsafe handoffs and transitions safety ratings were entered individually. In the adjusted models, both were entered simultaneously. Good/excellent safety grades and safe handoff and transitions ratings were used as comparison groups in both unadjusted and adjusted models. For each adverse event, scores were dichotomized as "seldom" (never to several times per year) or "frequent" (daily to at least once per month).

RESULTS
Staff Nurse Perceptions of Safety in Dialysis Units

Nurse responses to the four items on the Handoffs and Transitions Scale reflect poor patient transition safety ratings by a majority of participants, as shown in Table 2. Moreover, only 39% of nurses positively endorsed safe patient transitions during

TABLE 2. Percent of Nurses Who Positively Endorse Patient Transitions Safety and Overall Patient Safety (Safety Grade) in Dialysis Units

Handoffs and Transitions Safety Items	Sample Who Disagreed (Positive Response) With Scale Item (%)
Things fall between the cracks during patient shift change.	28.4
Important patient care information is often lost during patient shift change.	41.7
Patient shift changes are often problematic for patients in this dialysis unit.	44.8
Problems often occur in the exchange of information during patient shift changes.	42.4
Mean composite score (% of sample with positive response)	
Overall handoffs and transitions safety	39
Safety grade	% of respondents
F (failing)	0.5
D (poor)	1.4
C (fair)	12.2
B (good)	48.4
A (excellent)	37.5
Overall patient safety	Mean composite score (% of sample with positive responses) 86

patient shift change in their dialysis units. On the other hand, 86% of nurses positively graded patient safety in their dialysis unit as either good or excellent.

Relationship Between Nurse-Rated Patient Transition Safety and Nurse-Reported Adverse Patient Events

The unadjusted and adjusted odds ratios for the associations between nurses' ratings of unsafe patient transitions during patient shift change, compared to nurses who rated patient transitions as safe, and the 13 adverse events are listed in Table 3. The unadjusted regression models revealed significant associations between nurse reports of unsafe patient transition during patient shift change and an increased likelihood of their reports of frequent occurrences (i.e., daily to once a month) of nine adverse events. When estimating the adjusted effects, controlling for the effect of patient safety grade ratings, nurse reports of unsafe patient transitions, compared to nurses who reported safe patient transitions, was independently associated with an increased likelihood of nurse reports of frequent occurrences of six adverse events, including shortened and skipped dialysis treatments by patients, vascular access thrombosis and infection, unexplained bleeding from the vascular access site, and complaints from patients and their families.

Relationship Between Nurses' Patient Safety Grade and Nurse-Reported Adverse Patient Events

The unadjusted and adjusted odds ratios for the associations between nurses' fair to failing patient safety grades for their unit, compared to nurses who graded patient

TABLE 3. Odds Ratios Associated With Significant Effects of Unsafe Patient Transitions and Poor to Failing Safety Grade on Adverse Events

	Unsafe Patient Transitions		Poor to Failing Patient Safety Grade	
Adverse Event	Unadjusted Model	Model Adjusted for Safety Grade	Unadjusted Model	Model Adjusted for Patient Transition Ratings
Dialysis hypotension	ns	ns	ns	ns
Skipped dialysis treatments	2.36***	1.96**	6.54**	4.65*
Shortened dialysis treatments	2.59***	2.06**	ns	ns
Vascular access infection	1.87**	1.59*	2.52**	2.20**
Vascular access infiltration	1.59*	ns	ns	ns
Vascular access thrombosis	2.16***	2.07***	ns	ns
Bleeding from vascular access	1.77**	1.61*	2.10*	ns

(continued)

TABLE 3. Odds Ratios Associated With Significant Effects of Unsafe Patient Transitions and Poor to Failing Safety Grade on Adverse Events (*continued*)

Adverse Event	Unsafe Patient Transitions		Poor to Failing Patient Safety Grade	
	Unadjusted Model	Model Adjusted for Safety Grade	Unadjusted Model	Model Adjusted for Patient Transition Ratings
Complaints from patient/family	3.16***	2.72***	4.33***	2.85**
Medication error	2.08*	ns	3.07***	2.72**
Emergency room use	1.77**	ns	2.10*	1.96*
Hospital admission	ns	ns	2.15**	1.82*
Falls without injury	ns	ns	2.92*	ns
Falls with injury	ns	ns	ns	ns

*$p = .05$.
**$p = .01$.
***$p = .001$.

safety as good to excellent, and the 13 adverse events are listed in Table 3. The unadjusted effects of nurses' fair to failing grade for patient safety in their dialysis units were significantly associated with an increased likelihood of their reports of frequent occurrences of eight adverse events. The adjusted effects nurses' fair to failing hemodialysis dialysis unit patient safety grades, controlling for the effects of patient transitions safety, were independently associated with their reports of frequent occurrences of six adverse events, including patient emergency room admissions, hospital admissions, medication errors, skipped dialysis treatments by patients, vascular access infection, and patient and family complaints.

DISCUSSION

There is a growing body of evidence that demonstrates the existence of serious health care quality problems for patients undergoing transitions across sites of care such as primary care to specialty care or hospital to subacute care (AHRQ, 2007). However, research in hospital settings has shown that safe patient handoffs and transitions across inpatient units or during staff shift changes within patient units can facilitate positive patient outcomes and the reduction of adverse patient events (Mardon et al., 2010). Patient transition during patient shift change in outpatient hemodialysis units is a unique type of care transition that occurs within a dialysis unit multiple times a day rather than across sites of care. During these periods, a series of essential care processes are performed by nursing staff such as dialysis machine setup, predialysis patient assessment, vascular access cannulation and care, discontinuation of dialysis treatments, and postdialysis patient assessments. These patient transition care processes have a high potential for interruptions of care, miscommunication, and error. Indeed, findings from this study revealed that only 39% of nurses positively endorsed safe patient transitions during patient shift change in their dialysis units. These findings are similar to recent data from 653 U.S. hospitals that revealed only 47% of hospital staff, on average, positively endorsed safe patient handoffs and transitions across hospital units and during staff shift changes (Sorra et al., 2014). Moreover, patient handoffs and transitions were deemed in this report as an area for improvement. Unlike patient handoffs and transitions in hospitals, the findings from this study point to a unique period of patient transition during the patient shift change period in outpatient dialysis units, and nurses' ratings of safety during this period indicate a particular aspect of safety culture in outpatient dialysis units that warrants attention.

There was a striking difference in nurses' perceptions of safety during the specific period of patient transitions in their dialysis units compared to their overall perceptions of safety policies, procedures, and practices in their workplace, as reflected in their safety grade ratings. Specifically, in contrast to the low percentage of nurses who reported safe patient transitions in their dialysis units, 86% of nurses graded overall patient safety in their dialysis units as good or excellent. These differences in staff perceptions of particular aspects of patient safety in the workplace also exist in acute care hospital settings. Recent data from the AHRQ 2014 comparative database of 653 U.S. hospitals reveal that, although only 47% of hospital staff positively endorse safe handoffs and transitions, 76% of staff grade overall safety in their workplace as excellent or very good (Sorra et al., 2014). Thus, research findings in both inpatient and outpatient health care settings underscore the multidimensional nature of safety culture and need for broad safety assessments because some aspects of safety can be very good or excellent whereas other aspects may require attention and improvement.

Nurses' negative ratings of patient safety culture in this study, that is, unsafe patient transitions and fair to failing safety grades, were independently associated with their reports of frequent adverse patient events in the adjusted regression models (Table 3). Specifically, compared to nurses who endorsed safe patient transitions during patient shift change in dialysis units, nurses' ratings of unsafe patient transitions were independently associated with nurse reports of frequent occurrences (i.e., daily to monthly) adverse patient events assessed in this study. These findings are consistent with hospital-based research that reveals an independent association between positive ratings by staff of patient handoffs in hospitals and positive patient assessments of the quality of their inpatient care (Sorra, Khanna, Dyer, Mardon, & Famolaro, 2012). Likewise, an analysis of data from 179 U.S. hospitals revealed that positive ratings of patient handoffs and transitions by hospital staff were independently associated with lower rates of inpatient complication and adverse events (Mardon et al., 2010).

Fair to failing patient safety grades by nurses were also independently associated with multiple adverse patient events in this study. Similarly, hospital-based research revealed fair to failing safety grades were significantly related to patient complications and other adverse events (Mardon et al., 2010). The significant association between negative patient safety grades by nurses and the increased likelihood of their reports of adverse patient events in this study may reflect system issues such as inappropriate levels of staffing, a lack of procedural guidance, staff training, patient education procedures, or policy enforcement.

Implications for Clinical Practice and Future Research

Safety culture in the workplace reflects the way in which safety is managed. It also signals the attitudes, beliefs, values, and perceptions that employees share about the way "safety is done" in their job settings. The goal of patient safety culture in health care organizations is to lessen harm to patients and providers of care through system effectiveness and individual performance. The findings from this study indicate that outpatient dialysis units present potential threats to patient safety. The patient transition period during patient shift changes may be a starting point for improving patient safety culture in these settings. Specifically, there is a need to identify and improve high-risk and inefficient care processes during patient shift change. For example, a patient transition strategy of staggering the start of individual dialysis treatments in dialysis centers to limit the number of patients initiating and terminating therapy at one time may reduce distractions and facilitate safe care during the patient transition period (Holley, 2010). Also, dialysis unit *elasticity or slack* staffing models that accommodate variations in patient volume and workload that are typical during peak patient transition periods in dialysis units may assist in fostering safe care processes, minimizing error, and reducing adverse patient events during this time (IOM, 2004).

This study examined only two dimensions of patient safety culture in outpatient dialysis settings, and little is known of extent to which dialysis units foster other aspects of safety culture. AHRQ (2012) notes the following as key features of patient safety culture in health care organizations: (a) acknowledgement of the high-risk nature of their activities, (b) a determination to achieve safe operations, (c) an environment that is blame-free where individuals can report errors or near misses without fear of punishment, (d) collaboration across ranks and disciplines to find solutions to patient safety problems, and (e) a commitment of resources to address safety concerns. Crucial among these is the premise that a *safe* organization is not error-free (Garrick, Kliger, & Stefanchik, 2012). It is inevitable that people will make mistakes or some adverse events are likely to occur. In a culture of safety, a balance is achieved between not blaming individuals for errors and not tolerating egregious behaviors. In outpatient dialysis units and other ambulatory care settings, a strong safety culture should include individual peer review and accountability as well as root cause analyses to discover system and process issues that contribute to unsafe care processes and adverse events (Garrick et al., 2012). In addition, a promotion of safety culture through staff and patient education and training and a strong committed leadership is essential.

AHRQ (2013) recommends annual assessments of safety culture as 1 of its 10 top safety tips for hospitals. However, research is needed to develop valid and reliable safety culture assessment measures that are tailored for use in diverse ambulatory care settings. These tools can provide a basis for routine assessments of patient safety culture in ambulatory care to raise staff awareness about patient safety culture, assess the current state of patient safety culture, identify strengths and areas for improvement, examine trends in safety culture over time, and evaluate the impact of safety culture initiatives and interventions. The routine assessment of patient safety culture in outpatient dialysis and other ambulatory care settings may be a critical first step in efforts to identify threats to patient safety and improve the outcomes of patients who receive care in outpatient facilities that provide high-risk care. Finally, little is known regarding the full scope of patient safety culture in dialysis units and other ambulatory care settings such as ambulatory surgical centers and outpatient infusion centers. Further research is needed to address these gaps in knowledge.

Limitations

The occurrence of adverse events in this study was reported by nurses. Although research has shown that nurses are reliable informants regarding patient outcomes (Aiken et al., 2001; Sochalski, 2004; Thomas-Hawkins et al., 2008), research that aggregates patient safety assessments by staff to the facility level and links these assessments to actual facility-level patient outcomes is needed. In addition, the parent study sample was drawn from RNs who were members of a professional organization, the ANNA. Therefore, the staff nurse sample in this study may not be representative of staff nurses who work in outpatient hemodialysis units because, as ANNA members, they may possess characteristics that differ uniquely and significantly from nurses' work in hemodialysis units and are not members of this organization.

CONCLUSION

Little is known about the state of patient safety in ambulatory care settings such as outpatient dialysis units. Findings from this study suggest that, similar to inpatient hospital settings, a positive patient safety culture in ambulatory care is likely associated with lower adverse patient events. However, there is a crucial need for the development of valid and reliable measures of patient safety culture that are tailored to diverse ambulatory care centers. There is also a need for research in ambulatory care that links safety cultures with the outcomes of patients who receive care in these settings. The findings from patient safety research in ambulatory care will provide research-based evidence to build or expand a culture of patient safety in outpatient settings and, ultimately, to improve patient outcomes.

REFERENCES

Agency for Healthcare Research and Quality. (2007). *Closing the Quality Gap: A critical Analysis of Quality Improvement: Vol. 7. Care coordination.* Retrieved from http://www.ahrq.gov/downloads/pub/evidence/pdf/caregap/caregap.pdf

Agency for Healthcare Research and Quality. (2012). *Patient safety network (PSNet). Patient safety in ambulatory care.* Retrieved from http://psnet.ahrq.gov/primer.aspx?primerID=16

Agency for Healthcare Research and Quality. (2013). *Surveys on patient safety culture.* Retrieved from http://www.ahrq.gov/professionals/quality-patient-safety/patientsafetyculture/index.html

Agency for Healthcare Research and Quality. (2014). *Patient safety network (PSNet). Patient safety culture.* Retrieved from http://psnet.ahrq.gov/primer.aspx?primerID=5

Aiken, L. H., Clarke, S. P., & Sloane, D. M. (2002). Hospital staffing, organization, and quality of care: Cross national findings. *International Journal for Quality in Health Care 14*(1), 5–13.

Aiken, L. H., Clarke, S. P., Sloane, D. M., Sochalski, J. A., Busse, R., Clarke, H., ... Shamian, J. (2001). Nurses' reports on hospital care in five countries. *Health Affairs, 20*(3), 43–53.

Chang, Y., & Mark, B. (2011). Effects of learning climate and registered nurse staffing on medication errors. *Nursing Research, 60*(1), 32–39.

Clancy, C. M. (2011). New research highlights the role of patient safety culture and safer care. *Journal of Nursing Care Quality, 261,* 193–196.

DeVivo, R. (2001). *National ESRD patient safety initiative: Phase II report.* Retrieved from http://www.renalmd.org/WorkArea/DownloadAsset.aspx?id=515

Dillman, D. (2007). *Mail and Internet surveys: The tailored design method* (2nd ed.). Hoboken, NJ: John Wiley & Sons.

Flynn, L., Thomas-Hawkins, C., & Clarke, S. P. (2009). Organizational traits, care processes, and burnout among chronic hemodialysis nurses. *Western Journal of Nursing Research, 31,* 569–582.

Gandhi, T. K. (2005). Fumbled handoffs: One ball dropped after another. *Annals of Internal Medicine, 142*(5), 352–358.

Garrick, R., Kliger, A., & Stefanchik, B. (2012). Patient and facility safety in hemodialysis: Opportunities and strategies to develop a culture of safety. *Clinical Journal of the American Society of Nephrology, 7,* 680–688. http://dx.doi.org/10.2215/CJN.06530711

Himmelfarb, J. (2010). Optimizing patient safety during hemodialysis. *JAMA, 306*(15), 1701–1708.

Hofman, D. A., & Mark. B. (2006). An investigation of the relationship between safety climate and medication errors as well as other nurse and patient outcomes. *Personnel Psychology, 59,* 847–869.

Holley, J. L. (2006). A descriptive report of errors and adverse events in chronic hemodialysis units. *Nephrology News and Issues, 20*(12), 60–61, 63.

Holley, J. L. (2010). *Dangerous dialysis.* Retrieved from http://webmm.ahrq.gov/case.aspx?caseID=224

Institute of Medicine. (2004). *Keeping patient safe. Transforming the work environment of nurses.* Washington, DC: The National Academies Press. Retrieved from http://www.nap.edu/catalog/10851.htm

Mardon, R. E., Khanna, K., Sorra, J., Dyer, N., & Famolaro, T. (2010). Exploring relationships between hospital safety culture and adverse events. *Journal of Patient Safety, 6*(4), 226–232.

Port, F. K., Pisoni, R. L., Bragg-Gresham, J. L., Satayathum, S. S., Young, E. W., Wolfe, R. A., Held, P. J. (2004). DOPPS estimates of patient life years attributable to modifiable hemoalysis practices in the United States. *Blood Purification, 22*(1), 75–80.

Renal Physicians Association. (2007). *Health and safety survey to improve patient safety in end stage renal disease: Report of findings from the ESRD Professional Survey.* Retrieved from http://www.kidneypatientsafety.org/about.aspx

Saran, R., Bragg-Gresham, J. L., Rayner, H. C., Goodkin, D. A., Keen, M. L., van Dijk, P. C., … Port, F. K. (2003). Nonadherence in hemodialysis: Associations with mortality, hospitalizations, and practice patterns in the DOPPS. *Kidney International, 64,* 254–262.

Sochalski, J. A. (2004). Is more better? The relationship between nurse staffing and the quality of nursing care in hospitals. *Medical Care,42*(2, Suppl.), II67–II72.

Sorra, J., Famolaro, T., Yount, N. D., Smith, S. A., Wilson, S., & Li, H. (2014). *2014 User comparative database report* (AHRQ Publication No. 14-0019-EF). Rockville, MD: Agency for Healthcare Research and Quality.

Sorra, J., Khanna, K., Dyer, N., Mardon, R., & Famolaro, T. (2012). Exploring relationships between patient safety culture and patients' assessments of hospital care. *Journal of Patient Safety, 8*(3), 131–139.

Sorra, J. S., & Nieva, V. F. (2004). *Hospital survey on patient safety culture* (AHRQ Publication No. 04-0041). Rockville, MD: Agency for Healthcare Research and Quality.

Tapolyai, M., Fülöp, T., Uysal, A., Lengvárszky, Z., Szarvas, T., Ballard, K., & Dossabhoy, T. (2010). Regional differences in nonadherence to dialysis among southern dialysis patients: A comparative cross-sectional study to the dialysis outcomes and practice patterns study. *American Journal of the Medical Sciences, 339*(6), 516–518.

The Joint Commission. (2010). *Improving communications during transitions of care.* Oak Brook, IL: Joint Commission Resources.

Thomas-Hawkins, C., Flynn, L., & Clarke, S. P. (2008). Relationships between registered nurse staffing, processes of nursing care, and nurse-reported patient outcomes in outpatient hemodialysis units. *Nephrology Nursing Journal, 35*(2), 123–130, 145.

United States Renal Data System. (2013). *USRDS 2012 Annual data report: Atlas of chronic kidney disease and end-stage renal disease in the United States.* Bethesda, MD: National Institutes of Health and National Institute of Diabetes and Digestive and Kidney Diseases.

PATIENT SAFETY CULTURE AND NURSE-REPORTED ADVERSE EVENTS IN OUTPATIENT HEMODIALYSIS UNITS

Critique by *Julie Schexnayder, Mary A. Dolansky, and Karen Bauce*

OVERALL SUMMARY

Patient safety is an ongoing concern for nurses and health care providers. Establishing a culture of safety in care settings outside of the hospital, such as hemodialysis facilities, remains challenging due, in part, to limited empirical evidence regarding facilitators and barriers. This quantitative study addresses the gap through an analysis of hemodialysis staff nurse perceptions of patient safety and the association with nurse-reported adverse events. Study findings are clearly presented and emphasize the need for safe patient handoffs and transitions during shift change, when patients are most vulnerable for harm. All nurses, particularly those working in outpatient hemodialysis settings, will be able to utilize these research findings to improve patient safety culture and outcomes of care.

TITLE

Does the title include the key concepts/variables/phenomena of interest?

The title includes the variables of interest in the study—safety culture and nurse-reported adverse events.

Is it concise (12 words or less) and professionally stated?

The title is concise and professionally stated.

RESEARCHER(S) CREDIBILITY

Educational credentials?

The study authors have terminal research degrees and presumably are nursing faculty based on their academic affiliations.

Prior methodologic research experience of the authors (i.e., methodological expertise)?

An Internet search, as well as the text, revealed that the authors were the investigators of the larger parent study from which this study data was obtained. This indicates prior experience in conducting correlational research.

Subject matter content experience (prior research on the subject matter)?

An Internet search also revealed that both authors are hemodialysis nurses and therefore would have subject matter expertise.

ABSTRACT
Does it include the key components (objective/aim, background/rationale, methods, results, and conclusion)?

The abstract clearly describes the key components of the study. The research purpose/aim is stated at the beginning and a summary of methods highlights the cross-sectional correlational mailed survey design and sample (422 registered nurses who worked in outpatient dialysis facilities). Measurement strategies are provided for the main study variables. Results indicate that nurses rated their overall patient safety culture as good to excellent, but rated the safety of handoff and transitions in their units as poor. Adverse events were related to poor reports of safety culture. Notably, in the conclusion, the authors use inconsistent terminology, applying their findings to ambulatory care settings. Consistent language describing the population (outpatient hemodialysis units) would enhance clarity.

Does or does not include references?

The abstract appropriately does not include references.

Is it concise (150–200 words or less)?

The abstract significantly exceeds 200 words.

Does it entice you to read the rest of the article (interesting)?

The abstract would hold particular appeal to hemodialysis nurses and other nurses interested in patient safety culture.

INTRODUCTION/PROBLEM
Is the research problem or phenomenon of interest clearly stated?

The research problem is clearly described in the introduction. Safety gaps have been reported in outpatient hemodialysis settings, yet there is little understanding of the safety culture and whether the safety culture is related to adverse events.

Is it succinct?

The authors clearly and succinctly explicate the research problem.

Does it answer the "so what" question?

The authors address the "so what" question by explaining that outpatient hemodialysis units deliver high-risk, high-frequency procedures to large numbers of people with end-stage renal disease and safety gaps exist.

RESEARCH AIMS/OBJECTIVES
Is the research aim/objective clearly stated?

The aim is clearly stated in the Study Purpose section and three distinct research questions are listed.

Is it concisely written?

It is concisely written, described in two sentences.

Does it follow logically from the research problem/phenomenon of interest?

Each research question flows logically from the problem statement and research aim.

SIGNIFICANCE
Is the significance to nursing and health care clearly written?

Significance of the study to nursing and health care is included as part of the Background section. The authors summarize results of prior research indicating that a variety of adverse patient events occur in outpatient hemodialysis settings. They enhance the significance of the problem by citing Institute of Medicine and the Agency for Healthcare Research and Quality reports that highlight a need to address safety culture. The authors describe associations between a culture of patient safety and adverse events in hospital settings to support their hypothesis that safety culture is likely to be associated with adverse outcomes in outpatient hemodialysis units.

Does the significance follow from the research aim/objective?

The significance of the research problem follows from the aim of investigating relationships among variables that may contribute to adverse patient events in outpatient hemodialysis units.

BACKGROUND
Is there an explicit description of a theoretical perspective or conceptual framework? If not, is it implied?

In the Theoretical Framework section, the authors briefly describe the nursing organization and outcomes model by Drs. Aiken, Clarke, and Sloane (2002). The model incorporates two implicit study concepts: high-quality work environment and quality nursing care processes.

Are there clear theoretical/conceptual definitions of the concepts?

The concepts are represented in the theoretical definitions of patient safety culture and patient transitions safety. The authors also provide a theoretical definition of patient outcomes.

LITERATURE REVIEW
Primary sources only?

The literature review is contained within two background sections. The authors include primary literature on adverse events in hemodialysis units and patient safety culture.

Current (within the past how many years)?

The majority of citations were older than 5 years at the time of the study's publication, with a few older than 10 years. The authors previously referred to limited research on the research problem which may explain the inclusion of older literature.

Is the search strategy included?

No description of the search strategy is provided.

Is literature relevant to the research aims/objectives?

The literature cited was relevant to the study's aim of investigating patient safety in outpatient hemodialysis settings.

Is it chronologically presented (old to current)?

> There is no chronological ordering of the information but this does not detract from the reader's ability to understand what is currently known about the research problem.

Is it comprehensive? If not, is sufficient background literature provided?

> Though brief, the literature review is successful in presenting gaps in knowledge regarding safety culture and adverse patient events in hemodialysis units.

RATIONALE FOR THE STUDY

Is there a gap in the literature that this study will fill (will it extend prior knowledge)? Is the rationale clearly stated?

> The authors adequately articulate the gap, that not much is known about safety culture and adverse events in hemodialysis units in the United States.

Is this a follow-up or replication study?

> This is a follow-up of a parent study conducted by the authors.

RESEARCH QUESTION(S) AND/OR HYPOTHESES

Are these explicitly and clearly stated?

> The three research questions are laid out clearly under the heading "Study Purpose." Check to see if all headings/sections are enclosed within quotation marks.

Do they include the variables/phenomenon of interest?

> The questions include the variables of interest, patient transition and safety, patient safety (grades for patient safety), and adverse patient events.

Do they follow from the research aim/objective?

> The research questions follow logically from the research aim.

METHODS

Research Design/Paradigm

Is the research design clearly stated?

> The research design is clearly described within the Methods section as a cross-sectional, correlational survey design using secondary data obtained from a related parent study.

Is there consistency between the research design and paradigm?

> There is consistency between the use of a quantitative correlational survey design to examine relationships among variables of interest and the positivist paradigm, which seeks to generate knowledge from objective empirical data.

Is this the best choice of design to address the research problem/phenomenon of interest?

> This is an appropriate design considering the state of the science of our current understanding of safety culture and adverse events in outpatient hemodialysis units.

Is there rigor in the design?

> Cross-sectional studies are useful for determining whether relationships exist among outcome variables of interest and therefore there is rigor in the design choice.

SETTING
Is the setting clearly described?

> The setting is the natural environment of the study participants.

What biases are introduced as a result of this particular setting?

> It cannot be determined what bias may be introduced as a result of receiving surveys at home.

SAMPLING PLAN AND SAMPLE
Is the sampling plan clearly identified?

> The sampling plan is outlined within the Methods section and describes the simple random selection of nurses from the American Nephrology Nurses' Association membership list in the parent study. A simple random sampling methodology is useful for obtaining a representative sample while reducing bias in sample selection.

Does it represent the population of interest?

> The sampling plan is consistent with obtaining the population of interest as it targeted recruitment of nurses working in hemodialysis settings. It is not clear whether the parent study limited recruitment specifically to nurses working in ambulatory hemodialysis settings, however, the authors do state that the nurses receiving the survey packets self-identified as working in hemodialysis settings.

Is the sampling plan consistent with the research aim/objective?

> The sampling plan is consistent with the research aim of understanding the relationship between nurse-reported adverse events in outpatient hemodialysis units and patient safety outcomes.

Is the sample size sufficient (e.g., power analysis or data saturation)?

> No power analysis is provided therefore it is difficult to determine whether the sample size is sufficient. The sample is biased in that it only includes nurses who are members of the nephrology organization. Nurses who participate in their professional organizations may be different than nurses who do not participate. Similarly, the sample may be biased if there are differences in the nurses who chose to participate in the survey.

VARIABLES
Are variables clearly identified?

> The variables of nurse-reported adverse events and safety culture are clearly identified.

Are variables operationally defined and consistent with theoretical concepts?

> The outcome variables of interest are operationalized as follows: nurse-reported adverse events were measured as a series of items designed to capture the frequency of 13 adverse patient events occurring in the dialysis unit in the past year. Patient safety culture is operationalized in two ways: patient transition safety (four items of the Handoff and Transitions Scale of the Hospital Survey on Patient Safety Culture [HSOPS]) and patient safety grade (a single item on the HSOPS).

Are independent and dependent variables are identified, if applicable?

As this is a correlational study, the authors do not label the variables as dependent or independent. However, from the description of the nursing organization and outcomes model, it can be assumed that safety culture is the independent variable and adverse events is the dependent variable.

METHOD OF DATA COLLECTION

What are the methods of data collection?

The procedure for survey distribution is described in the Sample section. Nurses from the Nephrology Nurses Association were randomly selected to have survey packets mailed to their homes.

Are validity and reliability clearly addressed for prior research and current study, if applicable?

A Cronbach alpha of 0.91 was reported for the Handoff and Transitions Scale, providing evidence for its internal consistency reliability in this study sample. No information on reliability was provided for the patient safety grade nor is there any discussion of the instruments' validity to measure the constructs of interest. As this was a secondary data analysis, the authors could have referred readers to the original parent study publication for additional information on the study measures.

Do the measures/instruments address the underlying theoretical concepts or phenomenon of interest?

The study instruments do address nurse-reported adverse events and patient safety culture.

Were human rights protected?

Protection of human rights was assured as the study was approved by an institutional review board.

Are other ethical issues identified?

Although the researchers included a letter with the mailed surveys stating that completion of the questionnaires indicated consent to participate in the study, it is unknown whether the participants provided any identifiable information, particularly as demographic data was collected. If the data collected was anonymous, the authors should describe how it was ensured.

Is the data-collection method appropriate for research design?

The data collection was appropriate for this survey design.

Is there bias in data collection?

Bias may result from collecting data at only one defined period in time.

What is the fidelity of intervention addressed, if applicable?

As this was not an intervention study, fidelity was not addressed.

DATA ANALYSIS

Are data analysis techniques described (e.g., statistical tests, methodology for qualitative analysis)?

The data analysis is described in its own section and includes descriptive statistics, frequency distributions, and the use of unadjusted and adjusted logistic regression models.

Does the analysis answer the research question?

> The data analysis addresses each of the three research question.

Is it appropriate?

> The analysis plan is appropriate to answer the research questions.

Is the analysis comprehensive? Are themes identified?

> The analysis was comprehensive and described in both the Results and Discussion sections.

Is there bias in the analysis (trustworthiness? credibility?)?

> There does not appear to be bias in the data analysis. The authors provide a detailed explanation of how the statistical analysis was performed in the section Data Analysis and fully report study findings.

RESULTS

Are sample characteristics described and fully reported?

> The study sample is described in Table 1 and summarizes the characteristics of the 422 nurse participants.

Are findings presented related to research aim/objective?

> Study findings are clearly reported. Results for research question 1 are displayed in Table 2. Thirty-nine percent of the nurses reported safe patient transitions and 86% graded overall patient safety as good to excellent in the dialysis units where they worked. The relationship between nurse-rated patient transition safety and nurse-reported adverse patient events (research question 2) is found in Table 3. In the adjusted model (controlling for safety grade), as compared to nurse reports of safe transitions, nurse reports of unsafe transitions were independently associated with an increased likelihood of nurse reports of frequent adverse events. Similarly, for research question 3, in the adjusted model (controlling for safe transitions), nurse reports of fair to poor safety grade were independently associated with increased reports of adverse events. Though not identified as a specific research question, it would have been helpful for the authors to include a description of the frequency of adverse patient events.

Are all outcome variables addressed, if applicable?

> The outcome variables of patient transition and safety, patient safety (grades for patient safety), and adverse patient events are addressed.

Are results clearly presented in text and/or tables/figures?

> The authors clearly present the results both in the text and in tables.

Is significance of results reported, if applicable?

> Statistically significant findings between the outcome variables of interest are reported in the text and displayed in Table 3.

DISCUSSION OF RESULTS

Do the authors link the findings to the previous research studies?

> The authors link their findings to previous research studies, specifically comparing them to findings in hospital environments indicating a similarly low percentage of

staff endorsing safe patient transitions while reporting overall unit patient safety as positive.

Are the conclusions comprehensive, yet within the data?

The findings are interpreted appropriately and do not go beyond the data.

Do the authors interpret the results in the discussion?

The authors interpret the results in the Discussion section. They describe safety culture as multifaceted, which can lead nurses to report some aspects as positive and others as needing improvement.

Are the findings generalizable or transferable?

Generalizability is discussed briefly as a limitation related to the sampling strategy (recruitment of professional organization members).

LIMITATIONS
Identified? Accurate? Inclusive?

There is a specific Limitation section in which the authors focus on two limitations. First, measurement of adverse events is self-reported by the nurses. Objective measurements of safety performance would enhance the validity and reliability of the study. The authors also commented on the biased sample of nurses from the nephrology association as a limitation of generalizability. In addition, within the Implications section, the authors acknowledge that only two components of safety culture were included within the study. The authors describe other dimensions of safety culture from the literature that may be useful to further characterizing the phenomenon. The cross-sectional design is an additional limitation not identified in the text.

IMPLICATIONS
Are there implications for practice, education, research?
Are there implications for clinical practice?

In the section, "Implications for Clinical Practice and Future Research," the authors propose that hemodialysis units present a potential threat to patient safety. Specifically, they state that nurses can identify and improve care processes during shift change as one step to improving safety of care. This is salient given the proportion of nurses reporting suboptimal transitions safety in their study. The authors also state that improved understanding of patient safety culture dimensions will require development of valid and reliable instruments to measure patient safety culture in diverse ambulatory settings. It is unclear why the authors provide this comment as the study is focused on a uniform population—outpatient hemodialysis units. Check whether use of quotation marks for sections is consistent through each chapter.

RECOMMENDATIONS
Recommendations for future study/study replication?

Recommendations for future study are described but do not include study replication. The authors recommend research to address two distinct knowledge gaps: the lack of valid and reliable measures of patient safety culture in diverse outpatient care settings and an incomplete understanding of patient safety culture within hemodialysis units and other high-risk outpatient settings.

CONCLUSION
Is it succinct and does it tie everything together?

The conclusion is succinct and summarizes the data appropriately. The authors reiterate the association between a positive safety culture in outpatient hemodialysis units and fewer reported adverse patient events as well as the need for additional research to enhance understanding of the dimensions of patient safety culture in order to provide evidence-based care.

QUALITATIVE STUDIES

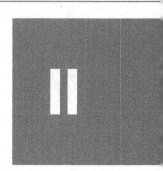

HYPERTENSIVE BLACK MEN'S PERCEPTIONS OF A NURSE PROTOCOL FOR MEDICATION SELF-ADMINISTRATION

12

Ophelia Thomas, DNP, RN,
is a registered nurse who completed her Doctor of Nursing Practice degree at Regis University in Denver, Colorado.

Pamella Stoeckel, PhD, RN, CNE,
is an associate professor of Nursing at Regis University who teaches in the Master's and DNP nursing programs.

ABSTRACT

A factor contributing to uncontrolled hypertension in older persons is medication nonadherence. Older Black men in a rural cardiology clinic were not taking blood pressure medication as prescribed resulting in uncontrolled hypertension. A nurse protocol to assist with self-administration of hypertensive medication was proposed to address the problem. This qualitative key informant study identified a purposive sample of 10 hypertensive Black men who were 65 to 70 years of age and nonadherent in taking their medication. The nurse conducted teaching sessions using the protocol to review evidence-based strategies for improving medication adherence. A follow-up phone call was done after 1 week. Participants were interviewed about their perceptions of taking hypertensive medication. The interviews were recorded, transcribed, and coded for themes using constant comparative analysis. Six themes emerged: *Medication Bottle Guides Medication Usage, Confusion about Side Effects, Reasons for Not Taking Medications, New Behavior, Unchanged Behavior,* and *Discovery of Other Problems.* The results showed that the nurse-administered protocol resulted in participants' changed attitudes about taking medication.

KEY WORDS: medication nonadherence; hypertension; Black men; nurse protocol; qualitative

Nonadherence to hypertension medication in older persons is a serious problem that requires consideration by nurses. There are approximately 65 million adults in the United States that have hypertension (Welch et al., 2011). The older population is rapidly growing, and data show that the prevalence of hypertension increases with age (Lionakis, Mendrinos, Sanidas, Favatas, & Georgopoulou, 2012). Older Black patients are particularly at risk of hypertensive disease (Sanne,

Thomas, O., & Stoeckel, P. (2016). Hypertensive black men's perceptions of a nurse protocol for medication self-administration. *Care Management Journals, 17,* 37–46. doi:10.1891/1521-0987.17.1.37. Republished with permission of Springer Publishing Company.

Muntner, Kawasaki, Hyre, & DeSalvo, 2008). According to Thomas-Kvidera (2005), managing hypertension continues to be a major challenge for health care providers even with advances in the prevention and treatment of cardiovascular disease. An important factor contributing to uncontrolled hypertension in older persons is medication nonadherence. According to Klootwyk and Sanoski (2011), blood pressure remains uncontrolled in 46% of patients with hypertension despite the use of antihypertensive medication. Nurses cannot assume that patients are taking their medication as prescribed. Poor adherence by older Black patients taking hypertensive medication is common and contributes to worsening of disease, death, and increased health care costs (Osterberg & Blaschke, 2005). This study addresses the issue of nonadherence of hypertensive medication in older Black men.

HYPERTENSION MEDICATION NONADHERENCE

This research study grew out of an issue identified at a cardiology clinic in Southern Georgia where Black men 65 to 70 years old were treated for hypertension. The cardiologist in charge of the practice observed that this group of patients was not taking their prescribed blood pressure medication and shared this with the nurse researcher. Although instructions were given by the physician, patients acknowledged that they were not taking their medication and their blood pressure remained high. Uncontrolled blood pressure has detrimental consequences for overall health (American Heart Association, 2013). Older Black men risk coronary artery disease and possible heart attacks, so the problem needed attention (Hyre, Krousel-Wood, Muntner, Kawasaki, & DeSalvo, 2007).

It was proposed that a nurse protocol on self-administration of hypertensive medication could improve adherence in taking medication by older Black male patients. A protocol was designed based on current evidence-based practice to engage each patient on a personal level and give tools that enabled patients to remember how and when to take their medication. An important aspect of the study was that it addressed the needs of a specific high-risk group of older adults in a rural area. The nurse researcher for this project was a master's-prepared nurse with experience working with hypertensive patients and was familiar with the clinic setting.

A factor contributing to uncontrolled hypertension in older persons is medication nonadherence.

Conceptual Framework

This study was based on a conceptual framework that included a combination of two theories: Dorothy Orem's self-care deficit theory and Albert Bandura's social learning theory. Dorothea Orem's self-care deficit theory is a self-care model that addresses the nurse's role in assisting a client in maintaining a functioning level of self-care (Orem, 2001). Self-care is described by Orem as the practice of activities that individuals initiate and perform on their own to maintain life, health, and well-being. Orem's theory guides and instructs persons in self-care actions to sustain life, health, and recover from disease or injury, as well as cope with their effects (Orem, 2001). In this study, patients lacked the ability to take medications independently and as a consequence had uncontrolled hypertension. The nurse-administered protocol was initiated to assist the patient in self-care. The strength of Orem's self-care deficit theory in this study was that it supported the development of actions to help participants be more self-sustaining.

Bandura's social learning theory also had relevance to this study. Bandura (1977) stated that observational learning has a powerful effect when observers believe that the person demonstrating the behavior is similar to them. In this study, the nurse nurtured relationships with the participants to help them observe, participate, and practice new skills in taking their hypertensive medications.

Review of the Literature

Studies reveal that hypertensive medication adherence in older adults is a challenge for health care providers who develop and manage programs for this population (Krousel-Wood, Muntner, Islam, Morisky, & Webber, 2009). Along with the increase of average life expectancy, older patients experience an increased incidence of chronic diseases. This produces a negative effect on elderly patients faced with treatment regimens that involve long-term drug therapy (MacLaughlin et al., 2005). The development of working relationships between patients and caregivers was suggested as a necessary part of improving medication adherence. A suggested method of assessing medication adherence in the older population was through interviews using open-ended, nonthreatening, and nonjudgmental questions to connect with patients (MacLaughlin et al., 2005).

Self-care is described by Orem as the practice of activities that individuals initiate and perform on their own to maintain life, health, and well-being.

Black men have lower rates of controlled hypertension than men of other racial groups (Sanne et al., 2008). Physiological differences were not believed to be the primary contributors to higher levels of hypertension between these groups. Although some differences such as medication side effects might contribute in some cases to higher rates of hypertension, it is believed that psychosocial issues are the primary contributors to disparities (Martins & Norris, 2004). Modifiable causes of uncontrolled hypertension in Black male patients were identified as obesity, high dietary intake of sodium and fat, low dietary calcium, missed office appointments, and low adherence to treatment plans (Martins & Norris, 2004).

Lewis, Schoenthaler, and Ogedegbe (2012) confirm a serious problem of medication nonadherence by Black men with hypertension. Hyre et al. (2007) found that Black men were less likely to be adherent to antihypertensive medications compared with Black women, White women, or White men. Evidence supports that medication nonadherence is a significant problem for older Black men (older than 60 years of age) showing them to be 2.45 times more likely to be less adherent (Hyre et al., 2007). Schlomann and Schmitke (2007) researched the reasons for medication nonadherence by Black men and found that personal beliefs and experiences including those of racism and financial struggles contributed to nonadherence. It was also noted that poor relationships and lack of communication between patients and health care providers were barriers to medication adherence. Kim, Han, Hill, Rose, and Roary (2003) found that depression was significantly associated with poor medication adherence.

Patient education was noted as an important approach to addressing nonadherence to prescribed medication in hypertensive patients. According to Karaeren et al. (2009)

to achieve higher adherence rates, it was important to improve the patient's knowledge about hypertension medications and understanding of the side effects of medications. The authors contended that it was especially important to educate patients about the significance or insignificance of side effects of their medications (Karaeren et al., 2009). A qualitative study by Bennett (2015) supported the need for hypertension education for Black males and found that men who understood the impact of high blood pressure were more likely to take their antihypertensive medications.

Karakurt and Kaşikçi (2012) suggested that patients with hypertension should have necessary knowledge of their diagnosis to successfully address their illness. Types of knowledge included being able to define hypertension, evaluate risk factors, and understand the importance of taking medication. Hekler et al. (2008) posit that understanding the consequences of their illness can positively affect medication adherence by patients with chronic illness.

Habit forming and habit changing occurred by altering the sequencing of steps that lead to desired outcomes.

Uses of different interventions, tools, and protocols to address medication adherence were addressed in the literature. Krulish (2005) described different types of medication compliance aids. A standardized approach was suggested in evaluating patients' ability to self-administer medication based on strengths and deficits. Tools recommended by Krulish included medication lists, medication schedules, pillboxes, and telephone reminders. Using these tools according to the authors affected the participants' perceptions of their ability to take hypertensive medication and contributed to forming new habits.

According to Lally and Gardner (2013) supporting habit formation involved three main behaviors: focusing on strategies to initiate a new behavior, supporting context-dependent repetition of behavior, and facilitating the development of automaticity. Techniques for disrupting existing unwanted habits such as restructuring the personal environment and initiating alternative responses to situational cues were discussed. Lowman (2013) described how habits are formed and changed. Habit forming and habit changing occurred by altering the sequencing of steps that lead to desired outcomes. It involved changing the behavioral sequences that connected cues, routines, and rewards.

Rose, Kim, Dennison, and Hill (2000) concluded from their study on adherence that the relationship between Black men and their health care providers was critical to success. They identified mutual goal setting and communicating with an attitude of respect and understanding as being significant factors that improved adherence to hypertensive treatment recommendations. O'Neill and Feldman (2009) also encouraged building effective relationships with patients as an important approach to improving medication adherence.

PURPOSE

The purpose of this study was to determine if the introduction of a nurse protocol on self-administration of hypertensive medication could improve perceptions of taking hypertensive medication by Black men 65 to 70 years of age with hypertension. The intention was to improve adherence of taking hypertensive medication. The development of a nurse protocol on self-administration of hypertensive medication was proposed as a means of addressing the problem of medication nonadherence.

The research question was as follows: In Black men, 65 to 70 with high blood pressure does implementation of a nurse protocol on self-administration of hypertensive medication affect patients' perceptions of their ability to take hypertensive medication?

METHOD

This study was a response to a specific problem noted in this cardiology practice. A qualitative approach was chosen to address this problem using the key informant method. Merlo, Goodman, McClenaghan, and Fritz (2013) contend that qualitative research provides a unique opportunity for patients to express opinions and provide valuable insights into intervention processes. The key informant method gathers "rich, varied, and textured words from informants selected for their specialized knowledge and unique perspectives on the topic" (Polit & Beck, 2010, p. 237). This approach was appropriate in gaining understanding of the impressions of a vulnerable group of patients concerning their experience of taking hypertensive medication. Open-ended questions were asked with relevant follow-up questions to explore participants' thoughts and feelings.

The collaborative institutional training initiative course was completed by both nurse researchers. Institutional review board approval was approved as an "exempt" study. A letter of intent was signed by the cardiologist giving permission for the research to be conducted at the clinic. After thorough explanation of the project, participants signed informed consent prior to participating in the study. Confidentiality and anonymity were assured related to study participation. Participants could withdraw at any time. Information gathered had no identifiers. Only the nurse researchers and the transcriptionist viewed the results. All data were secured and password protected.

Sample

The nurse researcher used a purposive sample of participants obtained from office records at the cardiology clinic. Black men were chosen because this group was a predominate group in the cardiology practice, and office records revealed poor control of hypertension in this vulnerable group. Review of the literature supported that Black men's antihypertensive medication adherence was often poor and the reasons for adherence were not fully known (Hyre et al., 2007). This supported the need for investigation into what factors impacted older Black men's medication adherence. Criteria for inclusion included Black men 65 to 70 years old in a cardiology clinic with a primary diagnosis of hypertension taking different medications for high blood pressure. Participants could have secondary diagnoses. High blood pressure was defined as systolic above 140 and diastolic above 90. Participants had to read, write, and speak English. They could not have dementia and had to have an adequate level of psychomotor skills to manipulate the adherence tools. Ten prospective participants were identified through the clinic records. The nurse researcher met individually with each patient at their clinic visits to request their participation in the study. All 10 participants signed consent forms.

Treatment Protocol

One-hour individual teaching sessions were scheduled with each participant using the protocol developed by the nurse researcher. Appointments were set over a 1-month period following their routine clinic visits for blood pressure checks. The protocol on self-administration of hypertensive medication was developed from a thorough review of the literature. It was based on educational information about hypertension obtained from the Agency for Healthcare Research and Quality (AHRQ, 2011) developed by Krulish (2005). Other literature related to providing patient education was adapted from Esposito (1995). The studies of Kannampallil, Waicekauskas, Morrow, Kopren, and Fu (2013) identified tools that were used as part of the protocol to improve self-administration of hypertensive medication. These included the use of pillboxes supplied by the researcher and forms to record self-administration of medication.

An important part of the nurse protocol was the emphasis on trust building. Research by Yendelela et al. (2013) suggested that interventions to improve medication adherence could be enhance by incorporating trust-building components. The nurse's role was to gain trust from the patient by making effort to understand the patient's belief system and then working within the patient's belief system to develop skills to improve medication adherence.

An additional part of the protocol was the focus on successful nurse–patient communication. Patient education alone has not shown to improve adherence, but change can occur when education is combined with regimen simplification and effective provider/patient communication (American College of Preventive Medicine, 2011). A caregiver's style of communication was identified as one of the strongest predictors of a patient's trust in his or her caregiver.

An important part of the nurse protocol was the emphasis on trust building.

There were four steps in the implementation of the nurse protocol (Table 1). The first step was the initial assessment of the patient's knowledge of his or her illness, medication regimen, and adherence. This included taking time to initiate a trusting relationship. The nurse made an effort to get to know the patients by sitting down to achieve eye level and creating a safe place where patients could feel comfortable talking openly. Extra time was taken to specifically ask about attitudes, beliefs, and cultural norms about taking medication. It should be noted that throughout the teaching session the

TABLE 1. Nurses' Hypertensive Protocol

Steps	Hypertensive Protocol	Performed by	Tasks
1	Risk assessment and teaching tools	The nurse	Conducts an initial assessment of patient's knowledge, beliefs, and cultural norms
			Develops a trusting nurse–patient relationship and open communication
2	Education	The nurse	Provides education regarding self-administration and side effects of medication
			Demonstrates use of tools and forms
3	Evaluation	The patient	Demonstrates medication administration using new tools; Restates knowledge of prescribed medication and side effects
4	Follow-up phone call after 1 week	The nurse	Checks in on progress; Asks if there are questions

nurse researcher remained open to participants' questions and answered them as they were asked. An open and accepting approach was used to encourage participation. Active listening was employed with the intent of listening for meaning and careful attention to what the patient was saying. Techniques that were used included careful attention to verbal and nonverbal cues to show understanding and empathy.

A second step was the education of the patient. Each patient was asked about his expectations, needs, and experiences taking medication. The patient's medication regimen was reviewed and explained. Simple language without medical jargon was used to place emphasis on the importance of taking medication as prescribed and the consequences of not taking medication. This approach was based on adherence being enhanced when patients understand their condition and the benefits of treatment. Clear instructions were provided on how to use tools to assist in taking medication. The nurse demonstrated the use of the pillboxes to organize medication and the forms for self-recording. Supplemental information about drug side effects was provided. Patients were encouraged to ask questions. The nurse provided respectful responses and watched for patients' signs of frustration or confusion to address them immediately.

A third step was the evaluation of learning and observation of the patient using the new tools. Patients were given the opportunity to demonstrate how to use the pillbox and forms. They were asked to express understanding of the concepts related to medication self-administration by "teaching back" the information. The nurse had patients restate the positive benefits of taking their medication. The role of the nurse was to empower patients to self-manage their medication administration by giving positive reinforcement.

A fourth step was a follow-up phone call after 1 week to assess progress of each participant and answer questions. This gave the nurse the opportunity to assess further if patients needed additional help and to give encouragement. Patients were asked simply and directly if they were using the new tools and if they were following their drug regimen. An appointment was made over the phone to interview participants within 2 weeks.

Data Collection

The method of data collection for this study was individual interviews completed at the clinic or in the participants' homes at their convenience within 2 weeks after the teaching sessions. Forty-five-minute face-to-face interviews were conducted and digitally recorded. Participants signed consent to be recorded. The researcher sat across form the participants at eye level in a quiet place and conducted the interviews in an unhurried manner. To build rapport, the researcher talked informally with the participants before beginning the interview. The primary interview questions included the following: What was your perception of taking your blood pressure medication before receiving the nurse-administered protocol? What was your perception of taking your blood pressure medication after the nurse-administered protocol? Follow-up questions were drawn from the participants' responses and were used for clarification. Examples of follow-up questions included the following: Describe when you take your medication. Describe what causes you not take your medication. What effect did using the pillbox have on taking your medication?

Data Analysis

The process of data analysis for this study included transcribing the interviews and grouping the responses by questions in Word files. The data were reviewed multiple times by the researchers with notes made about the content. After reading the data and making notes, common ideas and concepts were identified through line-by-line coding as per Creswell's (1998) process of open coding. Beliefs about medication adherence were highlighted. Codes were combined and refined. Reflexive notes on physical expressions and behavior during the interviews were used to supplement the digital recordings. Major categories with themes emerged through a process of constant comparative analysis to identify similarities and differences (Patton, 2002). Themes and subthemes emerged from two broad categories that included perceptions before the nurse protocol and perceptions after the nurse protocol.

Trustworthiness

The aim of trustworthiness in this qualitative study was to support the argument that the inquiry's findings were "worth paying attention to" (Lincoln & Guba, 1985, p. 290). The researcher set aside biases about the topic at the beginning of the study. Four issues of trustworthiness were addressed: credibility, transferability, dependability, and confirmability (Lincoln & Guba, 1985). Credibility was achieved through setting aside biases at the beginning of the study and using peer debriefers who were two doctorally prepared qualitative researchers. Debriefers reviewed the research process and resulting codes, categories, and themes. They provided observations, and suggestions, and posed questions throughout the study. To address transferability, dependability, and confirmability, a complete audit trail provided a detailed accounting of the research process which included a reflexive journal with extensive field notes to establish rigor (Lincoln & Guba, 1985). Reflexive notes gave further insights into participants' responses.

RESULTS

Study participants were 10 Black men age 65 to 70 years, diagnosed with hypertension who met criteria for the study. Three of the participants were diagnosed with hypertension for 4 years or less, and seven were diagnosed with hypertension for more than 10 years. Based on information obtained from the cardiology clinic, all men were nonadherent in taking their hypertension medication. Nine of the participants were functionally independent. One participant required assistance from his mother with taking medication and meals preparation. Participants were interviewed about their perceptions of taking hypertensive medication. The data from the study revealed two broad categories: perceptions of taking hypertensive medication before the nurse intervention and perceptions of taking hypertensive medication after the nurse intervention. Themes for each category are presented as they emerged from the interviews (Table 2).

Credibility was achieved through setting aside biases at the beginning of the study and using peer debriefers who were two doctorally prepared qualitative researchers.

Perceptions of Taking Medication Before the Nurse Intervention

Bottle Guides Medication Usage. An important theme that came from the participants' interviews was the importance of the medication bottle as a guide for how and when to take hypertensive medication. They expressed that the *Bottle Guides Medication Usage.* They used the label on the bottle to determine how and when to take their medication. Only two of the 10 participants knew the names of their medication.

TABLE 2. Categories and Themes

Themes Before the Nurse Protocol	Themes After the Nurse Protocol
Bottle guides medication usage	New behavior
Confusion about side effects	Unchanged behavior
Reasons for not taking medications	Discovery of other problems

A participant stated, "No, I don't know the name [of the medication], but I can show you the bottles and which one I take." Another participant stated, "Yes, [I know the medication], if I am looking at the bottles, but I cannot just name them." Before the nurse intervention, it appeared that the medication bottle was particularly significant in helping all participants know the names and when to take their medication. Some participants also stated that they knew to take their medications when they ate. A participant expressed, "I take my medicine with food." Another said, "I don't ever take my medicine until I eat. I have to have something in my stomach." Additional cues to knowing when and how to take their medication included the time of day such as morning or evening and the color of the pills. Most of the participants, however, identified their medicine bottle as the main guide for knowing when and how to take their hypertensive medications.

Confusion About Side Effects. A second theme that emerged before the nurse intervention was *Confusion About Side Effects.* Of the 10 participants in this study, none were able to state a clear understanding of the side effects of their hypertensive medications. One participant stated, "Yes, all these medicines have some problems, the doctors just keep on giving us all this medicine that cause all of us to have other problems." Some of the participants knew they experienced side effects but were not sure what to do about it. One participant stated, "The water pill makes me go to the bathroom if I take it at night." Another participant noted that "the [medications] make me have dry mouth sometimes." Some acknowledged side effects and reported them but continued taking the medication. A participant reported, "One of the pills that I take makes me feel sleepy—I told the doctor when I was there last he did not change it, but I still am taking the medicine." A different perspective was offered by another participant who stated, "Some of this medicine was making me feel bad and I stopped taking the medicine until I got in to see the doctor." It was acknowledged that participants received written information about side effects, but it was not clear if they read or understood the information. A participant expressed "Yes, at the VA, they give me a piece of paper that have this information." Another participant stated, "Yes, the pharmacist gives me a sheet on it." They expressed minimal understanding of medication side effects.

Reasons for Not Taking Medications. A third theme noted before the nurse intervention was *Reasons for Not Taking Medications.* Participants acknowledged not taking their hypertensive medications and gave various reasons for why they failed to do so. One participant stated, "It is different time [each day] because sometimes I don't get out of bed until late. So I just wait until I can get me something to eat." Another participant clearly stated, "No, sometimes, I feel that I really don't need it [my medication], then I go to Walmart and take my blood pressure and it be up. Then I go back to take my medicines." One respondent stated, "It depends on how I am feeling when I get up, I am going to tell you the truth nurse, sometimes I feel so bad when I wake up and I will not take any medicine, I stay in bed."

Participants acknowledged that they sometimes did not take their medications on time. One stated, "No, you want me to tell the truths don't you, I miss taking it a lot, but I am going to get better." Another stated, "I really don't have a time [to take my medications]." "Sometime I skip taking my medication, for example, today be Thursday and I will have missed Wednesday." One person stated that "I fall asleep and forget." Only one participant stated that they took their medication on schedule. Several participants also stated that they did not take their medication on time because they had problems reading or seeing small print instructions on the medication bottles. One participant stated, "Yes, I had that surgery on my eyes; I can still see it [the medication label] some though." Another commented that "Yes [I have trouble seeing], I don't know why they make the writing so little." Eight out of 10 participants were able to see the small print instructions on the medicines bottles with the help of reading glasses.

Perceptions of Taking Medication After the Nurse Intervention

New Behavior. The theme of *New Behavior* was noted after the nurse met with each study participant following the nurse-administered protocol. New behaviors were identified that influenced the way they took their medications. Participants were able to clearly state the time to take their medication. One participant stated, "I take it [medications] once a day, once in the morning time about 6 o'clock every morning." Another said, "I take it, ah, around 9 in the morning, between 9 and 10, and then I take it between 9 and 10 in the evening. It is important that I take the medication to stay healthy."

The new behavior of using the pill container was noted with statements such as "what I have done is use the pill container you gave me … I set everything up in there; the first thing in the morning I get it." They stated, "I look at the container and take it from the container."

The participants also expressed using the medication chart to record taking their medication. One participant stated, "I have a chart that you left with me, I use that chart to know what day it is and when to take my medication—it helps me for the next day." Another stated, "I record every day; I see the calendar by my bed."

An additional new behavior was reading the pamphlets given to them by the nurse and asking questions. They expressed new understanding about the way they take their medication. Quotes included "I learned that the medication is to be taken as the doctor prescribed and it is not to be changed until talking with doctor." Another participant said, "If I miss, I don't double up and take two pills instead of one, like I use to do. I just make sure that I take the next dose."

Unchanged Behavior. There were participant behaviors that remained unchanged after the nurse intervention. Participants that received help taking their medication previously continued to require help. "My mama let me know when to take my medicine." *Unchanged Behavior* included that the medication bottle continued to play an important role in patients taking their medication. A participant stated, "I look at the bottles and put them [the pills] in the container and follow that each time." Some vague reasons for not taking medication persisted. One participant stated, "Ah, ah, I try to take my medication, but sometimes I just feel so bad, I don't know if it really works or not." Another participant responded, when asked what is difficult about taking your medication, that "Nothing difficult, just sometimes I just don't want to take it."

Discovery of Other Problems. A final theme that emerged following the nurse intervention involved *Discovery of Other Problems* that could affect patients' ability to take their medication. Each patient was asked about his ability to take his hypertensive medication. Some participants shared significant discouragement with their progress and gave comments such as "I am tired of taking so much medication" and "I don't know if it [my medication] is even working, my blood pressure is always up when I go to the doctor's office." Underlying feelings were revealed in statements such as "nothing helps; I just know that I need to take it and I take it."

DISCUSSION

This study revealed how 10 Black men 65 to 70 years of age with hypertension perceived a nurse protocol on self-administration of hypertensive medication. Before the nurse protocol, participants in the study indicated that they used their medication bottles as their primary guide in taking hypertensive medication. This finding was surprising in that participants were not newly diagnosed patients and were expected to have past knowledge of their medications from previous visits to the clinic and pharmacy. The importance of the design and readability of the medication label was emphasized by their focus on the information on the bottle. In addition, it was found that participants were not able to recall the name of their hypertensive medications or when to take them. They also expressed limited understanding of the side effects of medication even though they were given written information by the clinic and the pharmacy. A concerning finding was that previous to the nurse protocol, patients expressed experiencing side effects but had not reported them to their health care provider. These findings confirm a need for further patient education and align with Orem's theory of self-care deficit.

Before the nurse protocol, participants in the study indicated that they used their medication bottles as their primary guide in taking hypertensive medication.

Most participants in the study acknowledged not adhering to their medication regimen before the nurse protocol. The literature confirmed similar findings noting that older patients with hypertension had a low adherence rate (Uzun et al., 2009). Participants gave many reasons for not taking their hypertensive medication including "sometimes I don't need it." "It depends on how I feel ...," and "the writing on the bottle is so small." These findings were supported in the literature that stated that patients diagnosed with hypertension for a longer time fail to take their medication (Li, Kuo, Hwang, & Hsu, 2012). The small print on the medication bottles was an issue for the participants in the study. This finding was also noted by Cardarelli et al. (2011) who expressed the need for improving standardize medication labels with clearer text, larger font, and warning labels that would address safety measure for the older adults who rely on their medication bottles.

Participants did not take their medications on time for various reasons. In many cases, it was evident that they did not understand the importance of taking medications consistently. As a consequence, some of the participants perceived the medication were not needed or not working. Hong, Oddone, Dudley, and Bosworth (2006) supported this finding in stating that hypertension was an asymptomatic disease, thus causing a problem for antihypertensive medication adherence. It was also noted that participants did not take their hypertensive medication because of experiencing side effects. The literature confirmed that side effects of hypertensive medication play an important role in the asymptomatic disease and that the treatment may make individuals feel worse than the actual disease (Hong et al., 2006). Suggestions include carefully reviewing medication side effects at every clinic visit and asking if patients have experienced any new effects.

The literature confirmed similar findings noting that older patients with hypertension had a low-adherence rate.

Perceptions of taking hypertensive medication after the nurse intervention included that participants reported changes in their understanding of when and how to take their medications. Patients were more specific about the names of their medications and were clear about when they should be taken. The meeting with the nurse provided a face-to-face encounter that personalized the patient experience and initiated a nurse–patient relationship. The establishment of a relationship with improved communication was shown to be a means to improve medication adherence. Schoenthaler, Allegrante, Chaplin, and Ogedegbe (2012) strongly supported this finding by stating

> The quality of patient–provider communication has been identified as an important and potentially modifiable factor associated with improved patient outcomes. Patient–provider communication that is characterized by shared decision making and patient centeredness is associated with better self-reported adherence in patients with chronic diseases. (p. 372)

Participants continued to use medication bottles as guides after the nurse protocol, but they also used tools that were shared by the nurse. They spoke of using the pill container and the medication record as a means of confirming that they were taking their medication in the appropriate dose and at the right time. In addition, most of participants reported that interaction with the nurse helped increase their awareness of the importance of taking their hypertensive medication as prescribed. The concepts of Bandura's (1977) social learning theory were a framework used by the nurse in helping the participants observe, participate, and practice new skills to better adhere to taking their hypertensive medications.

Some of the participants' behaviors remained unchanged after the nurse's intervention. One participant expressed that his mother continued to manage his medication for him. Another participant in this study expressed that even though taking his medication was not difficult, he did not always take it as prescribed. Some of the reasons were nonspecific and vague. The literature noted that nonadherence of hypertensive medication in Black men could be related to psychosocial factors. Cené et al. (2013) supported continued investigation and intervention into the numerous psychosocial factors impacting the lives of Black men that adversely impact their ability to adhere to therapy. Findings confirm that nurses should consider additional factors when working with patients that are nonadherent in taking medication.

An important finding of the study was that participants had other health problems that contributed to nonadherence and serious health issues. One of the participant's words revealed a depression that needed further assessment. This was supported by Cené et al. (2013) who found that depressive symptoms were associated with medication nonadherence. It is proposed that by establishing a trusting relationship with patients, they will reveal more about themselves. Nurse should be attentive to these additional issues that contribute to nonadherence. The literature supported the idea that development of trusting relationship between the patient and health care provider leads to obtaining an accurate assessment of adherence that would most likely yield the most honest and accurate responses (Martin, Williams, Haskard, & Dimatteo, 2005).

Participants said that they appreciated the face-to-face time with the nurse during this study, and many expressed that they would like to have more visits to discuss their medications and health-related issues. Participants perceived that they were listened to and that they gained new knowledge about their disorder. In summary, the establishment of a relationship with the nurse provided a means of introducing new tools that supported adherence in taking hypertensive medication in older Black male patients.

LIMITATIONS AND RECOMMENDATIONS

A limitation of this study was that the sample was small and included only older Black men from the rural South. Additional studies could include a larger sample of Black men of different ages in urban areas and in other parts of the country. This would give insight into the impact of the protocol on age groups and types of communities. Future studies should also include Black women of different ages with hypertension to determine if the protocol works the same for different genders. Further studies are needed to investigate psychosocial factors that affect medication adherence in Black men and women. Future studies are recommended to determine if the protocol is appropriate with different ethnic and racial groups.

An additional limitation of the study was that it was conducted over a short period of several months. Future uses of the protocol need to be evaluated for longer periods to determine if there is consistent change in adherence behavior. Administration of the protocol presumes that the nurse will have time to build relationships with patients and maintain contact to encourage them in taking their medications.

IMPLICATIONS FOR CHANGE

The result of this research supported findings of past studies and contributes to nursing knowledge about medication adherence in a high-risk population of older Black men in a rural area. It presents an adherence approach based on the development and administration of a nurse protocol. The protocol was developed in response to a specific need within a cardiology practice experiencing problems with medication adherence. The implication of the success of the protocol in helping patients' take their medication is that it will be continued by nursing staff at the clinic as part of an ongoing process to improve medication adherence. Clinic staff was oriented to the protocol including the use of the pillbox and recording forms. Appropriate patient follow-up was added to the protocol to sustain adherence. An important implication of the study was the need for staff to take *time* to develop trusting relationships with patients in a culturally competent manner. Knowing that patients consistently used the prescription bottle even after the protocol makes it important to assess whether patients can read and understand instructions. The role of the nurse in administering the protocol was to empower the patient to self-manage medication administration and to be perceptive of factors that inhibit adherence. Based on future research, this nurse protocol may be effective in assisting diverse groups in various setting with self-administration of hypertensive medication.

Hypertension continues to be a major challenge for health care providers even with the advances in prevention and treatment of cardiovascular disease. An important factor that contributes to uncontrolled hypertension is medication nonadherence. This study demonstrates how a vulnerable group of patients revealed their impressions of how a nurse protocol supported medication adherence.

Hypertension continues to be a major challenge for health care providers even with the advances in prevention and treatment of cardiovascular disease.

REFERENCES

Agency for Healthcare Research and Quality. (2011). *ACEIS, ARBS, or DRI for adults with hypertension.* Retrieved from http://effectivehealthcare.ahrq.gov/index.cfm/search-for-guides-reviewsand-reports/?productid=759&pageaction=displayproduct

American College of Preventive Medicine. (2011). *Medication adherence time tool: Improving health outcomes. A resource from the American College of Preventive Medicine.* Retrieved from http://www.acpm.org/?MedAdherTT_ClinRef

American Heart Association. (2013). *Statistical fact sheet: 2013 Update. High blood pressure.* Retrieved from http://www.heart.org/idc/groups/heart-public/@wcm/@sop/@smd/documents/downloadable/ucm_319587.pdf

Bandura, A. (1977). *Social learning theory.* Englewood Cliffs, NJ: Prentice.

Bennett, J. (2015). Beliefs and attitudes about medication adherence in African American men with high blood pressure. *MedSurg Matters, 22*(3), 4.

Cardarelli, R., Mann, C., Fulda, K., Balyakina, E., Espinoza, A., & Lurie, S. (2011). Improving accuracy of medication identification in an older population using a medication bottle color symbol label system. *BMC Family Practice, 12,* 142.

Cené, C., Dennison, C., Hammond, W. P., Levine, D., Bone, L., & Hill, M. (2013). Antihypertensive medication nonadherence in Black men: direct and mediating effects of depressive symptoms, psychosocial stressors, and substance use. *Journal of Clinical Hypertension, 15*(3), 201–209.

Creswell, J. W. (1998). *Qualitative inquiry and research design: Choosing among five approaches.* Thousand Oaks, CA: Sage.

Esposito, L. (1995). The effects of medication education on adherence to medication regimens in an elderly population. *Journal of Advanced Nursing, 21*(5), 935–943.

Hekler, E., Lambert, J., Leventhal, E., Leventhal, H., Jahn, E., & Contrada, R. (2008). Commonsense illness beliefs, adherence behaviors, and hypertension control among African Americans. *Journal of Behavioral Medicine, 31*(5), 391–400.

Hong, T., Oddone, E., Dudley, T., & Bosworth, H. (2006). Medication barriers and anti-hypertensive medication adherence: The moderating role of locus of control. *Psychology, Health & Medicine, 11*(1), 20–28

Hyre, A., Krousel-Wood, M., Muntner, P., Kawasaki, L., & DeSalvo, K. (2007). Prevalence and predictors of poor antihypertensive medication adherence in an urban health clinic setting. *Journal of Clinical Hypertension, 9*(3), 179–186.

Kannampallil, T. G., Waicekauskas, K., Morrow, D. G., Kopren, K. M., & Fu, W. (2013). External tools for collaborative medication scheduling. *Cognition, Technology and Work, 15*(2), 121–131.

Karaeren, H., Yokuşoğlu, M., Uzun, S,., Baysan, O., Köz, C., Kara, B., ... Uzun, M. (2009). The effect of the content of the knowledge on adherence to medication in hypertensive patients. *Anadolu Kardiyoloji Dergisi, 9*(3), 183–188.

Karakurt, P., & Kaşikçi, M. (2012). Factors affecting medication adherence in patients with hypertension. *Journal of Vascular Nursing, 30*(4), 118–126.

Kim, M., Han, H., Hill, M. N., Rose L., & Roary, M. (2003). Depression, substance use, adherence behaviors, and blood pressure in urban hypertensive Black men. *Annals of Behavioral Medicine, 3*(26), 24–31.

Klootwyk, J. M., & Sanoski, C. A. (2011). Medication adherence persistence in hypertension management. *Journal of Clinical Outcomes Management, 18*(8), 351.

Krousel-Wood, M., Muntner, P., Islam, T., Morisky, D., & Webber, L. (2009). Barriers to and determinants of medication adherence in hypertension management: Perspective of the Cohort Study of Medication

Adherence among Older Adults (CoSMO). *Medical Clinics of North America, 93*(3), 753–769. http://dx.doi.org/10.1016/j.mcna.2009.02.007

Krulish, L. (2005). M0780: Oral medications. *Home Healthcare Nurse, 23*(2), 72–76.

Lally, P., & Gardner, B. (2013). Promoting habit formation. *Health Psychology Review, 7*(Suppl. 1), S137–S158.

Lewis, L., Schoenthaler, A., & Ogedegbe, G. (2012). Patient factors, but not provider and health care system factors, predict medication adherence in hypertensive Black men. *Journal of Clinical Hypertension, 14*(4), 250–255.

Li, W., Kuo, C., Hwang, S., & Hsu, H. (2012). Factors related to medication non-adherence for patients with hypertension in Taiwan. *Journal of Clinical Nursing, 21*(13–14), 1816–1824.

Lincoln, Y. S., & Guba, E. G. (1985). *Naturalistic inquiry.* Beverly Hills, CA: Sage.

Lionakis, N., Mendrinos, D., Sanidas, E., Favatas, G., & Georgopoulou, M. (2012). Hypertension in the elderly. *World Journal of Cardiology, 4*(5), 135–147. Retrieved from http://www.ncbi.nlm.nih.gov/pmc/articles/PMC3364500/pdf/WJC-4-135.pdf

Lowman, R. L. (2013). Habit forming, habit changing. *Psyccritiques, 58*(2).

MacLaughlin, E., Raehl, C., Treadway, A., Sterling, T., Zoller, D., & Bond, C. (2005). Assessing medication adherence in the elderly: which tools to use in clinical practice? *Drugs & Aging, 22*(3), 231–255.

Martin, L., Williams, S., Haskard, K., & Dimatteo, M. (2005). The challenge of patient adherence. *Therapeutics and Clinical Risk Management, 1*(3), 189–199.

Martins, D., & Norris, K. (2004). Hypertension treatment in African Americans: Physiology is less important than sociology. *Cleveland Clinic Journal of Medicine, 71*(9), 735–743.

Merlo, A. R., Goodman, A., McClenaghan, B. A., & Fritz, S. L. (2013). Participants' perspectives on the feasibility of a novel, intensive, task-specific intervention for individuals with chronic stroke: A qualitative analysis. *Physical Therapy, 93*(2), 147–157.

O'Neill, J. L., & Feldman, S. R. (2009). Practical ways to improve patients' use of their medications. *Current Medical Literature: Dermatology, 14*(4), 85–92.

Orem, D. E. (2001). *Nursing: Concept of practice* (6th ed.). St. Louis, MO: Mosby.

Osterberg, L., & Blaschke, T. (2005). Adherence to medication. *The New England Journal of Medicine, 353*(5), 487–497.

Patton, M. Q. (2002). *Qualitative research and evaluation methods* (3rd ed.). Thousand Oaks, CA: Sage.

Polit, D., & Beck, C. (2010). *Essentials of nursing research: Appraising evidence for nursing practice* (7th ed.). Philadelphia, PA: Lippincott Williams & Wilkins.

Rose, L., Kim, M., Dennison, C., & Hill, M. (2000). The contexts of adherence for African Americans with high blood pressure. *Journal of Advanced Nursing, 32*(3), 587–594.

Sanne, S., Muntner, P., Kawasaki, L., Hyre, A., & DeSalvo, K. (2008). Hypertension knowledge among patients from an urban clinic. *Ethnicity & Disease, 18*, 42–47.

Schlomann, P., & Schmitke, J. (2007). Lay beliefs about hypertension: An interpretive synthesis of the qualitative research. *Journal of the American Academy of Nurse Practitioners, 19*(7) 358–367.

Schoenthaler, A., Allegrante, J. P., Chaplin, W., & Ogedegbe, G. (2012). The effect of patient–provider communication on medication adherence in hypertensive Black patients: Does race concordance matter? *Annals of Behavioral Medicine, 43*(3), 372–382.

Thomas-Kvidera, D. (2005). Heart failure from diastolic dysfunction related to hypertension: Guidelines for management. *Journal of the American Academy of Nurse Practitioners, 17*(5), 168–175.

Uzun, S., Kara, B., Yokus͵oğ͘lu, M., Arslan, F., Yilmaz, M., & Karaeren, H. (2009). The assessment of adherence of hypertensive individuals to treatment and lifestyle change recommendations. *Anadolu Kardiyoloji Dergisi, 9*(2), 102–109.

Welch, L. K., Olson, K. L., Snow, K. E., Pointer, L., Lambert-Kerzner, A., Havranek, E. P., … Ho, P. (2011). Systolic blood pressure control after participation in a hypertension intervention study. *American Journal of Managed Care, 17*(7), 473–478.

Yendelela, C., Hargraves, J., Rosal, M., Briesacher, B., Schoenthaler, A., Person, S., … Allison, J. (2013). Reported racial discrimination, trust in physicians, and medication adherence among inner-city African Americans with hypertension. *American Journal of Public Health, 103*(11), e55–e62.

Correspondence regarding this article should be directed to Ophelia Thomas, DNP, RN, Regis University, 108 Travis Lane, Leesburg, GA 31763. E-mail: Ophelia2@msn.com

HYPERTENSIVE BLACK MEN'S PERCEPTION OF A NURSE PROTOCOL FOR MEDICATION SELF-ADMINISTRATION

Critique by *Deborah B. Fahs*

OVERALL SUMMARY

Black men experience a disproportionately higher burden of high blood pressure and its effects on overall health compared with other groups. Adherence to a prescribed hypertensive medication regimen is influenced by a variety of social, economic, and cultural factors, with evidence suggesting lower rates of controlled hypertension in older Black men. This study utilizes Orem's self-care deficit theory and Bandura's social learning theory to guide a qualitative approach for understanding factors that contribute to hypertension medication nonadherence as well as the influence of a nurse-developed protocol for medication self-administration. The key informants in this study, patients at a rural cardiology clinic, provided surprising reasons for medication nonadherence, which have implications for how nurses collaborate with this population to improve outcomes of care.

TITLE

Does the title include the key concepts/variables/phenomenon of interest?

The title of this manuscript contains the phenomenon of interest, the effectiveness of a nurse protocol for medication self-administration in older, Black men toward maintaining compliance with their prescribed antihypertensive medication(s).

Is it concise (12 words or less) and professionally stated?

The title is clearly stated and concise (12 words).

RESEARCHER(S) CREDIBILITY

Educational credentials?

Both the first and second authors are doctorally prepared nurses, and the second author serves as faculty at Regis University. During the time of investigation, the first author was a master's-prepared nurse who was familiar with both the population of interest and the clinic setting where the research was conducted.

Prior methodological research experience of the authors (i.e., methodological expertise)?

It is unknown whether either one of the authors has any previous methodological expertise in conducting qualitative studies.

Subject matter content experience (prior research on the subject matter)?

An Internet search revealed that the second author has multiple publications in the areas of client education, theory and practice, cultural diversity as well as studying DNP perceptions of the practice role in the care of older adults. Her research interests and publications establish her credibility as a content expert in the research phenomenon of interest.

ABSTRACT
Does it include the key concepts (objective/aim, background/rationale, methods, results, and conclusion)?

The opening sentence of the abstract explains the importance of the study and answers the "why" question or the reason this topic was chosen for investigation. The research participants were clearly identified according to age, gender, and ethnicity and the methodology was plainly defined. The basic findings were concisely reported in one sentence.

Does or does not include references?

The abstract is appropriately free of references.

Is it concise (150–250 words or less)?

The abstract is comprehensive yet concise with a word count of slightly less than 250 words.

Does it entice you to read the rest of the article (interesting)?

The abstract is interesting and is applicable to all health care settings, such as home care, clinic, or hospital venues. It is well prepared and enables the reader to review the article quickly and succinctly to determine whether it is of interest to his or her practice or literature search.

INTRODUCTION/PROBLEM
Is the research problem or phenomenon of interest clearly stated?

The research problem is introduced with some clarity in the opening sentences of the manuscript by referencing the serious nature of older person's nonadherence to antihypertensive medications. However, the specific population of interest, which is older Black men, is not introduced until the third sentence. It would improve the introduction with a statement outlining the specific phenomenon of interest, specifically, older Black men, in the opening sentence.

Is it succinct?

The research problem is succinctly stated in the last sentence of the Introduction section.

Does it answer the "so what" question?

The introduction, similar to the abstract, offers the rationale as to why this particular problem is worthy of investigation, relating nonadherence to antihypertensive medication(s) to increased morbidity, mortality, and health care costs.

RESEARCH AIMS/OBJECTIVES
Is the research aim/objective clearly stated?

The research question, aim/purpose is clearly and concisely stated. By administering a nurse protocol focused on self-administration of hypertensive medications, the researchers sought to improve perceptions of taking hypertensive medication in hypertensive, Black men, age 65 to 70 years old, with the ultimate goal of improving medication adherence.

Is it concisely written?

The research question is concisely written.

Does it follow logically from the research problem/phenomenon of interest?

> The objective of the research flows logically from the phenomenon of interest and the researcher makes the argument to support the reason the problem deserves new research.

SIGNIFICANCE

Is the significance to nursing and health care clearly written?

> The researchers clarify the significance of studying medication nonadherence as it relates to the negative impact on patient morbidity, mortality, and health care costs.

Does the significance follow from the research aim/objective?

> The researchers cite statistical evidence in supporting the importance of studying antihypertensive medication nonadherence. The study, however, was not meant to provide quantitative evidence related to the seriousness of the problem, but rather to qualitatively study the patient's perceptions of medication self-administration. The researchers aimed to offer valuable insight behind the "why" of patient nonadherence.

BACKGROUND

Is there an explicit description of a theoretical perspective or conceptual framework? If not, is it implied?

> The study is explicitly based on a conceptual framework and embodies two theories. The first, Dorothy Orem's self-care deficit theory, describes a self-care model addressing the role of the nurse in supporting the client in maintaining a functional level of self-care. This theory broadly reflects the phenomenon of interest and is both meaningful and appropriate to the study.
>
> The second theory is based on Bandura's (1977) social learning theory, which the researchers link to their study by describing how the nurse nurtured relationships with the participants to assist them in learning new skills related to medication compliance. Bandura (1977) theorized that when individuals believe the person demonstrating a behavior (nurse) holds similarities to them, observational learning can be effective. It is unclear, however, what the similarities are between the participants and the nurse since there is a distinct role difference between the two.

Are there clear theoretical/conceptual definitions of the concepts?

> Self-care as conceptualized by Orem is well described in the section on the Conceptual Framework. Bandura's theoretical concept of social learning, such as observational learning, is not defined.

LITERATURE REVIEW

Primary sources only?

> The researchers include a mix of primary and secondary sources. For example, in the first citation, statistical data was referenced from a secondary source rather than the original study.

Current (within the past how many years)?

> Some of the sources should have been more current, ideally within 5 years of publication. Taking into account historical and seminal sources, the manuscript cited

several sources older than 10 years. Because clinical management recommendations change rapidly, sources citing the guidelines for hypertensive management need to be updated.

Is the search strategy included?

The search strategy was not included in the review.

Is literature relevant to the research aims/objectives?

The literature review revealed relevant sources to the research purpose and aim.

Is it chronologically presented (old to current)?

Although the literature review was not chronologically presented from oldest to most current, the content flowed smoothly and effortlessly, making it simple for the reader to follow and understand.

Is it comprehensive? If not, is sufficient background literature provided?

The literature review content was comprehensive and focused on the key concepts related to the study. It included statistics related to morbidity and mortality as a result of nonadherence to medication regimens, personal struggles and beliefs of Black men related to nonadherence, patient education as an approach to addressing nonadherence, strategies to facilitate new behaviors, and relationship building between the client and the provider. There was a logical flow between previous and present works.

RATIONALE FOR THE STUDY

Is there a gap in the literature that this study will fill (will it extend prior knowledge)? Is the rationale clearly stated?

Although there has been research in the area of hypertension and compliance among older Black men, nonadherence continues to be detrimental to the patient's state of health and challenging for the nurse. Therefore, the study is useful in posing possible solutions to the ongoing conundrum of nonadherence toward developing a better understanding behind the "why" of patient nonadherence behaviors. The gap in knowledge is clearly stated.

Is this a follow-up or replication study?

The study was original research rather than a replication or follow-up study and was designed to address a particular problem with nonadherence to antihypertensive medication noted in a cardiology practice in a rural area.

RESEARCH QUESTION(S) AND/OR HYPOTHESES

Are these explicitly and clearly stated?

The research question was clearly stated and can be found in the last sentence of the purpose discussion. The study was qualitative in nature; therefore it was appropriate that there was no stated hypotheses.

Do they include the variables/phenomenon of interest?

The research question includes the population of interest, older hypertensive Black men, as well as the phenomenon of interest, which is their perception of a nurse protocol for medication self-administration and its effect on their ability to follow a prescribed medication regimen for hypertension.

Do they follow from the research aim/objective?

The research question directly follows from the purpose of determining the effect of a nurse protocol on self-administration of hypertensive medication on improving perceptions of taking hypertensive medication in the population of interest.

METHODS
Research Design/Paradigm
Is the research design clearly stated?

The research design is clearly stated in the Methodsection as a qualitative approach using the key informant method.

Is there consistency between the research design and paradigm?

There is consistency between this qualitative research design and the constructivist paradigm, as it allows the researchers to explore the participants' individual, subjective experiences with nonadherence to a prescribed medication.

Is this the best choice of design to address the research problem/phenomenon of interest?

The researchers choose this methodology wisely as it enabled them to "dig deeper" in an attempt to gather a depth of valuable information and insights about medication nonadherence not answered by one sentence or a simple response.

Is there rigor in the design?

Given that the reasons for Black men's often poor adherence to antihypertensive medication regimens are not fully understood, the key informant qualitative design can be considered rigorous.

SETTING
Is the setting clearly described?

The setting for the initial intervention was described as a cardiology practice in which older Black men, with poor hypertension control, were the predominate group of patients. Subsequent encounters occurred either in the clinic or in the patient's home.

What biases are introduced as a result of selecting this particular setting?

The researcher (presumably the lead author) states she was familiar with the cardiology clinic setting and that the cardiologist in charge of the practice had shared observations about older Black men's nonadherence to their antihypertensive medication regimen. The researcher's specific relationship with this clinic and/or its patients is unclear and would pose bias if she was familiar with the patients or was employed in the clinic. An additional source of bias results from limiting the study setting to one cardiology clinic in one particular location in one state.

SAMPLING PLAN AND SAMPLE
Is the sampling plan clearly identified?

The sample was defined as a purposive sample of participants obtained by the nurse researcher from office documentation at a rural cardiology clinic. According to office records, the demographics of the clinic were well suited to the research aim since Black men with uncontrolled hypertension predominated in that particular clinic.

Does it represent the population of interest?

The population of interest is older Black men with a primary diagnosis of hypertension for which they are taking medication(s) to control high blood pressure. The criteria for inclusion reflect this population. Individuals with a diagnosis of dementia were excluded as it was necessary for the men to manipulate the tools necessary for medication adherence.

Is the sampling plan consistent with the research aim/objective?

The purposive sampling methodology is consistent with the research aim because it focuses on selecting participants with specific characteristics of the population of interest.

Is the sample size sufficient (e.g., power analysis or data saturation)?

Because the study was of qualitative design, there was no power analysis. Data saturation was not described.

VARIABLES

Are variables clearly identified?

The study was a qualitative design; therefore, specific variables are not identified.

Are variables operationally defined and consistent with theoretical concepts?

Qualitative studies do not use operationally defined variables.

Are independent and dependent variables identified, if applicable?

Because this is a qualitative study, no independent and dependent variables are identified.

METHOD OF DATA COLLECTION

What are the methods of data collection?

Key informant interview was the method of data collection, which involved the nurse researcher conducting individual interviews with each participant, either at the clinic setting or in the patient's home, 2 weeks following the protocol-based teaching session.

Are validity and reliability clearly addressed for prior research and current study, if applicable?

Not applicable in this qualitative study.

Do the measures/instruments address the underlying theoretical concepts or phenomenon of interest?

As this is a qualitative study that utilized face-to-face interviews to collect data from key informants, there are no research instruments.

Were human rights protected?

The institutional review board approved the research as "exempt" and written permission (letter of intent) was signed by the cardiologist in the clinic where the research took place. Protection of human rights was adhered to with the participants signing consent forms agreeing to participate.

Are other ethical issued identified?

There do not appear to be any identifiable ethical issues. Confidentiality and anonymity were assured and the participants were told they could withdraw from the study at any time. Only the nurse researcher and transcriptionist viewed the interview results and the data was secured and password protected.

Is the data-collection method appropriate for research design?

The key informant interview is appropriate for obtaining in-depth information from individuals with particular knowledge about a problem or phenomenon of interest.

Is there bias in data collection?

In qualitative studies, the researcher collecting the data, either by conducting interviews or through direct observations of participants in the field, introduces an element of bias by virtue of his or her presence. The researcher's subjectivity can influence what is seen, asked, and heard, and participants' responses may be influenced by the researcher's presence. Although there is no explicit evidence of bias in data collection in this study, it is assumed to exist to some degree.

What is the fidelity of intervention addressed, if applicable?

Not applicable.

DATA ANALYSIS

Are data analysis techniques described (e.g., statistical tests, methodology for qualitative analysis)?

Although not explicitly stated, the researcher appears to have used thematic analysis, which involves transcribing data obtained from interviews, grouping participant responses, and forming common ideas and concepts from the data through line-by-line open coding. The process of coding involves labeling data for meaning, which allows for the discovery of interrelated themes.

Does the analysis answer the research question?

The analysis provides greater insight into the participants' perceptions of taking hypertensive medications as well as their perceptions of a nurse protocol to assist with self-administration of hypertensive medication.

Is it appropriate?

Thematic analysis is appropriate for identifying, analyzing, and interpreting patterns or themes within data, in order to gain greater understanding of a particular phenomenon of interest.

Is the analysis comprehensive? Are themes identified?

The analysis was comprehensive and categories with themes and subthemes emerged through constant comparative analysis, outlining similarities and differences in responses. Two main themes identified were perceptions of taking medication before the nurse intervention and perceptions of taking medication after the nurse intervention. From the two main themes, three subthemes also emerged. The themes are clearly explained with supporting data.

Is there bias in the analysis (trustworthiness? credibility?)?

The researcher(s) describe the aim of trustworthiness in the study, identifying credibility, transferability, dependability, and confirmability as crucial elements to their investigative process. The interviews were digitally recorded, which facilitates accuracy of transcription. The researchers further explain that they maintained a complete audit trail of the research process, including a reflexive journal with extensive field notes, to establish rigor. Although the researcher referred to setting aside bias at the beginning of the study, it is impossible to eliminate all forms of human subjectivity. In addition, there is no mention of a reflexive journal developed for the purpose of reflecting on the ways in which the researcher's preconceived ideas, perceptions, or beliefs may have influenced the interpretation of the data.

RESULTS

Are sample characteristics described and fully reported?

The researcher (s) described the study participants as 10 Black men, age 65 to 70 years, who were diagnosed with hypertension and based on medical records from the cardiology clinic, nonadherent in taking their antihypertensive medication. Three participants were diagnosed with hypertension 4 years or less and seven were diagnosed for more than 10 years. No other sample characteristics are provided, such as marital status, or years of education completed.

Are findings presented related to research aim/objective?

The findings on participants' perceptions of taking hypertensive medications both before and after the nurse intervention were presented and themes and categories were supported by participants' comments. The researchers acknowledged that some participants' behaviors remained unchanged after the intervention and that other problems posing barriers to patient medication adherence were discovered.

Are all outcome variables addressed, if applicable?

Not applicable in a qualitative study.

Are results clearly presented in text and/or tables/figures?

The themes were clearly labeled with supporting explanations outlined in both the text and in table form, so that the reader might quickly scan the manuscript to determine major study results.

Is significance of results reported, if applicable?

Not applicable.

DISCUSSION OF RESULTS

Do the authors link the findings to previous research studies?

The study contains an extensive discussion of the findings related to previous studies. For example, prior to the nurse protocol, participants acknowledged their medication nonadherence, which is consistent with other findings on low adherence rates in older individuals with hypertension. The small print used on the medication bottles was found to be a contributor to nonadherence in the current study, which has also been previously reported in the literature. Both Orem's theory of self-care deficit and Bandura's social learning theory were discussed and linked with the study findings.

Are the conclusions comprehensive, yet within the data?

> The discussion was comprehensive and does not go beyond the data. It provided added value for nurses in determining reasons underpinning patient nonadherence.

Do the authors interpret the results in the discussion?

> The authors interpret the results, that is, discern what is important and what can be learned, throughout the Discussion section. They highlight, in particular, the need for further patient education on self-administration of hypertensive medication grounded in Orem's self-care deficit theory.

Are the findings generalizable or transferable?

> Although the sample size was small and the setting was limited to a rural, southern region of the United States, results can be used as a basis for studying larger sample sizes in other areas of the country.

LIMITATIONS
Identified? Accurate? Inclusive?

> The researcher(s) accurately identified some study limitations, noting that the small sample of older Black men from a southern, rural town, could be extended to investigating a larger sample of Black men, as well as including Black women of all ages in urban areas and other parts of the country. The researchers also recognized the need for additional studies related to psychosocial factors contributing to nonadherence of antihypertensive medication (s). It was acknowledged that the study was conducted over a short time period (several months) and should be evaluated over a longer time frame to better understand changes in nonadherence behaviors.

IMPLICATIONS
Are there implications for practice, education, research?

> The section Implications for Change describes the benefit of incorporating the nurse researcher-developed hypertensive protocol in practice. The researcher also cited the importance of a culturally competent approach to developing trusting patient relationships and a need to ascertain whether patients can read and fully understand the prescription directions. Implications for future research are discussed in the section Limitations and Recommendations.

Are there implications for clinical significance?

> Implications for clinical significance are not addressed. However, the study findings may help nurses to develop interventions based on a new understanding of the behaviors, needs, and challenges of older Black men self-administering hypertensive medications.

RECOMMENDATIONS
Recommendations for future study/study replication?

> Recommendations for future research include expanding the use of this particular nurse-developed medication adherence protocol to diverse groups in various settings to improve self-administration of hypertensive medications.

CONCLUSION
Is it succinct and does it tie everything together?

Although the conclusion was not identified in a separate section of the manuscript, the investigator ended the manuscript by reinforcing the importance of patient antihypertensive medication adherence to prevent, manage, and treat cardiovascular disease. The study demonstrated the perceptions of a vulnerable group of patients, explaining their nonadherence behaviors and how a nurse protocol targeted at nonadherence may mitigate these behaviors. The conclusions drawn by the researcher (s) were clear, succinct, and aligned well with the research aim and objectives.

PRIMARY CARE EXPERIENCES OF PEOPLE WHO LIVE WITH CHRONIC PAIN AND RECEIVE OPIOIDS TO MANAGE PAIN: A QUALITATIVE METHODOLOGY

13

Barbara St. Marie, PhD, ANP, GNP, ACHPN (Associate Faculty)
College of Nursing, The University of Iowa, Iowa City, Iowa

ABSTRACT

Background and purpose: The prevalence of chronic pain continues to rise and the majority of patients with chronic pain are managed in primary care. The purpose of this research was to provide the perspectives of patients who live with chronic pain and receive opioids to help manage their pain from primary care.

Methods: In this qualitative study, 12 participants from a Midwest primary care clinic described their primary care experiences with receiving opioids for chronic pain. Thematic and interpretive analyses were used to understand the issues.

Conclusions: Participants receiving opioids for pain management through primary care feared losing access to opioids, wanted to protect sobriety when they had histories of substance use disorder, experienced stress at their jobs with frequent appointments, identified inconsistencies in health care prolonging their suffering and increasing substance misuse, and identified improvement in coping with pain when they had confidence in health care providers.

Implications for practice: Providing patient-centered care while managing patients with pain and unknown risk for prescription opioid misuse is possible. Understanding influences that create prescription opioid risk for misuse can help nurse practitioners improve their delivery of care by providing consistent and convenient health care encounters, and help patients protect themselves from risk of prescription opioid misuse.

KEY WORDS: pain management; pharmacotherapy; primary care; substance abuse

INTRODUCTION

There is growing evidence that the harms of opioid therapy for the treatment of chronic pain outweigh the benefits of treating the most complex presenting symptom found in primary care. One hundred sixteen million Americans live with chronic pain costing $560 to $635 billion annually (Institute of Medicine of the National Academies, 2011), and nearly 25 million live with substance use disorder (SUD) costing over 467

St. Marie, B. (2016). Primary care experiences of people who live with chronic pain and receive opioids to manage pain: A qualitative methodology. *Journal of the American Association of Nurse Practitioners*, *28*(8), 429–435. doi:10.1002/2327-6924.12342 billion dollars annually, with prescription opioid abuse or dependence affecting approximately 2 million people (U.S. Department of Health and Human Services, 2010; Substance Abuse and Mental Health Administration, 2014). Studies have shown an increase in misuse or overdose associated with opioid use and the National Institute on Drug Abuse attributes this to the increased availability of prescription opioids for the treatment of pain (Bohnert et al., 2011; Compton & Volkow, 2006; Dart et al., 2015; Edlund, Steffick, Hudson, Harris, & Sullivan, 2007; Gomes, Mamdani, Dhalla, Paterson, & Juurlink, 2011; Jena, Goldman, Weaver, & Karaca-Mandic, 2014; Palouzzi, Kilbourne, Shah, Nolte, Desai, Landen . . . Loring, 2012). Moreover, the prevalence of chronic pain also continues to rise and opioids are foundational to treatment, yet analysis of the medical literature has shown insufficient evidence for long-term effectiveness of opioids, and insufficient evidence for safety and harms of opioids for the treatment of chronic pain (Chou et al., 2015; Nuckols et al., 2014). Chronic pain carries significant burden, negatively impacting the biological, psychological, and social domains of people's lives, and cannot be ignored.

This study was carried out following the release of the Institute of Medicine's report titled, *Relieving Pain in America: A Blueprint for Transforming Prevention, Care, Education, and Research*. This transformative approach included changing the method of undergraduate and graduate education of pain; changing the culture of care delivery through interprofessional teams; delivering a balanced approach to pain including opioids, nonopioids, and nonpharmacological therapies; and concentrating on efforts for patient-centered care (Institute of Medicine of the National Academies, 2011). Moreover, in July 2012, the Food and Drug Administration (FDA) approved a strategy of Risk Evaluation and Mitigation for extended released and long-acting opioid medications to improve safety and reduce harm of opioids prescribed by health care professionals (U.S. FDA, 2012). These federal initiatives focus on the societal problems of rising prescription opioid misuse and chronic pain and offer recommendations for change. Nurse practitioners can gain understanding by looking at the problem through the lens of patient narratives, and are well positioned to promote changes guided by these perspectives to reduce vulnerability to collateral problems when pain is treated with opioids.

The majority of people with chronic pain are managed in primary care, and when opioids are used there is an inherent ambiguity for misuse or abuse of prescription opioids. A study by Morasco and Dobscha (2008) showed patients receiving opioid therapy in primary care had a four times higher incidence of SUD than patients in the general population who did not receive chronic opioid therapy (3.8% vs. 0.9%). Primary care providers are faced with competing mandates endeavoring to balance moral and ethical obligation to treat pain while feeling vulnerable to deceptions, misuse, or diversion of prescribed medications by their patients (Merrill, Rhodes, Deyo, Marlatt, & Bradley, 2002). These circumstances create a need to investigate the problem by asking the patients in primary care about their experiences and underlying influences while managing chronic pain with opioids.

A preliminary study of 34 individuals living with coexisting SUD and pain who received methadone for opiate addiction found when they entered the health care arena they were disturbed by the inability of health care providers to help their painful conditions, and recommended that health care providers manage pain with vigilant watch for misuse and relapse to SUD (St. Marie, 2014a). In this preliminary study, participants had known opiate addiction; however, patients in primary care settings may have less-defined SUD histories or unknown risk for opioid misuse. Studying the perspectives of patients receiving long-term opioids for chronic pain in this setting may guide change in the way we deliver safe and effective pain management.

PURPOSE

The purpose of this study was to provide a deeper understanding of the experiences, issues, and challenges that people face who live with chronic pain and received opioids to help manage their pain in primary care. The following research questions were addressed: (a) What are the experiences of individuals who live with chronic pain and receive opioid pain medications to manage their pain in primary care? and (b) What have been their health care experiences as they strive to manage their pain? There are gaps in the literature on exploring the experiences of patients receiving opioids in primary care.

METHODS

Narrative inquiry was used to explore how these participants made sense of experiences living with chronic pain and receiving opioids in primary care. The investigator's experiences as a nurse practitioner specializing in pain management in primary care, pain clinics, and hospitals for over 30 years afforded assumptions about the study design and interpretations of the results. The assumptions are as follows: (a) persons who live with SUD and chronic pain are reliable narrators of their experiences, (b) listening to patients' narratives allows health care providers to view the problem through the patient's eyes, and (c) patients often have insights that only those who have experienced pain and opioid exposure can have.

Sample and Setting

Two institutional review boards (IRBs) from different institutions approved this study and all participants gave written informed consent. Recruitment and interviews took place in a Midwest metropolitan primary care clinic until data saturation occurred. Flyers were posted in the primary care lobby with a phone number of the investigator. When potential participants called the phone number, screening took place by the principal investigator. Inclusion criteria used in this study included male or female, 18 years of age or older, any race or ethnicity, and conversant in English. The participants experienced persistent or chronic pain longer than 6 months and receive prescribed opioids while under the care of a primary care provider for a health problem that caused pain. They understood their participation in the interview was voluntary, agreed to be audiotaped, and were able to get to the interview at a designated location. The participants were reimbursed for their time participating in the study.

Data Collection

The data-collection methods included a demographic questionnaire, field observation notes, and semistructured interviews. Field observations noted participants' nonverbal cues, assistive equipment or braces, and tonal inflections. The interview guide consisted of open-ended questions about their experiences relating to living with chronic pain and receiving opioids from primary care and is shown in Table 1. The questions were developed from the investigator's clinical experience and past research experience, and relevant literature. One investigator conducted the interview in a private room at the primary care clinic, lasted approximately 60 to 90 minutes,

TABLE 1. Interview Guide

The Following Questions Were Used as a Guide in the Interview Process
1. What has it been like for you to live with persistent or chronic pain?
2. Has your pain ever been out of control? If so, can you tell me what happened?
3. What has it been like for you to live with treating pain with opioids/narcotics?
4. What kind of support do you receive?
5. What kind of nonmedicine ways do you use to manage your pain?
6. Have you needed opioids/narcotics to treat pain before coming into primary care?
7. Have you had problems with opioids/narcotics previously, for example, using more than prescribed?
8. Has your family or employer had concern over you taking opioids for pain?
9. I would like to hear about health care that has gone well for you and about health care that has not gone so well (Stevens, 1998).
10. What did you find was the best way to get pain relief?
11. Has a physician or nurse practitioner or physicians' assistant ever withheld treatment you needed to control your pain? Tell me what happened.
12. What should your health care team know about you in order to care for you in the best possible manner?
13. If you could design your pain management what would it look like?
14. Is there anything you would like to ask me?
15. Is there anything I should have asked you?

and each participant was interviewed once. The interviews were audio recorded on a digital file, sent to transcription service via a secured link, and stored in hard copy in a locked file cabinet at the researcher's work site.

Analysis

Thematic and interpretive analyses were used (Bloomberg & Volpe, 2008; Denzin & Lincoln, 2005). The interviews were analyzed iteratively as data collection was occurring. Steps in data analysis included reading the narratives and listening to the audio recordings while making notes in the narratives from the field notes. Narrative summaries were written on each participant to determine the emphasis of the narrative and to gather verbatim quotes. Ultimately, comparisons were made between participant narratives to determine similarities and differences, and themes were identified through the underlying relevant patterns of experiences. Interpretive analysis occurred through a lens shaped by the investigator's experiences as nurse practitioner caring for patients with chronic pain and at times prescribing long-term opioid therapy. Scientific rigor was established through dependability and validity. Dependability was assured by stability in participants' themes and no self-contradictory statements occurred within the time frame (Hall & Stevens, 1991). Validity occurred through an outside reviewer examining the interviews and judging if the coding and themes reflected the content of the interviews (Cohen & Crabtree, 2008).

RESULTS

Twelve participants were recruited and their demographic summary is shown in Table 2. There was no specific recruitment for SUD; however, in their interviews nine of 12 of the participants revealed a history of SUD.

TABLE 2. Demographic Data

Age, Mean (SD), Year	42(10.8)
Male, no. (%)	6(50)
Race/ethnicity, no. (%)	
White	7(58.3)
Black/African American	4(33.3)
Hispanic/Latino	1(0.1)
Employed, no. (%)	3(25)
Relationship, no. (%)	8(66.6)
Attended college, no. (%)	9(75)

There were four major themes found in the participants' narratives. These themes were as follows: (a) health care experiences while seeking relief for their pain, (b) fears of SUD, relapse, or losing access to opioids for pain, (c) low-or high-risk behaviors for misuse of opioids, and (d) use of nonmedicine methods of managing pain.

Health Care Experiences While Seeking Relief for Their Pain

All the participants experienced pain on a daily basis and there were expectations to attend frequent health care appointments to comply with the chronic opioid therapy agreement. Additionally, they described positive and negative experiences while receiving health care.

Frequent health care appointments. All the participants in this study were receiving chronic opioid therapy for treatment of their chronic pain and signed opioid therapy agreements. To comply with expectations of the agreement, it was required that they participate in rehabilitation therapies, counseling, and follow-up appointments with their health care provider. This often meant two to three appointment times per week. Three of 12 participants were employed and had to leave work on the days of their appointments, leading to work reprimands or working extra hours to make up for lost time. One person stated he had to drive a great distance from his job to reach his appointments and this was especially difficult in winter. Frequent health care appointments created hardships in their jobs and added stress.

Positive health care experiences. Participants described positive experiences of open communication, and feeling confidence in their health care providers. One participant's pain created restrictions in work and relationships, and his psychologist advocated receiving opioids for pain relief. Once he started prescription opioids he stated, ". . . my world opened up, it's insane how much it changed." This participant described 2 years of compliant use of prescribed opioids while he maintained sobriety from former alcohol and drug abuse. His prescribed opioids managed his pain so he could continue to work in the 2-year time period. Open communication with a caring health care team about pain, past SUD, or fear of SUD helped create a milieu where the participants took better care of themselves. One participant stated, ". . . because they care, I care." These participants defined caring as supportive validation of their pain, and receiving education about pain, pain medications, and addiction potential. When confident in health care, the participants felt less stress about their ability to cope when pain intensity was high and they were able to enjoy staying active.

Negative health care experiences. Participants described negative health care encounters when feeling stigmatized and receiving inconsistent communication or care. Participants felt stigmatized by their history of SUD and one participant stated, ". . . it's hell being somebody . . . [with] drug and alcohol problems, then walk into a doctor and say, 'I need narcotics' [for pain], because they do not wanna give them to you." Another participant explained how he went to the emergency room for a flare of chronic abdominal pain, was told to go to his primary care provider, went to his primary care provider who told him to go to the emergency department, in his frustration he went home, drank alcohol, and was admitted to the hospital with acute pancreatitis. These participants stated they received pain management from the opioids; however, when they experienced inconsistencies in care or felt stigmatized, their suffering was prolonged and some would abuse substances out of desperation or frustration.

Fears of SUD, Relapse, or Losing Access to Opioids for Pain

Fear of SUD or relapse. Nine of 12 participants in this study had a history of SUD and all of them were prescribed chronic opioid therapy for persistent pain. They feared losing sobriety and were very intentional about protecting their sobriety. One participant stated, "I don't wanna screw up my sobriety, I don't wanna get addicted, I was very frightened about getting addicted and frightened about craving [the drug of abuse]." Another participant who obtained additional illicit opioids while taking prescription opioids stated, "[I] won't use heroin because I'm more scared of that than anything, you know what I'm saying?" This individual was afraid of losing control and relapsing to heroin, yet was not afraid of losing control of his prescription opioids or the oxycodone he bought illicitly. These participants protected their sobriety and managed their pain to the best of their ability.

Fear of losing access to opioids. Many participants believed that individuals who misused their prescription opioids were "wrecking it for those who need it for pain." They reflected that media coverage of people overdosing was why health care providers were "cracking down" on prescribing opioids for those with chronic pain. One participant stated, "If I'm not getting it [prescription opioids] from my doctor, then I gotta find other ways to get it." This fear of losing access to prescription opioids led some of the participants to find illicit opioids.

Low- and High-Risk Behaviors for Misuse of Opioids

The investigator interpreted the comments within the narratives to reveal a range of low-risk to high-risk behaviors with use of prescription opioids. The participants with low-risk behaviors were compliant with their medication regimen, did not take more than prescribed, did not combine illicit substances with their prescription opioids, nor divert their prescription opioids. One low-risk participant stated, "Ever since I had the pain, I've always had my sobriety in the back of my mind." To ensure her safety from relapse and harm, she developed a protocol for taking medication with predetermined opioid amounts so she would not overconsume when pain changed. High-risk behaviors included taking more opioids than prescribed, calling in for early prescription refills, losing opioid prescriptions, or consuming illicit substances (Compton, Darakjian, & Miotto, 1998). Four of 12 participants described high-risk behaviors at some time while receiving prescription opioids for pain. One participant's narration revealed a level of desperation using manipulative strategies with his health care provider, leading to consumption of hundreds of milligrams of opioids per day. He used a strategy to direct the provider's attention away from his SUD with prescription opioids:

> I took that article [on abusing opioid] from [the newspaper] in to my doctor. I said, "Hey look," showing the newspaper article, "people have problems with this. I don't but here's a good article that you may wanna read." I mean there was some subtle things I was doing to try to block the noise of, "Hey [I] got a problem."

At the health care encounter, he thought his health care provider was suspicious of his overuse of prescription opioids, but found this distraction successful in receiving early refill. He revealed wanting to be stopped from overusing, yet was fearful about stopping because he saw no other options other than prescription opioids for his SUD or pain. This participant eventually received help at the clinic where recruitment occurred for this study.

Using Nonmedicine Methods to Manage Pain

Participants consistently spoke about how they manage pain that did not involve prescription opioids. They took pride as they described the strategies they created that brought them pain relief and peace. One participant stated, "You can't just treat yourself with drugs." The strategies these participants used for managing pain are listed in Table 3. Some of these methods were learned through health care encounters, some were learned on their own. Either way, the participants described executing these methods to manage pain instead of or in addition to opioid therapy.

DISCUSSION

Key findings were determined from the narratives of people receiving opioids for chronic pain in the primary care setting with known or unknown risk for SUD.

TABLE 3. Nonmedicine Strategies Used by Participants for Pain Management

The Following Are Nonmedicine Strategies That the Participants Selected on Their Own
Massage
Physical therapy
Counseling for their mental health
Walking their dogs
Generally being more active
Changing their diet to healthy foods
Exercise and stretching on their own
Sitting and walking with good posture
Swimming in a pool
Keeping company with healthy people ("if you hang with people that use, you're a user")
Fishing
Distractions by working at their job
Background noise
Meditation

These findings were as follows: (a) frequent health care appointments created hardships when participants held jobs, (b) participants want to protect their sobriety, (c) participants on prescription opioids for pain felt desperation and feared losing access to their opioids, (d) when advocacy and confidence in health care occurred, the participants were better able to cope with their pain, and (e) inconsistencies in health care and feeling stigmatized prolonged suffering and misuse of substances. There are opportunities for changing the way health care is delivered to this patient population.

Experiencing chronic pain leads to problems of maintaining employment. Studies show strong correlations between chronic pain and unemployment (Elliott, Smith, Penny, Smith, & Chambers, 1999; Johannes, Le, Zhou, Johnston, & Dworkin, 2010); however, these participants were trying hard to maintain employment despite pain and multiple health care appointments. Finding ways of delivering care so patients can receive opioids for pain, work at their jobs, and receive pain rehabilitation may enable job retention.

Participants reported trying to protect their sobriety in the context of chronic pain and chronic opioid therapy. These participants acknowledged fear of relapse when they had a history of SUD. Studies indicated that uncontrolled pain may precipitate relapse in people with history of SUD (St. Marie, 2014b; Trafton et al., 2004), yet chronic opioid therapy also creates risk (Jamison, Kauffman, & Katz, 2000; Rhodin, Gronbladh, Nilsson, & Gordh, 2006; Rosenblum et al., 2008). Care must be given to immediately address this when initiating opioids, establish a plan to prevent relapse, and, if needed, intervene early with referral for SUD treatment support.

Participants who overused prescription opioids felt a need to withhold information for fear of losing access to their prescription opioids needed for pain. One participant related, "a doctor's gonna know what I only let him know." While 9 of 12 participants disclosed history of SUD, only four participants described behaviors consistent with high risk for misuse of opioids (Compton et al., 1998). One participant openly identified risk to sobriety and was receiving help from an addiction specialist at the time of the study. Three participants did not reveal nor feel there was a need for addiction support or help at the time of this research study.

When participants had confidence in health care, they were better able to cope with their pain and were compliant with their opioid medication regimen. This was confirmed through other studies where patients on chronic opioid therapy improved function, quality of life, and remained stable without signs of misuse (Arnaert & Ciccotosto, 2006; Blake, Ruel, Seamark, & Seamark, 2007; Vallerand & Nowak, 2009).

Conversely, inconsistencies in care and feeling of stigmatization prolonged suffering and for some led to misuse of substances. This finding confirmed experiences of other participants, where degrading treatment from the health care team made them want to use again (St. Marie, 2014a).

LIMITATIONS

The limitations of this study involved the validity of the data analysis. The analysis occurred throughout the study by the principal investigator. The validation occurred through an audit by an external reviewer after the principal investigator completed the analysis process. Having a team of analysts involved in an ongoing process throughout the study would have improved validity.

CONCLUSIONS

The participants revealed changes that could improve pain management in primary health care practice. Nurse practitioners can advocate for change, such as (a) shifting the delivery of multidisciplinary care from clinic-to web-based monitor, education, and support to help reduce absenteeism from work and offer convenient health care encounters (Heapy et al., 2015), (b) providing system-based education of health care providers and systems coordinators that the negative consequences of inconsistent care and poor communications are severe and need to be taken as seriously as postsurgical complications or adverse drug reactions, and (c) providing education to health care providers so they understand that patients may withhold information vital to their care when there is lack of trust. A participant in a study of people with chronic pain in a methadone clinic maintained "secrets keep you sick," and recommended that patients be truthful with their health care provider in order to receive the best care (St. Marie, 2014a). While it may appear that motivation for withholding truth is about obtaining opioids, it may actually be the fear of losing pain-relieving tools. Nurse practitioners can also expedite early identification of overuse and misuse of opioids so that treatment evaluation and SUD support can be achieved. However, resources are not always available to provide appropriate monitoring of urine toxicology screening, pill counts, and access to prescription drug monitoring databases. Social policy needs to change regarding reimbursement of appropriate monitoring and nonmedicine modalities for pain. In the meantime, nurse practitioners can identify important areas of concern for their patients, remain focused on the patients' perspectives of care, and understand the meanings of patients' perceptions of helpful elements of care. Future research should be directed toward implementing innovative systems of health care delivery that allow for appropriate monitoring, evaluating the effect of opioid misuse risk education, and improve and promote access to the use of nonmedicine strategies in this population.

ACKNOWLEDGMENTS

The author thanks Dr. Janet Williams, professor, College of Nursing, University of Iowa, Iowa City, Iowa, for her contribution in validating the analysis of the data through her role as external auditor of the data. The author obtained the funding, conceived and designed the research project, submitted through IRB, collected the data through interviews, analyzed and interpreted the data, prepared the tables, and wrote the manuscript for final submission. Dr. St. Marie is accountable for the integrity of all aspects of the work and in ensuring that questions related to the accuracy or integrity of any part of the work are appropriately investigated and resolved.

REFERENCES

Arnaert, A., & Ciccotosto, G. (2006). Response phases in methadone treatment for chronic nonmalignant pain. *Pain Management Nursing*, **7**(1), 23–30.

Blake, S., Ruel, B., Seamark, C., & Seamark, D. (2007). Experiences of patients requiring strong opioid drugs for chronic non-cancer pain: A patient-initiated study. *British Journal of General Practice*, **57**(535), 101–108.

Bloomberg, L. D., & Volpe, M. (2008). *Completing your qualitative dissertation: A roadmap from beginning to end.* Los Angeles, CA: Sage Publications.

Bohnert, A. S. B., Valenstein, M., Bair, M. J., Ganoczy, D., McCarthy, J. F., Ilgen, M. A., & Blow, F. C. (2011). Association between opioid prescribing patterns and opioid overdose-related death. *Journal of the American Medical Association*, **305**(13), 1315–1321.

Chou, R., Turner, J. A., Devine, E. B., Hanson, R. N., Sullivan, S. D., Blazina, I., . . . Deyo, R. A. (2015). The effectiveness and risks of long-term opioid therapy for chronic pain: A systematic review for a National Institute of Health Pathways to Prevention Workshop. *Annals of Internal Medicine*, **162**, 276–286.

Cohen, D. J., & Crabtree, B. F. (2008). Evaluative criteria for qualitative research in health care: Controversies and recommendations. *Annals of Family Medicine*, **6**(4), 331–339.

Compton, P., Darakjian, J., & Miotto, K. (1998). Screening for addiction in patients with chronic pain and "problematic" substance use: Evaluation of a pilot assessment tool. *Journal of Pain and Symptom Management*, **16**(6), 355–363.

Dart, R. C., Surratt, H. L., Cicero, T. J., Parrino, M. W., Severtson, S. G., Bucher-Bartelson, B., & Green, J. L. (2015). Trends in opioid analgesic abuse and mortality in the United States. *New England Journal of Medicine*, **372**(3), 241–248.

Denzin, N. K., & Lincoln, Y. S. (2005). The discipline and practice of qualitative research. In N. K. Denzin & Y. S. Lincoln (Eds.), *The Sage handbook of qualitative research* (3rd ed., pp. 1–32). Thousand Oaks, CA: Sage Publications, Inc.

Dunn, K. M., Saunders, K. W., Rutter, C. M., Banta-Green, C. J., Merrill, J. O., Sullivan, M. D., . . . Von Korff, M. (2010). Opioid prescriptions for chronic pain and overdose. *Annals of Internal Medicine*, **152**(2), 85–92.

Edlund, M. J., Steffick, D., Hudson, T., Harris, K. M., & Sullivan, M. (2007). Risk factors for clinically recognized opioid abuse and dependence among veterans using opioids for chronic non-cancer pain. *Pain*, **129**(3), 355–362.

Elliott, A. M., Smith, B. H., Penny, K. I., Smith, W. C., & Chambers, W. A. (1999). The epidemiology of chronic pain in the community. *Lancet*, **354**(9186), 1248–1252.

Gomes, T., Mamdani, M. M., Dhalla, I. A., Paterson, J. M., & Juurlink, D. N. (2011). Opioid dose and drug-related mortality in patients with nonmalignant pain. *Archives of Internal Medicine*, **171**(7), 686–691.

Hall, J. M., & Stevens, P. E. (1991). Rigor in feminist research. *Advances in Nursing Science*, **13**(3), 16–29.

Heapy, A. A., Higgins, D. M., Cervone, D., Wandner, L., Fenton, B., & Kerns, R. D. (2015). A systematic review of technology-assisted self-management interventions for chronic pain: Looking across treatment modalities. *Clinical Journal of Pain*, **31**(6), 470–492. doi:10.1097/AJP.0000000000000185

Institute of Medicine of the National Academies (2011). *Relieving pain in America: A blueprint for transforming prevention, care, education, and research*. Washington, DC: The National Academies Press.

Jamison, R. N., Kauffman, J., & Katz, N. P. (2000). Characteristics on methadone maintenance patients with chronic pain. *Journal of Pain and Symptom Management*, **19**(1), 53–62.

Jena, A. B., Goldman, D., Weaver, L., & Karaca-Mandic, P. (2014). Opioid prescribing by multiple providers in Medicare: Retrospective observational study of insurance claims. *British Medical Journal*, **348**, g1393. doi:10.1136/bmj.g1393

Johannes, C. B., Le, T. K., Zhou, X., Johnston, J. A., & Dworkin, R. H. (2010). The prevalence of chronic pain in United States adults: Results of an internet-based survey. *Journal of Pain*, **11**(11), 1230–1239.

Merrill, J. O., Rhodes, L. A., Deyo, R. A., Marlatt, G. A., & Bradley, K. A. (2002). Mutual mistrust in the medical care of drug users: The keys to the "narc" cabinet. *Journal of General Internal Medicine*, **17**(5), 327–333.

Morasco, B. J., & Dobscha, S. K. (2008). Prescription medication misuse and substance use disorder in VA primary care patients with chronic pain. *General Hospital Psychiatry*, **30**(2), 93–99.

Nuckols, T. K., Anderson, L., Popescu, I., Diamant, A. L., Doyle, B., Di Capua, P., & Chou, R. (2014). Opioid prescribing: A systematic review and critical analysis of guidelines for chronic pain. *Annals of Internal Medicine*, **160**(1), 38–47.

Paulozzi, L. J., Kilbourne, E. M., Shah, N. G., Nolte, K. B., Desai, H. A., Landen, M. G. . . . Loring, L. D. (2012). A history of being prescribed controlled substances and risk of drug overdose death. *Pain Medicine*, **13**(1), 87–95.

Rhodin, A., Gronbladh, L., Nilsson, L. H., & Gordh, T. (2006). Methadone treatment of chronic non-malignant pain and opioid dependence—A long-term follow-up. *European Journal of Pain*, **10**(3), 271–278.

Rosenblum, A., Joseph, H., Fong, C., Kipnis, S., Cleeland, C. S., & Portenoy, R. K. (2008). Prevalence and characteristics of chronic pain among chemically dependent patients in methadone maintenance and residential treatment facilities. *Journal of the American Medical Association*, **289**(18), 2370–2378.

Stevens, P. E. (1998). The experiences of lesbians of color in health care encounters: Narrative insights for improving access and quality. *Journal of Lesbian Studies*, **2**(1), 77–94.

St. Marie, B. (2014a). Healthcare experiences when pain and substance use disorder coexist. *Pain Medicine*, **15**(12), 2075–2086.

St. Marie, B. J. (2014b). Coexisting addiction and pain in people receiving methadone for addiction. *Western Journal of Nursing Research*, **36**(4), 535–552.

Substance Abuse and Mental Health Administration. (2014). Results from the 2012 National Survey on Drug Use and Health: Summary of national findings. Retrieved from http://www.samhsa.gov/data/NSDUH/2012-SummNatFindDetTables/NationalFindings/NSDUHresults2012.htm#fig 5.1

Trafton, J. A., Oliva, E. M., Horst, D. A., Minkel, J. D., & Humphreys, K. (2004). Treatment needs associated with pain in substance use disorder patients: Implications for concurrent treatment. *Drug and Alcohol Dependence*, 73(1), 23–31.

U.S Department of Health and Human Services. Substance Abuse and Mental Health Services Administration. Office of Applied Studies. (2010). Treatment Episode Data Set—Discharges (TEDS-D)—Concatenated, 2006 to 2011. ICPSR30122-v5. Ann Arbor, MI: Inter-university Consortium for Political and Social Research [distributor], 2015-11-23. doi:10.3886/ICPSR30122.v5

U.S Food and Drug Administration (FDA) (2012). Blueprint for prescriber education for extended-release and long-acting opioid analgesics. Retrieved from http://www.fda.gov/downloads/Drugs/DrugSafety/Postmarket-DrugSafetyInformationforPatientsandProviders/UCM311290.pdf

Vallerand, A., & Nowak, L. (2009). Chronic opioid therapy for nonmalignant pain: The patient's perspective. Part I—Life before and after opioid therapy. *Pain Management Nursing*, **10**(3), 165–172.

PRIMARY CARE EXPERIENCES OF PEOPLE WHO LIVE WITH CHRONIC PAIN AND RECEIVE OPIOIDS TO MANAGE PAIN: A QUALITATIVE METHODOLOGY

Critique by *Nadine M. Marchi*

OVERALL SUMMARY

The topic of this research is timely as treatment of chronic pain with opioids continues to be an important health challenge. The report was clearly written. The qualitative approach revealed rich data in the narrative reports of the experiences of people who live with chronic pain. The setting of the study was appropriate for the problem being explored as most patients with chronic pain are treated in primary care. The study methods were described in detail so the reader could easily identify the processes used by the researcher. The results were presented thoroughly with many examples from narrative interviews obtained from patients. Overall, this report was interesting and provides important information for clinicians regarding the current problems with opioid abuse or dependence.

TITLE

Does the title include the key concepts/variables/phenomenon of interest?

The title was clear and reflected the significant aspects of the research. The title delineated the group of people who were studied and the nature of their problem, such as those individuals who are receiving primary care and who live with chronic pain and receive opioids. The keywords were *pain management, pharmacotherapy, primary care,* and *substance abuse.* The researcher could include the word *qualitative* as a keyword to assist others who are particularly interested in qualitative methodology.

Is it concise (12 words or less) and professionally stated?

The title is long at 19 words and could be shortened by omitting the study design methodology as the methodology is identified in the abstract. The title is professionally stated.

RESEARCHER(S) CREDIBILITY

Educational credentials?

The educational credentials of the sole author are clearly stated and are appropriate for conducting the study. The researcher is a nurse practitioner with a PhD. The researcher is certified in nursing specialties appropriate for the topic (adult, geriatric, and advanced hospice and palliative care). These are all areas where pain medication is prescribed by nurse practitioners. In addition, the researcher is a faculty member at a major, national, research-intensive university and has also practiced as a nurse practitioner for over 30 years in primary care, pain clinics, and hospitals.

Prior methodological research experience of the authors (i.e., methodological expertise)?

Based on a search of the literature, since 2011, the researcher has published six articles on this topic in peer-reviewed journals. Three more articles have been published by this researcher as second author. The researcher is also the principal investigator on a grant concerning opioid misuse.

Subject matter content experience (prior research on the subject matter)?

Based on all of the information noted previously, the researcher is well qualified to conduct this study, both in terms of subject matter and methodological expertise.

ABSTRACT

Does it include the key components (objective/aim, background, methods, results, and conclusions)?

The abstract includes the key components and is structured according to the requirements of the *Journal of the American Association of Nurse Practitioners*. It includes the background/purpose, methods, conclusions, and implications for practice. As specified, the abstract does not include references. The first line of the abstract entices the reader to learn more about the timely topic of pain management in primary care. The abstract is succinct, it identifies the purpose of the study, the qualitative data collection method, and how the data were analyzed. The conclusions of the study presented in the abstract are stated concisely.

Does or does not include references?

The abstract does not include references, as appropriate.

Is it concise (150–250 words or less)?

The abstract meets the word limit of 200 words and is concise.

Does it entice you to read the rest of the article (interesting)?

The implications for nursing practice are outlined in the abstract and include the positive statement that pain can be managed effectively using patient-centered care. This statement helps persuade the reader to delve into the article in more detail to find out the strategies used to confront an often frustrating problem for patients and health care providers.

INTRODUCTION/PROBLEM

Is the research problem or phenomenon of interest clearly stated?

The introduction to this article was well organized and began with statistics concerning the epidemic of substance abuse disorder in chronic pain patients who are prescribed opioids.

Does the problem have significance for nursing?

The problem is of great significance for nursing and especially for nurse practitioners who prescribe medications.

Is it succinct?

The problem statement is succinctly stated.

Does it answer the "so what" question?

> The "so what" question is answered as the researcher is very knowledgeable about the opioid crisis and the experiences of persons with chronic pain.

RESEARCH AIMS/OBJECTIVES

Is the research aim/objective clearly stated?

> The research aim is clearly identified. The introduction began with a broad approach and ended with a description of the researcher's preliminary study concerning substance abuse disorder and pain. The introduction includes presentation of the importance of studying chronic pain treatment in primary care and substance abuse disorder by emphasizing the current gravity of the problem for patients and society as a whole. The current facts about opioid substance abuse are presented followed by the research objective. This informs the reader as to the magnitude of the problem and flows logically.

Is it concisely written?

> The introduction that includes the research aims is concisely written.

Does it follow logically from the research problem/phenomenon of interest?

> The introduction is logical and flows directly from the research problem identified, such as the harm associated with opioid prescriptions for chronic pain.

SIGNIFICANCE

Is the significance to nursing and health care clearly written?

> Although there is no separate section in the article focused on the significance of the research to nursing and health care, in the article introduction there is ample evidence presented regarding the significance of the problem. The significance for nursing is identified and clearly written. First, the significance for nurse practitioners who prescribe opioids in primary care is described along with how this group can promote change to address the problem. Then, additional facts about the magnitude of the problem are provided. Lastly, the researcher presents how this study can influence the delivery of safe and effective health care.

Does the significance follow from the research aim/objective?

> The significance of the research follows directly from the problem statement.

BACKGROUND

Is there an explicit description of a theoretical perspective or conceptual framework? If not, is it implied?

> There is no explicit or implied description of a theoretical perspective or conceptual framework. The researcher mentions experiences as a nurse practitioner as the basis for the assumptions about the study. A review of recent manuscripts published in the *Journal of the American Association of Nurse Practitioners* reveals no conceptual framework or theoretical perspective presented in the Original Research section of other similar articles.

Are there clear theoretical/conceptual definitions of the concepts?

> There are no definitions of the concepts.

LITERATURE REVIEW

The literature review is presented in the Introduction rather than as a separate section of the paper. They were not chronologically presented but arranged as topics were presented in each paragraph for supporting evidence. Research from prominent public sources such as the National Institute on Drug Abuse, Institute of Medicine, and U.S. Department of Health and Human Services was presented to support the research aim. The review of the literature comprehensively informs the reader about the problem. The sources for the statistics were government agencies, other published research reports, and a preliminary study performed by the researcher.

Primary sources only?

The researcher uses primary sources only.

Current (within the past how many years)?

The research studies cited were published from 1999 to 2015, thus current research is included. When older research was cited, there was often a more current reference as well. There were some instances when older research was cited without an accompanying current reference. The majority of the research presented was within the previous 5 years of the publication of the article. This suggests the researcher has a thorough review of information discovered in the past as well as current knowledge.

Is the search strategy included?

The search strategy was not included.

Is literature relevant to the research aims/objectives?

All of the research was relevant to the research aims and revolved around substance abuse, chronic pain, opioid prescribing, and patient experiences. The research was summarized with a critical comment or appraisal after the citation.

Is it chronologically presented (old to current)?

The background literature was not presented chronologically but was presented in a logical manner to justify the research objectives.

RATIONALE FOR THE STUDY

Is there a gap in the literature that this study will fill (will it extend prior knowledge)?

The study is a preliminary study to explore the perspectives of patients in primary care with chronic pain who have received long-term opioids. These patient perspectives can guide pain management. A previous preliminary study was conducted by the same researcher involving chronic pain patients and methadone treatment. The researcher identified the gap in the literature as the patient in primary care who is receiving opioids and managing chronic pain.

Is the rationale clearly stated?

The rationale for the study is clearly stated.

RESEARCH QUESTIONS AND/OR HYPOTHESES

Are these explicitly and clearly stated?

The two research questions are clearly and explicitly stated. The first question follows the aim of the research study and relates specifically to patients with chronic pain receiving opioids in the primary care setting. The second research question is wider in scope and pertains to the total health care experiences of chronic pain patients receiving opioids.

Do they include the variables/phenomena of interest?

The variables of interest in the first research question are identified and congruent with the research aim. The second research question does not include the variable of interest and research aim related to primary care experiences. The second research question though is appropriate for the research study as it provides contextual background for the first research question.

Do they follow from the research aims/objectives?

The first research question is directly related to the study aim; the second research question is also related to the broader aim of the research but is broader in scope. These research questions are amenable to qualitative study as they align with patient experiences.

METHODS
Research Design/Paradigm
Is the research design clearly stated?

The research design is qualitative using narrative inquiry. This is clearly stated in the title of the article and text. The assumptions and frame of reference are explicitly stated. These are derived from the researcher's experiences as a nurse practitioner specializing in pain management for over 30 years. The researcher has conducted a body of research on the topic of pain management. This study augments other studies of the same topic but provides the additional perspective of patients in primary care. The method is feasible as the researcher interviewed patients at a primary care clinic recruiting patients who came to the clinic. By audiotaping, the investigator also allowed for additional analysis. The narrative research story evokes emotion as the researcher describes facts outlining the degree of the opioid problem and provides samples of patient interviews recounting their struggles with pain management.

Is there consistency between the research design and paradigm?

The narrative qualitative approach is consistent with the paradigm of understanding the patient's experience.

Is this the best choice of design to address the research problem/phenomenon of interest?

This narrative qualitative design is the best choice to obtain the patient's understandings of their personal experiences.

Is there rigor in the design?

Because the researcher was collecting data using narrative inquiry, the method for establishing rigor is by evaluating credibility and trustworthiness. The researcher established credibility and trustworthiness by including patient participants fully in the research process. In addition, all research procedures and steps in the process are fully described to the reader. Parameters of rigor for qualitative research (participant involvement, clarity in research procedures, and experiential interviews), regarding narrative inquiry are met. Narrative inquiry should also provide meaningful opportunities for the participants to review their transcripts and the researcher's retold story and their comments and reactions to the story of the research. This was not present in the research.

SETTING
Is the setting clearly described?

The setting is the primary care clinic where the researcher worked and where the patients received their primary care. The location is identified as a Midwest metropolitan primary care clinic. The investigator conducted the interviews in a private room at the primary care clinic. This is fully described.

What biases are introduced as a result of selecting this particular setting?

Only patients who are already received treatment at that primary care setting are eligible to participate in the study.

SAMPLING PLAN AND SAMPLE
Is the sampling plan clearly identified?

The sampling plan is clearly identified, and includes patients with chronic pain who are being treated with opioids at the particular setting. Fliers were posted directing potential participants to call the researcher. The researcher screened the participants to determine if they met criteria for participation based on exclusion criteria that are described in the article. The sample of patients also participated voluntarily, agreed to be audiotaped and was able to come to the clinic for the interview at a specified location and time.

Does it represent the population of interest?

The sample represents a population of chronic pain patients who have experienced pain for longer than 6 months and are under the care of a primary care provider.

Is the sampling plan consistent with the research aim/objective?

This is the same population of patients identified in the research questions.

Is the sample size sufficient (e.g., power analysis or data saturation)?

In this study, sample size was determined by data saturation at 12 participants as no new themes became apparent when new participants were interviewed.

VARIABLES
Are variables clearly identified?
Are variables operationally defined and consistent with theoretical concepts?
Are independent and dependent variables identified, if applicable?

There are no identified variables as the purpose of this research project is to learn about the patients in detail to identify patterns or themes from the narratives provided by the patients. The meaning of the research comes from the participants. This is consistent with qualitative research.

METHOD OF DATA COLLECTION
What are the methods of data collection?

The data-collection method was described; the researcher used a demographic questionnaire, field observation notes, and semistructured interviews. The researcher used an interview guide with open-ended questions developed from the literature, clinical experiences, and previous research to conduct the semistructured interview. A table with the interview questions is made available in the article. This is helpful and provides the reader with a glimpse of the narrative interview process. The researcher does not provide details about how the demographic questionnaire was administered or how the field notes were collected. The purpose of the field notes is described. The researcher was able to obtain a private room at the clinic where she worked and interview the participants at the clinic site for convenience of the patient. Each patient was interviewed by the investigator for 60 to 90 minutes and the interview was audiotaped. The interviews were then transcribed. Hard copies of the interviews were stored in a locked file at the researcher's work site. The researcher indicated that she reimbursed patients for their time, but no other details about the reimbursement ate presented.

Are validity and reliability clearly addressed for prior research and current study, if applicable?

Validity and reliability of the data are assumed, as the researcher states that patients often have insights that only individuals who have experienced pain and managed it with opioids can have.

Do the measures/instruments address the underlying theoretical concepts or phenomenon of interest?

The data-collection methods yielded data that addressed the phenomena of interest, that is, obtaining a deeper understanding of the experiences, issues, and challenges faced by persons who live with chronic pain and receive opioids for their pain.

Were human rights protected?

Permission was obtained by the researcher from two institutional review boards to conduct this study and all participants gave informed consent.

Are other ethical issues identified?

One ethical issue identified is that the researcher did not allow for the possibility of follow-up interviews to fill in gaps and check meanings. The follow-up interview also would allow the researcher to make sure the patient is not suffering any emotional trauma related to the interview No other ethical issues are identified.

Is the data-collection method appropriate for research design?

The primary data collection method of semistructured interviews was appropriate for the qualitative research design.

Is there bias in data collection?

The bias that is inherent in personal accounts is present in this study. Also, only patients being treated at this particular clinic may introduce a bias as they may be more familiar with the researcher.

What is the fidelity of intervention addressed, if applicable?

There is no intervention; therefore, this is not applicable.

DATA ANALYSIS
Are sample characteristics described (e.g., statistical tests, methodology for qualitative analysis)?

The methodology for analysis is described in detail. The method of data review is thematic and interpretive analysis. The analysis of each narrative interview enabled the researcher to answer the research questions. Each narrative interview was analyzed using an iterative process as is expected with qualitative research. The criteria for qualitative data analysis were met in this study. In this study, themes were analyzed and narrative summaries written on each participant. The interpretation of the data was performed using the researcher's own experiences as a nurse practitioner working with chronic pain patients and providing opioid medications. One area the researcher did not identify was whether inductive or deductive reasoning was used to analyze the themes. Also, there were no unexpected emergent themes identified or the issue addressed.

Does the analysis answer the research question?

The analyses answer both of the research questions of the study.

Is it appropriate?

The analyses were appropriate for the narrative qualitative study.

Is the analysis comprehensive? Are themes identified?

Both thematic and interpretive analyses were used. According to the author, the interviews were analyzed iteratively as the data collection was occurring. Details of the data analysis procedures are presented by the author. Validity and dependability of the research study was noted by the researcher and references were provided to support the measures used.

Is there bias in the analysis (trustworthiness? credibility?)?

Because the researcher and another expert were the only individuals to review the data for validity, the researcher lists this as a limitation and recommends a team of experts to establish more accurate validity.

RESULTS
Are sample characteristics described and fully reported?

The table used to present demographic data (sample characteristics) was organized and provided the reader with a picture of the participants.

Are findings presented related to research aim/objective?

Another table, with the questionnaire, enables the reader to visualize the instrument used when interviewing participants. The third table provides examples of nonpharmacological pain relief as described by participants. All three tables are helpful to the reader by providing more details about relevant aspects of the study. Main themes were identified. Then, the researcher organized the results into paragraphs related to each theme. Extensive information about the lived experiences of each participant was presented. This was particularly interesting and allowed the rich data obtained in the narrative interviews to be reviewed by the reader. The quotes from participants are authentic and represent the research findings.

Are all outcome variables addressed, if applicable?

> The key variables in the study, the patient experiences, are addressed in the results.

Are results clearly presented in text and/or tables/figures?

> Results are clearly presented in the text, and described in detail.

Is significance of results reported, if applicable?

> The results are clinically significant. As a qualitative study, there are no reports of statistical significance.

DISCUSSION OF RESULTS

Do the authors link the findings to previous research studies?

> The study findings were compared to previous research. The researcher clearly states when findings in this study confirm previous research on the topic or present an alternative. For example, one finding was that frequent health care appointments conflict with job attendance. The researcher presents the finding and then offers additional research sources with the same result. At the end of the paragraph, a solution to the problem is suggested. This method of review offers a clear presentation of the results with a proposal for change. There is no mention of the transferability of findings but the nature of the case study method implies transferability.

Are the conclusions comprehensive, yet within the data?

> The discussion is comprehensive but does not go beyond the data.

Do the authors interpret the results in the discussion?

> There is significant detailed interpretation of the results in the Discussion section of the article.

Are the findings generalizable or transferable?

> The researcher validates transferability by suggesting further questions for exploration and implications. Generalization is not possible since one group of chronic pain patients cannot represent all similar groups.

LIMITATIONS

Identified? Accurate? Inclusive?

> One limitation is identified by the researcher related to the validity of the data analysis. The limitation is appropriate for this study. Because only one limitation was described, the reader is left to consider whether there are others. A more inclusive analysis of the limitations would make the article more robust. For example, the self-reported data, researcher's presence during data gathering, issues of anonymity/confidentiality, and the potential influence of the researcher's own bias when analyzing data are a few limitations not mentioned in the article.

IMPLICATIONS

Are there implications for practice, education, research?

> The researcher provides implications for advanced nursing practice in primary care. A recommendation is made associated with a needed change in social policy regarding

reimbursement for appropriate monitoring and nonpharmacological modalities for pain. The researcher offers three recommendations for future research derived from the results of this research study. There are two recommendations for health care education: how to improve inconsistent care and working with patients who may be withholding information related to their care. Therefore, the researcher has met the criteria to include implications for nursing practice, research, and education.

Are there implications for clinical significance?

The clinical significance of the results is reviewed thoroughly and suggestions provided.

RECOMMENDATIONS

Recommendations for future study/study replication?

As noted previously, the researcher offers three recommendations for future research derived from the results of this research study.

CONCLUSION

Is it succinct and does it tie everything together?

The conclusion is well written but lengthy. There is a patient quote from a previous study interrupting the flow of implications and recommendations. This is a valuable quote but might have been placed somewhere else in the article to substantiate data. Except for the quote, the conclusion is well organized and presents a strong statement for changes in health care delivery to improve safety and the patient experience.

OLDER ADULTS' PERCEPTIONS OF USING iPADS FOR IMPROVING FRUIT AND VEGETABLE INTAKE: AN EXPLORATORY STUDY

14

Ivan Watkins, JD, MLS, BS,
is a doctoral student in the School of Information at the University of Texas at Austin. He holds degrees in economics, law, and library and information science. His research focuses on educational interventions promoting older adults' eHealth literacy and the design of eHealth resources for the aging population.

Bo Xie, PhD, MS, BMedSci,
is an associate professor in the School of Nursing and School of Information at the University of Texas at Austin. She holds degrees in medicine, psychology, and science and technology studies (PhD from Rensselaer Polytechnic Institute, 2006). Her research focuses on the intersection of aging, technology, and health. Her research on eHealth literacy is funded by the National Institutes of Health and the Institute of Museum and Library Services.

Fruit and vegetable (FV) consumption can improve older adults' health outcomes, but conventional interventions can be resource demanding and make it difficult to provide just-in-time intervention content. iPad-based interventions may help overcome these limitations, but little is known about how older adults might perceive and use iPads for FV consumption. To address this gap in the literature, we conducted a qualitative study to explore older adults' perceptions and use of iPads for improving FV consumption between February and August of 2012. Five focus group sessions each lasting 120 minutes were conducted with 22 older adult participants. During each session, participants received guided exposure and instruction on iPad use and then explored three iPad applications targeting FV consumption (MyFood, FiveADay Lite, and Whole Foods Market Recipes). Detailed notes from focus group interviews were analyzed with a grounded theory approach that applied a constant comparative method to enable themes to emerge from the data.

Three themes were identified from the data regarding participants' baseline perceptions of iPads. These included (a) limited knowledge on iPad's functions, (b) iPads were intended for younger users, and (c) iPads were too expensive. Themes identified regarding participants' perceptions of iPads after guided exposure included (a) the touchscreen was easier to use than a computer mouse, (b) tapping the interface required practice, (c) portability was an asset in conjunction with functionality, (d) portability and functionality supported personal interests, (e) the difficulty of learning an iPad's functions varied, and (f) practice and instruction helped overcome fear of the iPad. Finally, participants recommended iPad app

Watkins, I., & Xie, B. (2015). Older adults' perceptions of using iPads for improving fruit and vegetable intake: An exploratory study. *Care Management Journals, 16*, 2–13. doi:10.1891/1521-0987.16.1.2. Republished with permission of Springer Publishing Company.

features that could help them overcome barriers to their FV intake. These included (a) locating inexpensive FV from nearby sources, (b) providing tailored food and recipe suggestions, and (c) tracking and communicating FV intake with a doctor. These findings have important implications for future research on mobile app-based eHealth interventions to improve older adults' FV intake.

KEYWORDS: older adults; tablet computers; fruit and vegetable consumption; user-centered design; nutrition; healthy eating

For older adults, a diet rich in fruits and vegetables (FV) correlates with improved health outcomes (Nicklett & Kadell, 2013) and protects against cardiovascular disease (Wang, Manson, Gaziano, Buring, & Sesso, 2012; Zhang et al., 2011), cancer (Aune et al., 2012; Aune et al., 2011), diabetes (Carter, Gray, Troughton, Khunti, & Davies, 2010; Cooper et al., 2012), and obesity (Fakhouri, Ogden, Carroll, Kit, & Flegal, 2012). However, less than one-third of older adults in the United States consume recommended servings of FV (Grimm, Blanck, Scanlon, Moore, & Grummer-Strawn, 2010). Interventions can increase FV intake among older adults (Burke et al., 2013) but often rely on print materials, telephone, or in-home visits to reach participants (Clark et al., 2011). These methods require significant time and expense (Krukowski, Tilford, Harvey-Berino, & West, 2011) and cannot deliver just-in-time intervention content (Riley et al., 2011).

These barriers could be overcome with e-interventions, defined as "systematic treatment/prevention programs, usually addressing one or more determinants of health (frequent health behaviors), delivered largely via the Internet (although not necessarily web-based), and interfacing with an end user" (Bennett & Glasgow, 2009, p. 274). E-interventions can result in greater FV intake than non-web-based interventions (McCully, Don, & Updegraff, 2013), but participation in FV e-interventions decreases with age (McCully et al., 2013). Potential explanations include older adults' low e-health literacy (Czaja, Beach, Charness, & Schulz, 2013), slow adoption of health information technologies (Fox & Duggan, 2013), and inexperience using the Internet (Zickuhr, 2013b).

Tablet computers with a touchscreen interface could improve the usability of FV e-interventions for older adults. Older adults can perform certain tasks (e.g., selecting onscreen objects) on touchscreens quicker, and with greater precision, than with a keyboard and mouse (Findlater, Froehlich, Fattal, Wobbrock, & Dastyar, 2013; Jochems, Vetter, & Schlick, 2012), whereas other tasks, such as typing, may be more difficult (Barnard, Bradley, Hodgson, & Lloyd, 2013). Despite this potential, older adults' perceptions and use of tablet-based FV interventions remain unclear. Also, little is known about the features facilitating older adults' use of tablets.

Tablet computers with a touchscreen interface could improve the usability of FV e-interventions for older adults.

To address these gaps, this study investigates the benefits and barriers for tablets to promote FV intake among older adults, and identifies a set of recommended features for overcoming these barriers. Although previous studies examined the usability and accessibility of tablets for older adults (e.g., Findlater et al., 2013), this study extends this work to identify a set of tablet features that can promote FV intake among older adults. In addition, this study generated findings on older adults' perception of tablets before and after guided exposure. These findings can be used to guide educational interventions for older adults who lack the knowledge, skills, or experience necessary to use tablets. We held five focus group sessions each lasting 120 minutes with 22 older adult participants in a public library setting. Using guided exposure to existing iPad features and three FV-related apps, we solicited rich qualitative data from the participants. Detailed notes from focus group interviews were analyzed with a grounded theory approach that applied a constant comparative method and enabled themes to emerge from the data.

Three themes were identified from the data regarding participants' baseline perceptions of iPads. These included (a) limited knowledge on iPad's functions, (b) iPads were intended for younger users, and (c) iPads were too expensive. Themes identified regarding participants' perceptions of iPads after guided exposure included (a) the touchscreen was easier to use than a computer mouse, (b) tapping the interface required practice, (c) portability was an asset in conjunction with functionality, (d) portability and functionality supported personal interests, (e) the difficulty of learning an iPads' functions varied, and (f) practice and instruction helped overcome fear of the iPad. Finally, participants recommended iPad app features that could help them overcome barriers to their FV intake. These included (a) locating inexpensive FV from nearby sources, (b) providing tailored food and recipe suggestions, and (c) tracking and communicating FV intake with a doctor. These findings have significant implications to future research on mobile app-based eHealth interventions to improve older adults' FV intake.

LITERATURE REVIEW

E-interventions may offer several potential advantages for older adults. First, e-interventions facilitate remote intervention participation (Bennett & Glasgow, 2009). Optimal mobility, or "being able to safely and reliably go where you want to go, when you want to go, and how you want to get there" (Satariano et al., 2012, p. 1508) declines with age and correlates with reduced FV intake (Nicklett & Kadell, 2013). Almost 80% of older adults have a chronic condition and a large proportion of them endure functional limitations that decrease mobility (Centers for Disease Control and Prevention, 2010). Health interventions have typically reached less mobile older adults by mail (Greene et al., 2008), telephone (Clark et al., 2011), or in-home visits (Bernstein et al., 2002). E-interventions may offer a more cost-effective approach than these conventional approaches for disseminating health messages to older adults (Archer et al., 2012; Krukowski et al., 2011).

Second, e-interventions can support tailored interventions. Tailoring is "any combination of strategies intended to reach one specific person, based on characteristics that are unique to that person, related to the outcome of interest, and derived from an individual assessment" (Kreuter, Strecher, & Glassman, 1999, p. 277). The transtheoretical model (TTM) provides theoretical support for tailored interventions (Prochaska & Velicer, 1997), and tailored nutrition interventions typically outperform nontailored nutrition interventions (Broekhuizen, Kroeze, van Poppel, Oenema, & Brug, 2012). The older population contains significant diversity in terms of, for instance, education, income, ethnicity, and computer and Internet use (Administration on Aging, 2012; Zickuhr & Madden, 2012). Tailored content that addresses each individual's unique characteristics could improve the outcomes of FV e-interventions.

Third, e-interventions could promote FV intake with social support. Social support is behavior intended to aid; it includes emotional support, instrumental support, informational support, and appraisal support (Heaney & Israel, 2008). Social support can increase FV intake among older adults, but which type of social support is most effective remains unclear (Nicklett & Kadell, 2013). Online social support often occurs through informal support groups (e.g., message boards) that connect users over common health interests (Taylor, 2011). This support particularly benefits people with chronic conditions that limits their mobility, which can make connecting with others difficult (Taylor, 2011). The prevalence of chronic conditions and limited mobility among older adults (Centers for Disease Control and Prevention, 2010) suggests the sharing of online social support could be especially useful with the aging population.

E-interventions delivered by mobile devices such as tablet computers could offer distinct benefits. Tablets can collect data on users' location, health status, and activities (Liu, Zhu, Holroyd, & Seng, 2011). This data could be used to generate just-in-time tailored content (Riley et al., 2011). Despite this potential, interventions delivered by mobile devices have produced disappointing results. One recent review found benefits in only 30% of 21 randomized controlled trials delivered by a mobile device (Kaplan & Stone, 2013). A possible explanation is that the design of mobile health applications was not guided by any health behavior theory (Breton, Fuemmeler, & Abroms, 2011; Cowan et al., 2013; West et al., 2013; West et al., 2012). An analysis of 204 weight loss apps found most of those apps included fewer than two evidence-based features (Breton et al., 2011). A similar analysis of 58 nutrition-related apps found only 4% of them tailored the content and 3% facilitated social support (West et al., 2013). Theory provides an evidence-based foundation to guide the design of interventions (Rimer & Glanz, 2005) and is especially useful for new technologies on which little research exists (Riley et al., 2011). App developers' unfamiliarity with health behavior theory may explain the absence of theory in the vast majority of existing apps (Kaplan & Stone, 2013).

Theory provides an evidence-based foundation to guide the design of interventions and is especially useful for new technologies on which little research exists.

In addition to the lack of theory-based mobile health apps, no known study has investigated tablet-based FV e-interventions with older adults. Several recent studies investigated tablet-based apps in physical activity and medication management interventions for older adults. The Active Lifestyle app sought to increase exercise with features for self-monitoring attitude toward exercise, goal setting, and positive reinforcement (Silveira et al., 2013). A social version of the app added a message board for sharing emotional support. This version produced greater adherence to exercise plans and participant retention than the individual version (Silveira et al., 2013). The Colorado Care Tablet app sought to improve medication management for older adults with multiple chronic conditions (Siek et al., 2010). Participants performed medication management functions on an app developed during six participatory design sessions. Participants preferred apps to use linear navigation, images in place of text, and simple interfaces with fewer features (e.g., listing filled medications rather than filled and prescribed medications). Notably, the oldest participants (older than age 80 years) still found the simplest interfaces too complex. As a result, Siek et al. (2010) recommended tailoring the interface's complexity to match each individual's preferences.

In addition to apps, tablet characteristics, such as large touchscreens, could improve older adults' use of the technology for health. Tablets' touchscreen interface enables older adults to complete certain tasks quicker and more accurately than with a keyboard or mouse (Findlater et al., 2013; Kobayashi et al., 2011; Marques, Nunes, Silva, & Rodrigues, 2011). The type of task (e.g., entering text or selecting an onscreen object) and the gesture used to complete a task (e.g., spreading two fingers to zoom) can affect older adults' performance on touchscreen. For instance, one study found older adults completed pointing and dragging tasks 35% quicker on an iPad than a mouse (Findlater et al., 2013). However, typing can be more difficult on a touchscreen than a tactile keyboard (Jayroe & Wolfram, 2012; McLaughlin, Rogers, & Fisk, 2009). Matching tasks to a device's characteristics can attenuate this issue (McLaughlin et al., 2009). For example, limiting typing tasks on a touchscreen interface could help make an app easier for older adults to use.

Exploratory studies have found older adults can learn gestures without difficulty (Leonardi, Albertini, Pianesi, & Zancanaro, 2010; Piper, Campbell, & Hollan, 2010), but certain gestures can create challenges. Tapping, defined as "a precise and quick succession of 'press' and 'release'" (Leonardi et al., 2010, p. 847), and gestures using two fingers (e.g., spreading fingers to zoom) are particularly problematic (Piper et al., 2010). Issues can occur from moving fingers pressed to the screen or pressing fingers to the screen for too long (Leonardi et al., 2010). Making interfaces less touch-sensitive might resolve these issues. Alternately, "swabbing," where users drag a finger across the screen toward an onscreen target reduced errors committed by older adults with hand tremors (Wacharamanotham et al., 2011).

Despite the growing evidence suggesting tablet-based e-interventions' prospects for improving older adults' health, the literature on this topic is still sparse, and currently, there are at least three significant gaps in the literature. These include (a) the application of health behavior theory to mobile FV e-interventions, (b) the design of FV e-intervention apps to accommodate older adults' needs and preferences, and (c) factors influencing older adults' adoption of tablets in FV e-interventions. Addressing these gaps can help develop useful, effective FV e-interventions for older adults that may subsequently improve their health.

Despite the growing evidence suggesting tablet-based e-interventions' prospects for improving older adults' health, the literature on this topic is still sparse.

RESEARCH QUESTIONS

To address these gaps in the literature, we investigated the following research questions (RQs) in this study:

RQ1: What are older adults' perceptions of using iPads for improving their FV consumption?

RQ2: How do older adults want to use iPads for FV-related purposes?

RQ3: What iPad features can help overcome some of the major barriers to older adults' FV consumption?

METHOD
Participants

There were 22 older adults, who were members of our Older Adult Team, participated in this study. Participant characteristics are summarized in Table 1. Participant recruitment employed standard recruitment strategies. These strategies

TABLE 1. Participant Demographic Information

Demographics	n (%)
Age (years)	
60–69	12 (55)
70–79	8 (36)
80 or older	2 (9)
Race/ethnicity	
African American	17 (77)
Latino	2 (9)
Asian	3 (14)
Gender	
Women	14 (64)
Men	8 (36)
Education	
High school graduate	10 (45)
At least some college	2 (9)
Bachelor's degree	4 (18)
Advanced degree	6 (27)
Yearly household income	
Less than $20,000	3 (14)
$20,000–39,999	6 (27)
$40,000–59,999	6 (27)
More than $60,000	4 (18)
Do not know or wish to answer	3 (14)
Use computers every day	
Yes	6 (27)
No	16 (73)
Heard of iPads	
Yes	3 (14)
No	19 (86)
Used an iPad	
Yes	2 (9)
No	20 (91)

included placing recruitment flyers at the research site and advertising in local newspapers and the county library's newsletter. All recruitment materials specified participants must be "age 60 years and older" to participate.

Research Site

The Hyattsville Branch Library served as the study's research site. This library branch is part of the Prince George's Memorial Library System, which provides library services to more than 860,000 residents in Prince George's County, Maryland. Prince George's County, Maryland, is majority African American (65%), 27% White, 16% Hispanic/Latino, and 4% Asian (U.S. Census Bureau, 2012). The Hyattsville library provided free wireless Internet connection, staff aid, and a conference room for this study. Focus group sessions occurred in a quiet, private conference room that holds up to 10 people. The iPads were connected to the library's free wireless Internet during the sessions.

Procedure

We conducted five focus group sessions with 22 participants between February and August of 2012. Each session lasted 120 minutes. Participants first completed an informed consent form approved by the university's institutional review board before any data collection. During each session, a research team member, the moderator, facilitated the discussion while a second member, the note taker, took detailed notes.

Each focus group session included seven activities (see Table 2). First, the moderator introduced the session goals and asked for participants' names and prior computer experience. Next, participants shared their own experience and perceptions of iPads. Third, participants discussed their FV intake and perceived barriers to

TABLE 2. iPad Focus Group Protocol

Time	Activity	Sample Questions
5 min	Introduction	• What is your name? • Tell us about your experience with computers.
5 min	Prior iPad experience	• Have you heard of iPads? • What do you know about iPads?
10 min	FV consumption patterns	• How many fruits and vegetables do you eat per day? • What barriers prevent you from eating fruits and vegetables? • What would make it easier for you to eat more fruits and vegetables? • How could an iPad help you eat more fruits and vegetables?
30 min	iPad demonstration	• Do you have any questions about using the iPad's features? • What additional information or instruction would make the iPad easier for you to use?
30 min	iPad app demonstration	• What is helpful about this app? • What do you like about this app? • What would you change about this app?
30 min	Design an app activity	• What are the top five things you would want in an iPad app? Why? • What app features would make it easier for you to consume more fruits and vegetables?
10 min	Wrap-up discussion	• How did you feel about using the iPad? • What aspects of using the iPad were easy or difficult? • How else would you like to use the iPad to manage your health? • How would you like to use the iPad to make better health decisions? • What features would you like to see on iPads to make them easier for you to use?

FV, fruit and vegetable.

eating FVs. Fourth, the moderator demonstrated the iPad's features including the touchscreen interface, wi-fi Internet connectivity, and the camera. During this activity, participants explored using the iPad's features and practiced performing some basic tasks, such as opening an app or typing. Fifth, the moderators introduced the participants to three existing, free FV-related apps (MyFood, FiveADay Lite, and Whole Foods Market Recipes) and explained their features. Sixth, the moderator solicited participants' ideas for app features that would help them increase FV intake. Last, the moderator led a wrap-up discussion, asking about participants' perceptions of iPads and soliciting any additional design suggestions.

Data Analysis

We analyzed data with a grounded theory approach, using a constant comparative method that allowed themes to emerge from the data (Corbin & Strauss, 2008; Glaser & Strauss, 1967). First, we analyzed data line by line with open coding to determine initial themes, categories, and salient concepts. Next, we used axial coding to deduce codes into subcategories. This step reduces the number of categories by identifying similarities among the categories and makes data more clear and understandable (Lindlof & Taylor, 2011). Finally, we conducted selective coding to enrich and finalize the categories. When appropriate, we used in vivo codes to preserve participants' words (Corbin & Strauss, 2008). The results reported in the following section use pseudonyms to protect participants' privacy and confidentiality.

RESULTS

Themes

We identified major themes that can be organized into three categories: (a) baseline perceptions of iPads, that is, participants' initial perceptions of iPads prior to using an iPad; (b) perceptions of iPads after guided exposure, that is, participants' perceptions after we demonstrated iPads' functions and guided participants to gain firsthand experience using iPads; and (c) how iPad apps can help older adults overcome barriers to FV intake, that is, participants' perceptions of major barriers to their FV intake, along with features they recommended for using iPads to help overcome some of these barriers. These categories and their subcategories are illustrated in Figure 1.

Baseline Perceptions of iPads

All participants had heard of iPads prior to participating in our study but lacked knowledge of iPad's functionality. Prior exposure to iPads came mainly from three sources: (a) family and friends, (b) church, and (c) advertising. For instance, Beth stated, "My son told me [an iPad is] a computer that is more compact. You can communicate with someone with it," whereas Suzy said, "My grandson has one but he goes through it so fast." Edward said his son "came back for Christmas with one and it sparked my interest and curiosity." Bea said, "I've seen some friends use the iPad" and "a lot of them use them for photo albums and graduation pictures as a camera." Church also emerged as a location that exposed older adults to iPads. Samantha mentioned, "At church, some of the people ... have iPads," whereas Jill said, "There are two people in the church who use [iPads]." Several participants first saw iPads at stores or in advertisements. Arthur had "seen [iPads] in stores," whereas John first saw an iPad "just on TV."

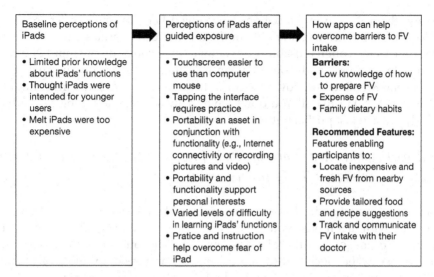

Baseline perceptions of iPads	Perceptions of iPads after guided exposure	How apps can help overcome barriers to FV intake
• Limited prior knowledge about iPads' functions • Thought iPads were intended for younger users • Melt iPads were too expensive	• Touchscreen easier to use than computer mouse • Tapping the interface requires practice • Portability an asset in conjunction with functionality (e.g., Internet connectivity or recording pictures and video) • Portability and functionality support personal interests • Varied levels of difficulty in learning iPads' functions • Pratice and instruction help overcome fear of iPad	**Barriers:** • Low knowledge of how to prepare FV • Expense of FV • Family dietary habits **Recommended Features:** Features enabling participants to: • Locate inexpensive and fresh FV from nearby sources • Provide tailored food and recipe suggestions • Track and communicate FV intake with their doctor

FIGURE 1. Major themes and characteristics. FV, fruit and vegetable.

Despite this prior exposure, participants did not understand iPads' functionality. They compared iPads to other devices when explaining the iPads' functions. Michelle asked, "What's the difference between the telephone and the iPad?" Jane responded, "It's kind of like a phone." Pumphrey commented that "the touch screen kind of reminds me of my phone." Tammy then asked, "It's kind of like a computer?" To clarify the difference between an iPhone and an iPad, the moderator held up the two devices, highlighting size and shape differences. This demonstration provoked follow-up questions on whether iPads can perform the same functions as iPhones. A participant asked, "You can watch things in this [iPad]?" whereas another asked, "You can actually talk to each other [via iPads]?"

Inadequate knowledge of the iPad's functionality influenced the participants' perceptions of iPads. Several participants felt iPads were designed for younger people. Jane stated, "I don't think I need an iPad. It's for younger people. I have a laptop ... I think [iPads are] for kids." Matt's family purchased an iPad, but he lacked knowledge about iPad functions that could be helpful for older adults, stating, "But it was like a toy I couldn't use, I asked them to return it for me." Pumphrey had the option to choose an iPad or laptop for work. He chose the laptop because "the laptop [is] familiar" and he knew little about iPads. Combined, these comments indicate participants perceived iPads as a device primarily intended for younger people.

Participants perceived iPads' expensive retail price as a barrier to adopting iPads. Carl stated, "It seems like [iPads] would be good ... [but] definitely the price would have to come down." Another participant noted that iPads cost "a lot of money!" whereas Walt stated his knowledge of iPads was limited to "the [high] cost and that it was a touchscreen." When told that an iPad costs between $500 and $700 (when the study was conducted), Benjamin stated, "That's too expensive for me!" Kevin asked if an AARP discount existed for iPads.

Perceptions of iPads After Guided Exposure

In the next activity, the moderator demonstrated the iPads' functionality and each participant explored using an iPad. Several themes emerged from this activity.

These themes include participants' perceived benefits and challenges of different iPads features, such as portability or the touchscreen interface. Most participants felt the touchscreen offered usability advantages over conventional input devices such as computer keyboard and mouse. Samantha's initial experience using an iPad included exploring MedlinePlus. gov, a health website from the National Institutes of Health. She stated, "Oh I like it! You don't have to always type anything in. With this [the iPad] you can just push a button and there it is!"

All participants had heard of iPads prior to participating in our study but lacked knowledge of iPad's functionality.

Similarly, Bob stated, "It's very impressive. You just don't need that mouse ... because with that mouse you gotta learn how to tip it just right. No wonder the old computers are going out!" Yolanda preferred, "The touch[screen] more so than using the mouse ... the touch and scrolling is quicker and easier for those of us can't type." After the moderator showed Vivian how to select links using her finger, she stated, "[iPads are] easier than [a] laptop! You do less work to find where you want to go. And with the laptop I have to use that little pad to move the cursor and sometimes that's hard to use." Similarly, Jim stated, "It's just striking how incredibly easy it is. What's the word—'user-friendly'? ... and you don't have to use a mouse, you just use your fingers." These statements indicate these participants found the touchscreen simple to operate because users can complete tasks with fewer steps and in less time.

Likewise, one participant found that an important benefit of the touchscreen was the ability to enlarge onscreen objects with simple finger gestures. By spreading two fingers apart, a user can enlarge onscreen text and images. After watching the moderator demonstrate this gesture on an iPad, Veronica said she loved that "you just touch [the touchscreen and have] the ability to make text large." Similarly, Henry stated that he "like[d] how you can zoom in and out." This feature especially benefited participants such as Veronica that had difficulty reading small type–size text on the MedlinePlus website.

Although the participants found the touchscreen provided advantages, they felt tapping the interface required practice. Vivian had difficulty "pressing something and it not going—you have to have a magic touch." Typing a web address with his finger, John accidentally tapped the same button twice and misspelled the address. John complained, "This [touchscreen] is sensitive to the touch." We also observed several participants press app icon too firmly while launching an app, and the app did not launch as a result. The moderator asked the participants to apply a lighter touch but the issue persisted. In addition, Bea used her fingernails, rather than the soft tissue on the tip of her finger, to click icons. The touchscreen did not respond. After the moderator explained that she should use the tip of her finger, not her nails, to use the touchscreen, Bea successfully tapped an icon to launch an app. These observations suggest that even though the touchscreen has usability advantages, older adults likely need guidance and practice to master tapping.

Next, participants perceived iPads' portability as an asset, especially when combined with iPads' functionality, such as Internet connectivity or recording pictures and videos. Vivian stated, "You can take it anywhere out of the country and have your information." Hairston added, "I like the smaller part. Say, if I was on a trip, I could just take this and be all set." Maria became interested in how portability could work with iPads' functionality, asking, "So if I am in Hawaii, I can show people what I am doing?" Barry explained, "My daughter and I ... were at the beach and she was using her iPad to take pictures." Similarly, Viola described a picture her daughter took, stating, "I was so amazed that she had [the picture] on [the iPad] ... I think [iPads are] better because you can take it with you." Viola also valued Internet connectivity and stated, "I think that's fascinating if you take a picture and then can share it." Despite these positive perceptions, participants felt portability could make iPads targets for theft. One participant mentioned a recent newspaper article about an iPad theft on a subway train.

Participants also felt iPads' portability and functionality could support their personal interests, such as religion or music. Malik found information about the beginning of Ramadan on the iPad and stated, "I am reading about Ramadan. Today, I start fasting." Similarly, Janis stated, "[A]t church, one of my deacons [uses] an iPad to pull up the Bible scripture." Maria agreed, stating, "People have [iPads] at church. They hold [iPads] up to record the service." Other interests included music. Adam stated, "You can listen to songs from Fats Domino and old guys like that [or] hear music from people like James Brown." Viola summarized these remarks, stating, "I'd like to use it as a little friend" that supports personal interests. These statements contrast with the participants' perceptions at baseline, when they felt iPads lacked relevance to their personal interests.

Notably, participants varied in their perceptions about the difficulty of learning to use iPads. Some participants felt iPads needed little instruction. Jane stated, "It's easy to use, as long as it gives you basic introductory information. But it is easy." Lester compared iPads to desktop computers, stating, "I just think [iPads are] easier to operate on 'Day one.'" Conversely, John felt "this [iPad] class needs to be three or four sessions ... I would need more time to really learn it." Similarly, Kevin stated, "[iPads have] been difficult [to learn]. But it seems the more you play with it, the more you're used to it ... by playing with it I got used to it." These statements suggest the amount of instruction on iPads older adults need varies greatly, with some participants needing little instruction, whereas others need multiple instructional sessions.

In addition, instruction and practice emerged as tools to overcome fears about iPads. Brenda noted, "The biggest obstacle is fear of the machine," whereas Henry stated, "There is some intimidation at first, but when you get your hands wet, you can explain it and feel better." Similarly, Kevin stated, "There was a sense of 'fear,' but with a class I ... feel better." Vivian summarized these statements, stating, "It's about conquering the fear through practice." These statements indicate practice and instruction helped participants overcome initial fears of using iPads.

The amount of instruction on iPads older adults need varies greatly, with some participants needing little instruction, whereas others need multiple instructional sessions.

How Apps Can Help Overcome Barriers to FV Intake

In the next activity, the moderator asked the participants to describe the barriers to consuming FV. Several themes emerged: (a) low knowledge of how to prepare FV, (b) concerns about FV expense, and (c) family dietary habits.

Participants felt inadequate knowledge of FV preparation impeded their FV intake. Yolanda stated, "It's the preparation ... I do not enjoy oranges and apples anymore, unless I put it in the microwave, so I'm hoping to find out other ways to prepare [oranges and apples]." Similarly, Jane noted, "[A challenge is] sometimes knowing how to prepare it differently and still get the values that you need from consuming, knowing new recipes and ways to cook." Michelle felt preparation could help her plan meals with FV, stating, "I always plan ahead, I think planning ahead is very helpful for me, planning on what you eat."

Expense also emerged as a barrier. Hairston stated, "Fruit is so expensive! Grapes are like $3.99 a pound." Eldridge continued, "It costs you to eat good vegetables and it's going to go higher because of the drought." When asked what would help him eat more FV, Caldwell stated, "Well, have the price come down." Viola noted, "Everything fresh tends to be more expensive." London added, "I'll agree with that. In fact, the price might be going up." These statements indicate the perceived expense of FV served as a barrier to FV intake.

Participants also felt their family's dietary habits influenced their FV intake. John stated, "I guess it is just upbringing. I didn't really eat a lot [of fruits and vegetables] growing up and my family doesn't talk about it much." Darlene stated, "I am from the islands and so we eat a lot of brown rice." London stated, "Yeah well, you know [my family has] southern roots [and eat dishes like] old fashioned chicken and dumplings."

With these barriers in mind, participants practiced using three existing iPad FV apps: MyFood, FiveADay Lite, and Whole Foods Market Recipes. During this practice, the moderator encouraged participants to critique the apps and suggest app features that could eliminate barriers. Participants made several recommendations, such as features that (a) locate inexpensive and fresh FV from nearby sources, (b) provide tailored food and recipe suggestions, and (c) track and communicate FV intake records to a doctor.

First, participants wanted an app feature that could locate nearby sources for inexpensive FV. When asked about desired app features, Viola stated, "I would like to know … where you can go to get inexpensive, fresh FV [from] community gardens or farmers' markets. And when they were open, and where they were located. How would I know where to go to get all that?" Henry agreed and added, "There are roadside gardeners that have fresher and cheaper stuff but that they are difficult to locate." Notably, none of the apps participants used during the session had a feature identifying the price, location, or hours of nearby FV sources.

Second, participants wanted an app feature providing food and recipe suggestions tailored to their dietary needs and taste preferences. While exploring the Whole Foods Market Recipes app, Mr. Brown stated, "This is neat! Sometimes if you don't know what to fix (for a meal), this gives the recipe and tells you how to cook it." Similarly, while using the MyFood app, Eldridge stated, "When you touch [an icon for a vegetable], it gives you things you normally wouldn't look for." The Whole Foods Market Recipes app allows users to select their favorite recipes from a list provided by the app but does not recommend recipes to users. Likewise, the MyFood app offers nutritional information for different FV but gives no recommendations tailored to a user's unique characteristics and preferences.

Third, participants wanted to track and communicate their FV intake with their doctor. Viola wanted "[a feature] I could use so that if I have to go to the doctor, I could just hand it to him and say 'here—read it.'" Likewise, Betty proposed a feature where "you could record what you eat and then the doctor could read it. Is that possible?" Rita added, "[If] you would do it that way instead of dealing with all that paper, you could take it with you [to the doctor], [after you] record what you've … eaten." In addition, Rita felt this feature could promote accountability and increase FV intake. She stated, "You [would] know that you had the total amount [of FV servings] … [and] you can't cheat" by eating fewer servings. Notably, none of the app participants used during the sessions had a feature enabling users to track their FV intake.

DISCUSSION

This study examined the benefits, barriers, and desired features for using tablets to promote FV intake among older adults. The findings identified app features older adults perceive as helpful to increasing their FV intake. Although prior studies investigated the usability of tablets for older adults (Findlater et al., 2013; Jayroe & Wolfram, 2012), this study provides a new perspective and identifies features specific to increasing FV intake. These features include (a) locating inexpensive FV from nearby sources, (b) providing tailored food and recipe suggestions, and (c) tracking and communicating FV intake records with their doctor. Identifying these features is an important initial step for developing tablet-based interventions that promote FV intake among older adults. In addition, using health behavior theory to guide the design of these features could improve their efficacy (West et al., 2013).

Social support could be incorporated in several of the recommended features. The Active Lifestyle app study suggested emotional support can improve outcomes in health behavior interventions with older adults (Silveira et al., 2013). Likewise, the ability to track and communicate FV intake with a doctor could facilitate social support. For example, if participants share their FV intake records with a doctor, the doctor could provide them with informational support, that is, the "provision of advice, suggestions, and information that a person can use to address problems" (Heaney & Israel, 2008, p. 190). With a record of a patient's FV intake, doctors could provide a patient with tailored suggestions for increasing FV intake that account for the patient's current diet.

Tailoring could also provide an effective approach to the features' design that has both theoretical and empirical support. Data on users' location and activities could be used to tailor messages. For example, an app could inform a user about nearby, inexpensive sources of FV that are consistent with the user's dietary preferences. Motivational messages could use data from the tracking feature to tailor messages that match a user's current FV intake. This feature would be consistent with the TTM, which asserts health messages better promote behavior change when they match the individual's current behavior (Prochaska & Velicer, 1997). For example, a motivational message targeted to individuals who eat no FV could encourage these individuals to begin considering how to add more FV to their diet. Individuals already consuming two or three servings of FV per day could receive messages with encouragement and information on how to further increase their intake to meet the recommended levels of consumption.

In addition to generating a set of features participants perceived as useful for promoting FV intake, this study produced findings on older adults' perception of tablets before and after guided exposure to tablets. These findings extend the literature on tablets' usability for older adults and provide insight on strategies for increasing tablet adoption among older adults in FV intake interventions. First, we found practice and instruction promoted a positive perspective of tablets and reduced anxiety about tablets. At baseline, participants perceived tablets as expensive devices designed for younger adults. After some practice and instruction, participants perceived tablets' portability and functionality as assets and felt that tablets could support their personal interests. This transition is consistent with existing work indicating exposure and training reduce the initial stress of using an eHealth technology and promotes adoption of that technology (Czaja et al., 2013). The practice and instruction process from this study could be integrated into interventions where older adults are unfamiliar with iPads.

Tailoring could also provide an effective approach to the features' design that has both theoretical and empirical support.

We also found participants' perceived difficulty of learning tablets' functions varied. This is not a surprise given that the older population is diverse in terms of, for instance, prior computer experience, training expectations, and age-related physical or cognitive changes (Fisk, Rogers, Charness, Czaja, & Sharit, 2009). Notably, this study on designing the Colorado Care Tablet app suggested higher age correlated to preference for reduced functionality. Tailoring the amount of functionality to match a user's preference was recommended as a solution to this issue (Siek et al., 2010). A similar concept could apply to instruction by tailoring the amount of instruction for each user receives. This approach could involve using an intelligent tutoring system, which provides users with a tailored path through learning content based on their ability and performance (McLaren, DeLeeuw, & Mayer, 2011). A pilot study found web-based intelligent tutoring effective for increasing older adults' computer literacy (Watkins, Xie, Devanarayanan, & Kanal, 2012). In conjunction, tailoring the level of functionality (a design approach) and instruction (a pedagogical approach) could ensure tablet-based interventions best match user's skill and knowledge of tablets.

Our participants perceived the touchscreen interface as easier to use than keyboard and mouse, which is consistent with the growing evidence that touchscreens offer usability advantages for older adults (Findlater et al., 2013; Jochems et al., 2012). However, our findings suggest older adults had no difficulty with two-finger gestures to zoom, which differs from a past study that found such gestures confused older adults (Piper et al., 2010). One possible reason is the difference in size between the touchscreen interfaces. Whereas the Piper et al. (2010) study used a large, table-sized touchscreen, our study used an iPad with a 9.7-in. (diagonal) touchscreen. This smaller touchscreen may better support the two-finger zoom gesture. Future research should examine how touchscreen size influences older adults' ability to perform different gestures, especially with increasing range of tablet sizes available in the marketplace (Franklin, 2013).

Similarly, our findings correspond with prior work that found tapping onscreen objects can be problematic for older adults (Leonardi et al., 2010; Wacharamanotham et al., 2011). Proposed solutions-include using alternative gestures, such as swabbing (Wacharamanotham et al., 2011), or tailoring an interface's sensitivity and timing to each user's needs (Leonardi et al., 2010). The findings from our study suggest an additional solution might exist in guided instruction and practice. Training older adults to tap onscreen objects could increase their tapping skill and avoid complex design solutions such as adjusting an interface's sensitivity for each user. In addition, practice could attenuate the initial stress of tablet use, which in turn could promote increased adoption of tablets.

LIMITATIONS AND FUTURE RESEARCH DIRECTIONS

Several limitations may impact the generalizability of findings. The sample may not be representative of the older population. Participants were sufficiently mobile and motivated to attend sessions at a public library. Although participant characteristics do not necessarily generalize to the older population, they may be consistent with older adults likely to patronize the library. Future research could expand the sample to other groups of older adults in different geographic locations and institutional contexts to determine these findings' generalizability. Also, almost all participants of this study lacked experience with tablet computers. Although older adults lag behind other groups to adopt tablets (Zickuhr, 2013a), the findings may not generalize to older adults with more tablet experience.

CONCLUSION

This study investigated older adults' perceptions and use of tablets for increasing FV intake to identify the features that best support older users. It produced a set of features participants perceived as supportive for increasing FV intake, including features for locating inexpensive sources of FV, providing tailored food and recipe suggestions, and tracking and communicating FV intake with a doctor. Using these findings, we provide recommendations for incorporating two particular theoretical constructs from health behavior theories, that is, social support and tailoring, into these features' design to improve the apps' efficacy at increasing FV intake.

Similarly, we found that after practice and instruction on using tablet functionality, participants perceived tablets as a useful, portable device for supporting their personal interests despite initial fears about the device. Future research should systematically investigate how practice and instruction can promote tablet adoption in tablet-based FV intake interventions. Practice and instruction also proved effective at teaching the participants' gestures, such as zooming, which are necessary to use the touchscreen interface. Based on these findings, we recommend that apps designed for older adults include features that provide instruction and practice activities. Furthermore, we recommend that instruction and practice features are tailored based on each individual's skills, knowledge, and experience with tablet computers to improve the effectiveness of these features. Future directions include developing an iPad app with the recommended features and testing the app in a large-scale intervention with older adults.

ACKNOWLEDGMENTS

We thank the librarians for their assistance with logistics and recruitment and research assistants David Piper, Rowena Briones, and Sarah Webster for their assistance with the data collection. The Electronic Health Information for Lifelong Learners-Older Adult Team (eHiLL-OAT) research project is funded through a Faculty Early Career Development Award to Bo Xie from the Institute of Museum and Library Sciences.

REFERENCES

Administration on Aging. (2012). *A profile of older Americans: 2011*. Retrieved from http://www.aoa.gov/aoaroot/aging_statistics/Profile/2011/7.aspx

Archer, E., Groessl, E. J., Sui, X., McClain, A. C., Wilcox, S., Hand, G. A., … Blair, S. N. (2012). An economic analysis of traditional and technology-based approaches to weight loss. *American Journal of Preventive Medicine*, 43(2), 176–182. http://dx.doi.org/10.1016/j.amepre.2012.04018

Aune, D., Chan, D. S., Vieira, A. R., Rosenblatt, D. A., Vieira, R., Greenwood, D., & Norat, T. (2012). Fruits, vegetables and breast cancer risk: A systematic review and meta-analysis of prospective studies *Breast Cancer Research and Treatment, 134*(2), 479–493.

Aune, D., Lau, R., Chan, D. S., Vieira, R., Greenwood, D. C., Kampman, E., & Norat, T. (2011). Nonlinear reduction in risk for colorectal cancer by fruit and vegetable intake based on meta-analysis of prospective studies. *Gastroenterology, 1,* 106–118.

Barnard, Y., Bradley, M. D., Hodgson, F., & Lloyd, A. D. (2013). Learning to use new technologies by older adults: Perceived difficulties, experimentation, behaviour and usability. *Computers in Human Behavior, 29*(4), 1715–1724. http://dx.doi.org/10.1016/j.chb.2013.02.006

Bennett, G. G., & Glasgow, R. E. (2009). The delivery of public health interventions via the Internet: Actualizing their potential. *Annual Review of Public Health, 30,* 273–292.

Bernstein, M. A., Nelson, M. E., Tucker, K. L., Layne, J., Johnson, E., Nuernberger, A., ... Singh, M. F. (2002). A home-based nutrition intervention to increase consumption of fruits, vegetables, and calcium-rich foods in community dwelling elders. *Journal of the American Dietetic Association, 102*(10), 1421–1427.

Breton, E. R., Fuemmeler, B. F., & Abroms, L. C. (2011). Weight loss—There is an app for that! But does it adhere to evidence-informed practices? *Translational Behavioral Medicine, 1*(4), 523–529.

Broekhuizen, K., Kroeze, W., van Poppel, M. N., Oenema, A., & Brug, J. (2012). A systematic review of randomized controlled trials on the effectiveness of computer-tailored physical activity and dietary behavior promotion programs: an update. *Annals of Behavioral Medicine, 44*(2), 259–286. http://dx.doi.org/10.1007/s12160-012-9384-3

Burke, K., Lee, A. H., Jancey, J., Xiang, L., Kerry, D. A., Howat, P. A., ... Anderson, A. S. (2013). Physical activity and nutrition behavioural outcomes of a home-based intervention program for seniors: A randomized controlled trial. *International Journal of Behavioral Nutrition and Physical Activity, 10,* 14. http://dx.doi.org/10.1186/1479-5868-10-14

Carter, P., Gray, L. J., Troughton, J., Khunti, K., & Davies, M. J. (2010). Fruit and vegetable intake and incidence of type 2 diabetes mellitus: Systematic review and meta-analysis. *BMJ, 341,* c4229.

Centers for Disease Control and Prevention. (2010). *Improving and extending the quality of life among older Americans: At a glance 2010.* Retrieved from http://www.cdc.gov/chronicdisease/resources/publications/aag/pdf/2010/healthy_aging1.pdf

Clark, P. G., Blissmer, B. J., Greene, G. W., Lees, F. D., Riebe, D. A., & Stamm, K. E. (2011). Maintaining exercise and healthful eating in older adults: The SENIOR project II: Study design and methodology. *Contemporary Clinical Trials, 32*(1), 129–139.

Cooper, A. J., Sharp, S. J., Lentjes, M. A. H., Luben, R. N., Khaw, K. T., Wareham, N. J., & Forouhi, N. G. (2012). A prospective study of the association between quantity and variety of fruit and vegetable intake and incident type 2 diabetes. *Diabetes Care, 35*(6), 1293–1300.

Corbin, J. M., & Strauss, A. (2008). *The basics of qualitative research: Techniques and procedures for developing grounded theory* (3rd ed.). Thousand Oaks, CA: Sage.

Cowan, L. T., Van Wagenen, S. A., Brown, B. A., Hedin, R. J., Seino-Stephan, Y., Hall, P. C., & West, J. H. (2013). Apps of steel: Are exercise apps providing consumers with realistic expectations? A content analysis of exercise apps for presence of behavior change theory. *Health Education & Behavior, 40*(2), 133–139. http://dx.doi.org/10.1177/1090198112452126

Czaja, S. J., Beach, S., Charness, N., & Schulz, R. (2013). Older adults and the adoption of healthcare technology: Opportunities and challenges. In A. Sixsmith & G. Gutman (Eds.), *Technologies for active aging* (pp. 27–46). New York, NY: Springer Publishing.

Fakhouri, T. H. I., Ogden, C. L., Carroll, M. D., Kit, B. K., & Flegal, K. M. (2012). *Prevalence of obesity among older adults in the United States, 2007–2010* (National Center for Health Statistics Data Brief No.106). Hyattsville, MD: National Center for Health Statistics.

Findlater, L., Froehlich, J. E., Fattal, K., Wobbrock, J. O., & Dastyar, T. (2013, April). *Age-related difference in performance with touchscreens compared to traditional mouse input.* Paper presented at the CHI 2013, Paris, France.

Fisk, A. D., Rogers, W. A., Charness, N., Czaja, S., & Sharit, J. (2009). *Designing for older adults: Principles and creative human factors approaches* (2nd ed.). Boca Raton, FL: CRC Press.

Fox, S., & Duggan, M. (2013). *Health online 2013.* Washington, DC: Pew Internet & American Life Project.

Franklin, A. (2013). Tablets buying guide. *CNET.* Retrieved from http://www.cnet.com/topics/tablets/buying-guide/

Glaser, B., & Strauss, A. (1967). *The discovery of grounded theory*. Chicago, IL: Aldine.

Greene, G. W., Fey-Yensan, N., Padula, C., Rossi, S. R., Rossi, J. S., & Clark, P. G. (2008). Change in fruit and vegetable intake over 24 months in older adults: Results of the SENIOR project intervention. *The Gerontologist, 48*(3), 378–387.

Grimm, K. A., Blanck, H. M., Scanlon, K. S., Moore, L. V., & Grummer-Strawn, L. M. (2010). State-specific trends in fruit and vegetable consumption among adults—United States, 2000–2009. *Morbidityand Mortality Weekly Report, 59*, 1125–1130.

Heaney, C. A., & Israel, B. A. (2008). Social networks and social support. In K. Glanz, B. K. Rimer, & K. Viswanath (Eds.), *Health behavior and health education* (4th ed., pp. 189–210). San Francisco, CA: Jossey-Bass.

Jayroe, T. J., & Wolfram, D. (2012, October). *Internet searching, tablet technology, and older adults*. Paper presented at the American Society for Information Science and Technology Baltimore, MD.

Jochems, N., Vetter, S., & Schlick, C. (2012). A comparative study of information input devices for aging computer users. *Behaviour & Information Technology, 32*(9), 902–919. http://dx.doi.org/10.1080/01449 29X.2012.692100

Kaplan, R. M., & Stone, A. A. (2013). Bringing the laboratory and clinic to the community: Mobile technologies for health promotion and disease prevention. *Annual Review of Psychology, 64*, 471–498.

Kobayashi, M., Hiyama, A., Miura, T., Asakawa, C., Hirose, M., & Ifukube, T. (2011). Elderly user evaluation of mobile touchscreen interactions. *Human-Computer Interaction–INTERACT 2011*, 83–99.

Kreuter, M. W., Strecher, V. J., & Glassman, B. (1999). One size does not fit all: The case for tailoring print materials. *Annals of BehavioralMedicine, 21*(4), 276–283.

Krukowski, R. A., Tilford, J. M., Harvey-Berino, J., & West, D. S. (2011). Comparing behavioral weight loss modalities: Incremental costeffectiveness of an Internet-based versus an in-person condition. *Obesity, 19*(8), 1629–1635.

Leonardi, C., Albertini, A., Pianesi, F., & Zancanaro, M. (2010, October). *An exploratory study of a touch-based gestural interface for elderly*. Paper presented at the NordiCHI '10 Proceedings of the 6th Nordic Conference on Human-Computer Interaction: Extending Boundaries, Reykjavik, Iceland.

Lindlof, T. R., & Taylor, B. C. (2011). *Qualitative communication research methods* (3rd ed.). Thousand Oaks, CA: Sage.

Liu, C., Zhu, Q., Holroyd, K. A., & Seng, E. K. (2011). Status and trends of mobile-health applications for iOS devices: A developer's perspective. *Journal of Systems and Software, 84*, 2022–2033. http://dx.doi. org/10.1016/j.jss.2011.06.049

Marques, T., Nunes, F., Silva, P., & Rodrigues, R. (2011). Tangible interaction on tabletops for elderly people. *Entertainment Computing—ICEC 2011, 6972*, 440–443.

McCully, S. N., Don, B. P., & Updegraff, J. A. (2013). Using the Internet to help with diet, weight, and physical activity: Results from the Health Information National Trends Survey (HINTS). *Journal of Medical Internet Research, 15*(8), e148. http://dx.doi.org/10.2196/jmir.2612

McLaren, B. M., DeLeeuw, K. E., & Mayer, R. E. (2011). A politeness effect in learning with web-based intelligent tutors. *International Journal of Human-Computer Studies, 69*(1–2), 70–79. http://dx.doi. org/10.1016/j.ijhcs.2010.09.001

McLaughlin, A. C., Rogers, W. A., & Fisk, A. D. (2009). Using direct and indirect input devices: Attention demands and age-related differences. *ACM Transactions on Computer-Human Interaction (TOCHI),16*(1), 1–15.

Nicklett, E. J., & Kadell, A. R. (2013). Fruit and vegetable intake among older adults: A scoping review. *Maturitas, 75*(4), 305–312. http://dx.doi.org/10.1016/j.maturitas.2013.05.005

Piper, A. M., Campbell, R., & Hollan, J. D. (2010, April). *Exploring the accessibility and appeal of surface computing for older adult health care support*. Paper presented at the CHI 2010 Proceedings of the 28th International Conference on Human Factors in Computing Systems, Atlanta, GA.

Prochaska, J. O., & Velicer, W. F. (1997). The transtheoretical model of health behavior change. *American Journal of Health Promotion,12*(1), 38–48. http://dx.doi.org/10.4278/0890-1171-12.1.38

Riley, W. T., Rivera, D. E., Atienza, A. A., Nilsen, W., Allison, S. M., & Mermelstein, R. (2011). Health behavior models in the age of mobile interventions: Are our theories up to the task? *Translational Behavioral Medicine, 1*(1), 53–71. http://dx.doi.org/10.1007/s13142-011-0021-7

Rimer, B. K., & Glanz, K. (2005). *Theory at a glance: A guide for health promotion practice* (2nd ed.). Washington, DC: U.S. Department of Health and Human Services.

Satariano, W. A., Guralnik, J. M., Jackson, R. J., Marottoli, R. A., Phelan, E. A., & Prohaska, T. R. (2012). Mobility and aging: New directions for public health action. *American Journal of Public Health, 102*(8),1508–1515. http://dx.doi.org/10.2015/AJPH.2011.300631

Siek, K. A., Ross, S. E., Khan, D. U., Haverhals, L. M., Cali, S. R., & Meyers, J. (2010). Colorado Care Tablet: The design of an interoperable Personal Health Application to help older adults with multimorbidity manage their medications. *Journal of Biomedical Informatics, 43*(5, Suppl.), S22–S26.

Silveira, P., van de Langenberg, R., van Het Reve, E., Daniel, F., Casati, F., & de Bruin, E. D. (2013). Tablet-based strength-balance training to motivate and improve adherence to exercise in independently living older people: A phase II preclinical exploratory trial. *Journal of Medical Internet Research, 15*(8), e159. http://dx.doi.org/10.2196/jmir.2579

Taylor, S. (2011). Social support: A review. In H. S. Friedman (Ed.), *The Oxford Handbook of Health Psychology* (pp. 189–214). New York, NY: Oxford University Press.

U.S. Census Bureau. (2012). *State and County QuickFacts.* Retrieved from http://quickfacts.census.gov/

Wacharamanotham, C., Hurtmanns, J., Mertens, A., Kronenbuerger, M., Schlick, C., & Borchers, J. (2011, May). *Evaluating swabbing: A touchscreen input method for elderly users with tremor.* Paper presented at the CHI 2011 Proceedings of the 2011 Annual Conference on Human Factors in Computing Systems, Vancouver, British Columbia, Canada. 25(2), 180–189.

Watkins, I., Xie, B., Devanarayanan, R., & Kanal, L. (2012). *Older adults, computer literacy, and web-based intelligent tutoring.* Paper presented at the International Conference of the International Society for Gerontechnology, Eindhoven, The Netherlands.

West, J. H., Hall, P. C., Arredondo, V., Berrett, B., Guerra, B., & Farrell, J. (2013). Health behavior theories in diet apps. *Journal of Consumer Health on the Internet, 17*(1), 10–24. http://dx.doi.org/10.1080/15398285.2013.756343

West, J. H., Hall, P. C., Hanson, C. L., Barnes, M. D., Giraud-Carrier, C., & Barrett, J. (2012). There's an app for that: Content analysis of paid health and fitness apps. *Journal of Medical Internet Research, 14*(3), e72. http://dx.doi.org/10.2196/jmir.1997

Zhang, X., Shu, X. O., Xiang, Y. B., Yang, G., Li, H., Gao, J., … Zheng, W. (2011). Cruciferous vegetable consumption is associated with reduced risk of total and cardiovascular disease mortality. *American Journal of Clinical Nutrition, 94*(1), 240–246.

Zickuhr, K. (2013a). *Tablet ownership 2013.* Washington, DC: Pew Internet & American Life Project.

Zickuhr, K. (2013b). *Who's not online and why.* Washington, DC: Pew Internet & American Life Project.

Zickuhr, K., & Madden, M. (2012). *Older adults and Internet use.* Washington, DC: Pew Internet & American Life Project.

OLDER ADULTS' PERCEPTIONS OF USING iPADS FOR IMPROVING FRUIT AND VEGETABLE INTAKE: AN EXPLORATORY STUDY

Critique by *Joseph D. Perazzo*

OVERALL SUMMARY

This qualitative study presents a novel intervention for older adults, the use of iPads to improve fruit and vegetable (FV) intake. Gaps in the literature are used to provide the study rationale. The aims of the study are not clearly stated in the paper, rather become clear when the researchers discuss the methodology. Although the authors state that they used a grounded theory approach for the study it is not clear what theory emerged from the study results. A more appropriate design would have been a qualitative descriptive design. The researchers report the rich data that emerged from the five focus groups that were conducted, and the resultant themes are logical and consistent with the data presented. The researchers also were aware of the study limitations, and recommend that further research regarding older persons' use of iPads be implemented, including instruction on the iPad use.

TITLE

Does the title include the key concepts/variables/phenomenon of interest?

The title of the article includes words that are descriptive of the population investigated by the authors as well as the phenomenon of interest.

Is it concise (12 words or less) and professionally stated?

The title is professionally stated but is slightly long at 15 words. The subtitle "an exploratory study" could be cut without diminishing the information available in the title as the nature of the study is presented in the abstract and the body of the article.

RESEARCHER(S) CREDIBILITY

Educational credentials?

The authors' educational backgrounds and previously published work demonstrate expertise related to the topics covered in the article. The first author's credentials include undergraduate work in economics and graduate work in library science with health informatics focus and a law degree. The second author, a nursing faculty member, has a PhD in science and technology studies, a master's degree in psychology, and a bachelor of medical science.

Prior methodological research experience of the authors (i.e., methodological expertise)?

Based on their prior research and their academic preparation the authors demonstrate the methodological expertise to conduct the study.

Subject matter content experience (prior research on the subject matter)?

The authors have research foci related to e-health literacy as well as previous published work in the area, including a systematic review of ehealth literacy interventions in older adults.

ABSTRACT

Does it include the key components (objective/aim, background/rationale, methods, results, and conclusions)?

The article's abstract includes the key components of the study, including their objectives, key background points, methods, results, conclusions.

Does or does not include references?

The abstract does not include any references.

Is it concise (150–250 words or less)?

The abstract is long (317 words) and could be shortened or structured to make it more concise.

Does it entice you to read the rest of the article (interesting)?

The authors provide an interesting overview of their study, which entices the reader to continue to read the entire article.

INTRODUCTION/PROBLEM

Is the research problem or phenomenon of interest clearly stated?

The introduction and discussion of the phenomenon of interest primarily is a discussion of the current state of the science regarding e-interventions and older adults. The authors discuss the paucity of e-health interventions available to older adults to help them to make informed health choices.

Does the problem have significance for nursing?

The primary focus in the introduction is demonstrating the potential utility of e-interventions for older adults and identifying a gap in the literature. This problem is of significance to nursing and health care, particularly as there is a growing population of older adults. New interventional modalities, especially those that rely on technology and at the same time encourage health promotion, are of particular interest.

Is it succinct?

The introduction is long and includes some components that would be better addressed later in the article. Part of the problem seems to be that the authors have two major areas of research, the feasibility of using iPads, and the tracking of FV intake using iPads. The authors only briefly touch on the issues associated with adequate FV intake in older adults, which ultimately weakens (though does not completely diminish) the argument they make for their research. The authors chose to restate information at the end of the introduction that describes methods and results, which generally would be placed later in the article. The introduction would be more succinct if the authors were to cut this information from this section and replace it with a reiteration of the purpose of the investigation.

Does it answer the "so what" question?

The introduction answers the "so what" question particularly in relation to the adoption of iPads by older adults.

RESEARCH AIMS/OBJECTIVES
Is the research aim/objective clearly stated?

Upon review of the authors stated aims, there are notable inconsistencies in the aims stated in different areas of the paper. In the abstract, the authors state: "To address this gap in the literature we conducted a qualitative study to explore older adults' perceptions and use of iPads for improving fruit and vegetable (FV) consumption."

At the end of the introduction, the authors add more information to the aims of the study in stating: "To addresses these gaps, this study investigates the benefits and barriers for tablets to promote FV intake among older adults, and identifies a set of recommended features for overcoming these barriers"

The authors also modify the stated purpose of the study in their presentation of the research questions that drove the investigation, which include questions about how older adults want to use iPads and an exploration of potential features. Ultimately the reader sees that the authors cover much more than perceptions and use of iPads in their investigation, which should be reflected in their purpose statements. Further, the purpose statements should be consistent throughout the paper.

Is it concisely written?

The introduction is not as concise but would be improved by eliminating the content on methods and results from this Introduction section.

Does it follow logically from the research problem/phenomenon of interest?

Although the introduction flows from the twofold research problem that the authors identified, based on the issues identified above regarding the change in the primary focus of the study.

SIGNIFICANCE
Is the significance to nursing and health care clearly written?

The significance to nursing and health care are addressed in a very limited manner. The authors make a very good case regarding the lack of knowledge related to e-interventions, but do not present a strong argument for its use in improving nutrition in older adults. The vast majority of the background and literature review are dedicated to e-intervention, with far less mention of the underlying health benefits and downstream impact of these interventions on the health of older adults. The authors' argument would be strengthened by discussing the significance of the health problem with equal weight to the proposed intervention delivery method.

Does the significance follow from the research aim/objective?

The authors do address significant gaps in the literature about iPad as an intervention delivery method with older adults, which is in line with their research aims.

BACKGROUND

Is there an explicit description of a theoretical perspective or conceptual framework? If not, is it implied?

The authors discuss theory as a deficit seen in the development of apps designed to promote health behavior. In particular, they make an argument for the integration of the theoretical constructs of social support and tailoring to improve iPad applications. However, a theoretical framework for their presented investigation is lacking. The choice of qualitative methods is appropriate for eliciting perceptions from participants, but the authors do not explicitly state a theoretical or conceptual framework for their investigation. Furthermore, while making their argument for the study, they use the term "just-in-time interventions," which remains undefined throughout the paper. The background provides an excellent justification for the use of iPads (e.g., the authors' discussion of the expense and feasibility of current interventions), but does not provide a theoretical rationale for the use of e-intervention in this population, nor the framework that guided their choice of methods and analysis.

Are there clear theoretical/conceptual definitions of the concepts?

There are no theoretical concepts included.

LITERATURE REVIEW

Primary sources only?

Apart from the aforementioned recommendation for a more thorough discussion of the significance of FV intake in older adults, the literature review is very well done. The authors were thorough, using primary references from literature.

Current (within the past how many years)?

The authors used literature published within the last 10 years, the majority of which was published within 5 years of this publication. It is notable that all references that are outside of the 5-year time frame (from the date of publication) referred to significant foundational works (e.g., theoretical foundation papers) that should be included despite not being published recently.

Is the search strategy included?

The authors do not discuss a specific search strategy, yet all of the literature they discuss is relevant to e-interventions, including discussions of e-interventions in older adults. The authors leave the reader with no question about the current state of the science of e-interventions, including what has worked, what has not worked, and what needs to be done next.

Is literature relevant to the research aims/objectives?

The majority of the literature cited is relevant to the use of technology for interventions for older adults. There is less attention to the older adults' lack of fruits and vegetables in their diet. The use of e-interventions seems to be of most interest to the researchers, and specifically the use of iPads.

Is it chronologically presented (old to current)?

The literature is not presented chronologically but rather is presented in clusters of related studies. This presentation is coherent and easy to follow.

RATIONALE FOR THE STUDY
Is there a gap in the literature that this study will fill (will it extend prior knowledge)? Is the rationale clearly stated?

A major strength of this article is a well-articulated rationale for the authors' desire to study the potential for iPad e-interventions in health care. The authors provide a rich literature review on current e-interventions, which included discussions of specific successes of these studies as well as gaps in the literature. The authors discuss three prominent gaps in the literature, specifically: (a) application of health behavior theory to mobile FV e-interventions (and potential application of theory in future research such as the Transtheoretical Model), (b) the design of FV e-intervention apps to accommodate needs and preferences of older adults, and (c) factors influencing older adults' adoption of tablets for and FV intervention. Further, the authors discuss the benefit of addressing these gaps in knowledge.

RESEARCH QUESTIONS AND/OR HYPOTHESES
Are these explicitly and clearly stated?

The authors do an excellent job clearly and explicitly stating their research questions.

Do they include the variables/phenomena of interest?

There are three specific research questions that include the variables of interest. Older adults' perceptions of using iPads, how they want to use iPads, and iPad features that can overcome barriers to FV intake.

Do they follow from the research aim/objective?

The first research question is most in line with the stated purpose of the paper. Further reading demonstrates that the authors also explored research questions specific to FV intake. Alhough it makes sense that exploring FV intake as part of their investigation of iPad perceptions, this aim was not as clear until the specific discussion of the focus group activities. There could have been two separate studies, one focused specifically on perceptions of iPad use and the other on use of iPads for increasing FV intake among older adults.

METHODS
Research Design/Paradigm
Is the research design clearly stated?

The authors collect qualitative data through five focus groups, and state the use of grounded theory as the research design. The use of a qualitative method is appropriate to obtain the specific and insightful data they wanted to collect.

Is there consistency between the research design and paradigm?

Grounded theory, however, does not fit as the best method to answer their research questions. The goal of a grounded theory study is to inductively produce a theory of a psychosocial process, particularly of a phenomenon in which there is an adaptation or change over time. In this case, there is no resultant theory and thus grounded theory was not executed. Rather, the authors analyzed qualitative data to produce descriptive themes that they present in plain language.

Is this the best choice of design to address the research problem/phenomenon of interest?

The best choice of design would be the qualitative descriptive design, which the researchers used. There is no need for grounded theory.

Is there rigor in the design?

There is rigor in the basic descriptive qualitative focus group design, but the use of grounded theory is lacking rigor.

SETTING
Is the setting clearly described?

The setting is very clearly described. The authors conducted data collection at a branch library that provided a private conference room for their data collection and wireless internet for demonstrating the utility of iPads.

What biases are introduced as a result of selecting this particular setting?

The authors state that one of the recruitment methods included flyers at the research site and in the county library newsletter.

This may introduce a bias to those who utilize the library and have transportation to get to the library for the study. Those who do not use or do not have transportation to the library would not be able to participate given this setting.

SAMPLING PLAN AND SAMPLE
Is the sampling plan clearly identified?

The authors discuss recruitment of older adults (aged 60 and older) who were members of the library's Older Adult Team, but provide no other inclusion/exclusion criteria. Planning for participants of this age group is appropriate given their objective to better understand the perceptions of older adults in their use of iPads for FV intake.

Does it represent the population of interest?

However, the authors made no provision for previous iPad use which could potentially bias their results. Furthermore, no inclusion/exclusion criteria related to current FV intake were specified. Their recruitment efforts included advertisements at the library, the library newsletter, and local newspaper ads. There is no description of which recruitment strategy was most successful in obtaining participants. Also, all participants were recruited from the Older Adult Team, which could introduce bias. These potential biases threaten representation of the population of interest, but helped the authors to obtain a sample with characteristics in line with their aims.

Is the sampling plan consistent with the research aim/objective?

The sampling plan is consistent with the research objectives as the sample of older adults is necessary to answer the research questions.

Is the sample size sufficient (e.g., power analysis or data saturation)?

As a qualitative inquiry, no power analysis or sample size was predetermined, with a final sample of 22 participants. No description of how many individuals attended each focus group is provided.

VARIABLES
Are variables clearly identified?

Embedded in the focus group protocol are the variables of interest, but they are not specifically identified as variables in the study.

Are variables operationally defined and consistent with theoretical concepts?

There are no operational definitions of variables, and there is no underlying theory presented as part of this exploratory study. This is appropriate for an exploratory study.

Are independent and dependent variables identified, if applicable?

Not applicable to a qualitative study.

METHOD OF DATA COLLECTION
What are the methods of data collection?

This qualitative study involved structured interview guide that corresponded to a 120-minute focus group. The authors conducted five focus groups that were facilitated by one researcher while another researcher took notes on the discussions. The focus groups followed a predetermined interview guide that is presented to the reader in tabular forma and described in the narrative. The authors do an excellent job of providing the reader with an outline of the focus group agenda both in the narrative and in a table. The researchers also present the interview guide with a corresponding timeline that guided the focus group discussion.

Are validity and reliability clearly addressed for prior research and current study, if applicable?

Validity and reliability are not explicitly discussed, but the interview schedule has face validity and the method of data collection is described in detail and would lead to reliable data as each session followed the same format. This method is appropriate for focus group studies. The authors do not mention audio recording and transcription of focus groups, suggesting that data analysis was of research notes. Although researcher notes and observations are a key component of qualitative methods, it may introduce a risk of missing data, thus affecting the reliability of the data.

Do the measures/instruments address the underlying theoretical concepts or phenomenon of interest?

Yes, the focus group questions address both of the key variables, the older adults' perceptions of iPad use and their use of iPads for FV intake.

Were human rights protected?

The authors indicated that institutional review board approval was obtained. They also note that informed consent was obtained prior to initiation of study procedures at each focus group.

Are other ethical issues identified?

The researchers do not indicate how the field notes will be protected, that is, where they will be stored. Also, the researchers did not note that the notes would be free of participant identifiers, but this is assumed in that none of the questions indicate reference to specific individuals. Training of the research team members who took the notes would guard against this concern.

Is the data-collection method appropriate for research design?

The focus group method is appropriate for a qualitative descriptive design.

Is there bias in data collection?

The bias introduced may be because the participants were selected from the Older Adult Team.

What is the fidelity of intervention addressed, if applicable?

The fidelity of the intervention is not directly addressed.

DATA ANALYSIS

Are data analysis techniques described (e.g., statistical tests, methodology for qualitative analysis)?

The authors describe their data analysis process as a constant comparison technique consistent with grounded theory methodology. The authors' description, although in line with basic qualitative analysis, lacks specific procedures they took during their analysis (e.g., no mention of analysis meetings, discussions, or consensus).

Does the analysis answer the research question?

The researchers were able to answer their research questions through the analysis they describe.

Is it appropriate?

The authors do identify themes from their data, but their presentation does not follow a set hierarchal qualitative analysis ranging from themes to categories. The researchers mix the grounded theory analytic method with an exploratory design that would imply a more descriptive qualitative analysis.

Is the analysis comprehensive? Are themes identified?

Themes were identified yet the description of the analysis was not comprehensive. Most notable, no constant comparison techniques are described in their analysis (e.g., theoretical sampling, inductive comparison beginning with first focus group to tailor further analyses).

Is there bias in the analysis (trustworthiness? credibility?)?

There is no mention of member checking or efforts to verify the trustworthiness of the analysis with participants. In general, this section lacks specific analytic detail.

RESULTS

Are sample characteristics described and fully reported?

Sample characteristics of the 22 participants are presented in detail in a comprehensive table.

Are findings presented related to research aim/objective?

The authors do a very good job of presenting their results related to the research aims of the study. They provide but do not overuse quotations and describe each of their reported themes. Rather, their results demonstrate a highly interpretive process which is much more useful to the reader. The quotations serve to provide specific and representative examples of each theme, but are not the primary focus throughout the presentation of results. The authors present categories with representative themes. Typically, themes are the highest level of abstraction in a qualitative analysis followed by subthemes or categories.

Are all outcome variables addressed, if applicable?

There are no specific outcome variables but the variables of interest are addressed.

Are results clearly presented in text and/or tables/figures?

The authors provide results in a figure and in the narrative. The figure is a summary of the results related to each of the research questions and appears to be a process figure with arrows, which does not align with the goals of the analysis. Removing this figure would not detract from the presentation of the results. A minor critique is that it appears there is a typo in the figure in the first block in which "Melt iPads were too expensive" should read "Felt iPads were too expensive." The only other thing missing from the Results section is an indication of frequency with which participants commented on the themes. No description of thematic saturation is presented, which directly corresponds to the sparse information provided in the analysis section. The majority of the results are in line with the research questions and stated purpose, with the exception of the FV barriers questions in the focus group interview (which do, however, add richness to the data). The results are provided in detail in the text.

Is significance of results reported, if applicable?

As this is an exploratory qualitative descriptive study, there is no reporting of significance levels that would characterize quantitative study results.

DISCUSSION OF RESULTS

Do the authors link the findings to previous research studies?

The Discussion section is very well done. The authors reiterate their purpose and provide a comprehensive interpretation of their findings. They link their findings to previous studies. In doing so, they are able to present how their study is consistent with previous studies and also how their study contributes to the current state of the science.

Are the conclusions comprehensive, yet within the data?

The Discussion section is very comprehensive but does not go beyond the data.

Do the authors interpret the results in the discussion?

The authors interpret their results in line with prior research in this area. They discuss specific ways that they tailored their iPad class to improve upon previous research and presented the specific results that demonstrate improvement.

Are the findings generalizable or transferable?

There is no specific mention of transferability of results in the Discussion section, but they do address generalizability in the limitations.

LIMITATIONS
Identified? Accurate? Inclusive?

The authors clearly state limitations to their findings, including generalizability based on participant characteristics and iPad experience. In general, qualitative studies are not conducted with a goal of generalizability but, rather, transferability to similar groups. The authors do not mention methodological limitations including a relatively small sample size and nontranscribed interview analyses. Overall the limitations are accurate but abbreviated.

IMPLICATIONS
Are there implications for practice, education, research?

The authors discuss useful and pragmatic implications and recommendations, primarily for future research. They discuss potential for their research to be taken in new directions, including the tailoring and testing of FV apps for older adults, and recommend the use of tablets in promoting health behavior in older adults. Their study provided rich insight on potential features that could be added to existing apps or tailored in new apps that would help older adults to overcome barriers to FV intake. There is no mention of specific practice recommendations in this section, likely due to the current state of the science (e.g., not being used regularly by this population thus not recommended in practice).

Are there implications for clinical significance?

The perceptions of iPad relevance in the lives of older adults has clinical significance. Adoption of technologically driven interventions among older adults may be premature.

RECOMMENDATIONS
Recommendations for future study/study replication?

The authors address recommendations for future research, including replication of the study with other groups of older adults, specifically those in other geographic sites and within other institutional arrangements. The authors do not mention specific institutional settings, but as this study was conducted In a library setting, a range of other settings is possible, for example, senior centers, churches, and so on.

CONCLUSION
Is it succinct and does it tie everything together?

The authors provide a succinct and comprehensive conclusion to their research findings that includes a reiteration of their results, implications for theoretically driven tailoring of iPad apps, and their recommendations for future research in this area (specifically the testing of tailored apps in larger, representative studies).

SUMMARY AND FUTURE DIRECTIONS

Joyce J. Fitzpatrick

15

Nursing is a developing science, with its early roots in both educational and clinical research. Building on a strong scientific foundation, during the past decade nursing has been part of an evidence-based practice (EBP) movement that has spread throughout the health care delivery system. Nurses in professional practice are expected to understand the research process, the EBP process, and quality-improvement (QI) processes. Further, they must differentiate the sources of evidence and methodologies used in the different processes and apply them to practice on a daily basis. All of this is expected while the nurse is caring for acute and critically ill patients in hospitals or carrying a heavy caseload of clients in outpatient and/or home care services. Thus, it is imperative for professional nurses at all levels to understand the distinctions and the similarities among and between these processes; both EPB and QI processes rely on knowledge generated in research (Fitzpatrick, 2016).

Scientific research forms the foundation for the evidence used in professional practice. In the absence of research evidence the nurse is expected to initiate studies to expand the knowledge base for practice. Most often the research initiated by clinical nurses is performed in collaboration with nurse researchers who are either available in the hospital's nursing research department or in partnership with an academic institution. As partners in this collaboration it is important for the clinicians to understand the basic elements of research. And in reviewing the research evidence while applying the EBP and QI models, nurses at all levels must be knowledgeable about the research process and able to critique the published research literature.

This is often not an easy task. Clinicians develop their expertise through clinical ways of knowing, a process that allows them to come to conclusions about clinical phenomena quickly through their expert assessments and clinical judgments (Fitzpatrick, 2002). The extent to which nurses are clinical experts may inhibit their skills as researchers. Yet it is imperative that they have basic understanding of the research process so as to make judgments about its relevance and applicability to their clinical practice.

According to the American Association of Colleges of Nursing (AACN) Essentials of baccalaureate education for professional nursing practice (2008) the BSN-prepared nurse is expected to demonstrate a basic understanding of the research process and models for evidence based practice (p. 16). The AACN Essentials document outlines the sample content that would be included to meet this criterion. The critiques included in this book are key components of the sample content described by AACN.

Since 2010 there has been a significant increase in the number of students entering BSN completion programs. This trend reflects the key recommendations in the Institute of Medicine (2010) report, *The Future of Nursing* regarding educational preparation of professional nurses. Although there are several recommendations in this Institute of Medicine (IOM) report that have shaped current nursing education, the recommendation to increase the percentage of RNs with baccalaureate degrees to 80% by 2020 is particularly relevant. There has been significant growth in BSN programs that prepare RNs who completed associate degrees and diplomas in nursing. The typical programs are RN to BSN or RN to MSN programs. One of the most important courses in these programs is the basic research course, as most often these students have not previously studied the research process. They may have been exposed to nursing research studies in their clinical courses but they most likely would not have been expected to critique or evaluate these studies.

According to the National Institute of Nursing Research (NINR), nursing research develops knowledge to build the scientific foundation for nursing practice, prevent disease and disability, manage and eliminate symptoms caused by illness, and enhance end-of-life and palliative care (NINR, 2017). In September 2016, NINR published its Strategic Plan focused on these key areas of research (NINR, 2016). Built on the "NINR mission to promote and improve the health and quality of life of individuals, families, and communities" (NINR, 2016, p.6), several priority areas for scientific focus emerged. These included symptom science, wellness, self-management, and end-of-life and palliative care. In addition, through programs and activities, NINR focuses on promoting innovation and preparing the next generation of nurse scientists (NINR, 2016).

All of the studies included for critique in this book add to the body of knowledge in nursing, including both the clinical science of patient care as delineated by the NINR priorities or the delivery of that care by expert nurses. Without a focus on the knowledge and skills of nurses, the clinical interventions cannot be substantiated as attributable to professional nurses. The studies were selected to highlight important components of the research process for students to learn to critique various types of research designs. As evidenced in the critiques that are included, none of the studies is perfect. Yet all contribute to the expanding knowledge base in nursing and guide future research initiatives.

With the expansion of BSN and graduate-prepared nurses, the future for the nursing discipline is bright. Professional nurses can be expected to contribute to the translational research models that are being advanced in clinical academic environments. It i important to note that because professional nurses are on the front lines of care delivery, they can contribute much to our understandings of patient outcomes, an important initiative in both the care delivery and research arenas. As we prepare the next generation of professional nurses it is particularly important that they develop their skills as clinical experts with a firm understanding of research and the research process.

REFERENCES

American Association of Colleges of Nursing. (2008). *The essentials of baccalaureate education for professional nursing practice*. Washington, DC: Author. Retrieved from http://www.aacnnursing.org/Portals/42/Publications/BaccEssentials08.pdf

Fitzpatrick, J. J. (2002). The balance in nursing: Clinical and scientific ways of knowing and being. *Nursing Education Perspectives*, 23(2), 57. Retrieved from https://journals.lww.com/neponline/Fulltext/2002/03000/The_Balance_in_Nursing__Clinical_and_Scientific.2.aspx

Fitzpatrick, J. J. (2016). Distinctions between research, evidence-based practice, and quality improvement. *Applied Nursing Research, 29*, 261. doi:10.1016/j.apnr.2015.12.002

Institute of Medicine. (2010). *The future of nursing: Leading change, advancing health.* Washington, DC: National Academies Press.

National Institute of Nursing Research. (n.d.). What is nursing research? Retrieved from https://www.ninr.nih.gov

National Institute of Nursing Research. (2016). The NINR Strategic Plan: Advancing science, improving lives. Retrieved from https://www.ninr.nih.gov/sites/www.ninr.nih.gov/files/NINR_StratPlan2016_reduced.pdf

INDEX

Printed in the United States
By Bookmasters